AF778726

BIOCHEMISTRY RESEARCH TRENDS

BUTYRATE

FOOD SOURCES, FUNCTIONS AND HEALTH BENEFITS

BIOCHEMISTRY RESEARCH TRENDS

Additional books in this series can be found on Nova's website under the Series tab.

Additional e-books in this series can be found on Nova's website under the e-book tab.

BIOCHEMISTRY RESEARCH TRENDS

BUTYRATE

FOOD SOURCES, FUNCTIONS AND HEALTH BENEFITS

CONG-JUN LI
EDITOR

nova publishers
New York

Copyright © 2014 by Nova Science Publishers, Inc.

All rights reserved. No part of this book may be reproduced, stored in a retrieval system or transmitted in any form or by any means: electronic, electrostatic, magnetic, tape, mechanical photocopying, recording or otherwise without the written permission of the Publisher.

For permission to use material from this book please contact us:
Telephone 631-231-7269; Fax 631-231-8175
Web Site: http://www.novapublishers.com

NOTICE TO THE READER

The Publisher has taken reasonable care in the preparation of this book, but makes no expressed or implied warranty of any kind and assumes no responsibility for any errors or omissions. No liability is assumed for incidental or consequential damages in connection with or arising out of information contained in this book. The Publisher shall not be liable for any special, consequential, or exemplary damages resulting, in whole or in part, from the readers' use of, or reliance upon, this material. Any parts of this book based on government reports are so indicated and copyright is claimed for those parts to the extent applicable to compilations of such works.

Independent verification should be sought for any data, advice or recommendations contained in this book. In addition, no responsibility is assumed by the publisher for any injury and/or damage to persons or property arising from any methods, products, instructions, ideas or otherwise contained in this publication.

This publication is designed to provide accurate and authoritative information with regard to the subject matter covered herein. It is sold with the clear understanding that the Publisher is not engaged in rendering legal or any other professional services. If legal or any other expert assistance is required, the services of a competent person should be sought. FROM A DECLARATION OF PARTICIPANTS JOINTLY ADOPTED BY A COMMITTEE OF THE AMERICAN BAR ASSOCIATION AND A COMMITTEE OF PUBLISHERS.

Additional color graphics may be available in the e-book version of this book.

Library of Congress Cataloging-in-Publication Data

ISBN: 978-1-63117-657-9

LCCN: 2014935911

Published by Nova Science Publishers, Inc. † New York

CONTENTS

Preface vii

Contributors ix

Chapter 1 Enhancing Butyrate Biosynthesis in the Gut for Health Benefits 1
Robert W. Li and Cong-Jun Li

Chapter 2 Butyrate and Intestinal Function 25
Jacqueline I. Alvarez-Leite, and Edenil Costa Aguilar

Chapter 3 Large Bowel Short Chain Fatty Acid Production, Immune Status and Immune Cell Function: Implications for Chronic Inflammatory Disease 51
Kim Y. C. Fung, Leah Cosgrove, Julie Clarke, Trevor Lockett, Tatsuya Morita, Koji Hase and David Topping

Chapter 4 Butyrate Actions on Carcinogenesis: Focus on Epigenetic Mechanisms 69
Aline de Conti

Chapter 5 Potential Beneficial Effects of Butyrate against Food Allergy 81
Margherita Di Costanzo, Lorella Paparo, Rosita Aitoro, Linda Cosenza, Rita Nocerino, Tommaso Cozzolino, Vincenza Pezzella, Gianfranco Vallone and Roberto Berni Canani

Chapter 6 Short Chain Fatty Acids in Regulation of the Immune System and Tissue Inflammation in the Intestine 91
Myung H. Kim and Chang H. Kim

Chapter 7 Biological Effects of Sodium Butyrate in the Regulation of Gene Expression on Astrocytoma Cell Lines and Improvement of Therapies 109
Monika Garrido-Armas and Francisco Arenas-Huertero

Chapter 8 Butyrate, WNT Signaling and Colorectal Cancer 133
Michael Bordonaro and Darina L. Lazarova

Chapter 9 Butyrate-Mediated Protection against Colonic Inflammation and Colon Carcinogenesis: Role of Butyrate Transporters and Butyrate Receptors **157**
Vadivel Ganapathy, Puttur D. Prasad, Muthusamy Thangaraju, Pamela M. Martin and Nagendra Singh

Chapter 10 Epigenetic Influence of Butyrate Producing Bacteria in Metabolic Syndrome **177**
Marlene Remely, Ines Tesar and Alexander G. Haslberger

Chapter 11 Butyrate Facilitates Epigenetic Reprogramming **189**
Justin E. Brier-Jones, Jason B. Kiroyan and Xiao-Bing Zhang

Chapter 12 Role and Function of Short Chain Fatty Acids in Rumen Epithelial Metabolism, Development and Importance of the Rumen Epithelium in Understanding Control of Transcriptome **199**
Ransom L. Baldwin, VI and Kyle R. McLeod

Chapter 13 Regulation of Cellular Processes by Epigenetic Mechanisms of Butyrate **219**
Kasturi Ranganna, Omana P. Mathew and Shirlette G. Milton

Chapter 14 Butyrate: A Dietary Inhibitor of Histone Deacetylases and an Epigenetic Regulator **233**
Cong-Jun Li, Robert W. Li, Ransom L. Baldwin and Theodore H. Elsasser

Index **259**

PREFACE

This is the first book specifically devoted to butyrate and its biological functions in the health of humans and animals. It is the result of the collective efforts of a group of international experts working on different aspects of butyrate.

It has been recognized for a long time that consumption of dietary fibers has positive metabolic health effects. These effects are directly associated with short-chain fatty acids (SCFAs), particularly butyric acids, formed by the microbial degradation of dietary fibers in the digestive tract. In the last decade, multiple beneficial effects of butyrate at the intestinal and extra-intestinal levels have been demonstrated. As nutrition research is transferring from epidemiology and physiology to the molecular mechanisms of biological effects, we have come to realize that nutrients, such as butyrate, are not simply food ingredients or metabolic elements. Butyrate not only plays an important role in fueling colonocytes and maintaining intestinal homeostasis, it also functions as an important epigenetic regulator through its inhibitory effects on histone deacetylases, thereby modifying the chromatin landscape.

Chromatin modification has evidently aroused as a very important mechanism in regulating the transcriptional status of the genome, and changing the functions of cells at the genetic and epigenetic levels. Butyrate-induced biological effects provide examples of epigenomic regulation induced by nutrient elements and provide a basis for understanding the full range of the biological roles and molecular mechanisms that butyrate may play in cell growth, proliferation, and energy metabolism. With the advances in researching and understanding the molecular mechanism of butyrate's biological functions, there is a mounting interest in butyrate because its impact on epigenetic mechanisms will lead to more specific and efficacious therapeutic strategies for the prevention and treatment of different diseases.

This book is a comprehensive collection of highly innovative research ideas, strategies, and crucial points related to butyrate and its biological functions. It assembles a body of work that covers a range of scientific fields such as cancer research, immunology, metabolism, stem cell study, genomics, epigenomics and metagenomics. The objective of this book is to promote molecular biology, functional genomics, metagenomics research and bioinformatics that serve as launching points for the systems biology and for future research into the functions and mechanisms of butyrate. With recent advances in different but intriguing research fields, this book is a great reference for biochemists, molecular biologists, biomedical scientists, animal scientists and clinical researchers. This book is also a great reference for graduate students working in the related fields of biomedical sciences and animal sciences.

I extend my great appreciation to all of the authors, who passionately committed themselves to this book and to their respective chapters. Their dedication makes this book possible.

Cong-Jun Li, Ph. D.
Epigenetics
Bovine Functional Genomics Laboratory,
Agricultural Research Service
US Department of Agriculture
Beltsville, MD 20705, USA
Tel: 301-504-7216
congjun.li@ars.usda.gov

Contributors

Edenil Costa Aguilar

Departamento de Bioquimica e Imunologia, Universidade Federal de Minas Gerais _ Caixa Postal 486 _ 30161-970 Belo Horizonte, Brazil.

Rosita Aitoro

Food Allergy Unit, Department of Translational Medical Science, Pediatric Section, University of Naples, Federico II, Italy.

Jacqueline I. Alvarez-Leite

Departamento de Bioquimica e Imunologia, Universidade Federal de Minas Gerais _ Caixa Postal 486 _ 30161-970 Belo Horizonte, Brazil

Francisco Arenas-Huertero

Laboratory of Experimental Pathology. Hospital Infantil de México Federico Gómez, Facultad de Ciencia y Tecnología, Universidad Simón Bolívar, México, D.F.

Marlene Remely Bakk

Department of Nutritional Sciences, University Vienna, Vienna, Austria.

Ines Tesar Bakk

Department of Nutritional Sciences, University Vienna, Vienna, Austria.

Ransom L. Baldwin, VI

Bovine Functional Genomics Laboratory, Agricultural Research Service, US Department of Agriculture, Beltsville, MD 20705, USA.

Roberto Berni Canani

Food Allergy Unit, Department of Translational Medical Science, Pediatric Section, University of Naples “Federico II” European Laboratory for the Investigation of Food Induced Diseases, University of Naples “Federico II”, Italy.

Michael Bordonaro
Department of Basic Sciences, The Commonwealth Medical College, 525 Pine Street, Scranton, PA 18509, USA.

Justine E. Brier-Jones
Division of Regenerative Medicine MC1528B, Department of Medicine, Loma Linda University. 11234 Anderson Street, Loma Linda, California 92350, USA;.

Julie Clarke
CSIRO, Preventative Health National Research Flagship, Australia; CSIRO, Animal, Food, and Health Sciences, Adelaide and North Ryde, Australia.

Linda Cosenza
Food Allergy Unit, Department of Translational Medical Science, Pediatric Section, University of Naples "Federico II", Italy.

Leah Cosgrove
CSIRO, Preventative Health National Research Flagship, Australia; CSIRO, Animal, Food, and Health Sciences, Adelaide and North Ryde, Australia.

Tommaso Cozzolino
Food Allergy Unit, Department of Translational Medical Science, Pediatric Section, University of Naples "Federico II", Italy.

Aline de Conti
National Center for Toxicological Research (NCTR), Food and Drug Administration (FDA), 3900 NCTR Road, Bld 14C, Room 105, Jefferson, Arkansas 72079, USA.

Margherita Di Costanzo
Food Allergy Unit, Department of Translational Medical Science, Pediatric Section, University of Naples "Federico II", Italy.

Theodore H. Elsasser
Bovine Functional Genomics Laboratory, Agricultural Research Service, US Department of Agriculture, Beltsville, MD 20705USA.

Kim Y.C. Fung
CSIRO, Preventative Health National Research Flagship, Australia, Life Sciences Centre, Riverside Corporate Park, 11 Julius Ave, North Ryde NSW, 2113;CSIRO, Animal, Food, and Health Sciences, Adelaide and North Ryde, Australia.

Vadivel Ganapathy
Department of Biochemistry and Molecular Biology, Medical College of Georgia, Georgia Regents University, Augusta, GA 30912, USA.

Monika Garrido-Armas

Laboratory of Experimental Pathology. Hospital Infantil de México Federico Gómez, Mexico, D. F.

Koji Hase

RIKEN Centre for Integrative Medical Sciences, Kanagawa 230-0045, Japan;The Institute for Medical Sciences, University of Tokyo, Tokyo 108-8639, Japan;PRESTO, Japan Science and Technology Agency, Saitama 332-0012, Japan.

Alexander G. Haslberger

Department for Nutritional Research and Fed. Ministry for Health, University Vienna, Vienna, Austria.

Myung H. Kim

Laboratory of Immunology and Hematopoiesis, Department of Comparative Pathobiology, Weldon School of Biomedical Engineering, Center for Cancer Research, Purdue University, West Lafayette, IN 47907, USA.

Chang H. Kim

Laboratory of Immunology and Hematopoiesis, Department of Comparative Pathobiology, Weldon School of Biomedical Engineering, Center for Cancer Research, Purdue University, West Lafayette, IN 47907, USA.

Jason B. Kiroyan

Division of Regenerative Medicine MC1528B, Department of Medicine, Loma Linda University. 11234 Anderson Street, Loma Linda, California 92350, USA

Darina L. Lazarova

Department of Basic Sciences, The Commonwealth Medical College, 525 Pine Street, Scranton, PA, USA

Cong-Jun Li

Bovine Functional Genomics Laboratory, Agricultural Research Service, US Department of Agriculture, Beltsville, MD 20705, USA.

Robert W. Li

Bovine Functional Genomics Laboratory, Agricultural Research Service, US Department of Agriculture, Beltsville, MD 20705, USA.

Trevor Lockett

CSIRO, Preventative Health National Research Flagship, Australia; CSIRO, Animal, Food, and Health Sciences, Adelaide and North Ryde, Australia.

Pamela M. Martin

Department of Biochemistry and Molecular Biology, Medical College of Georgia, Georgia Regents University, Augusta, GA 30912, USA.

Omana P. Mathew
Department of Pharmaceutical Sciences, College of Pharmacy, Texas Southern University, 3100 Cleburne St, Houston, Texas 77004, USA.

Kyle R. Mcleod
Department of Animal Sciences, University of Kentucky, Lexington 40546, KY, USA.

Shirlette G. Milton
Department of Pharmaceutical Sciences, College of Pharmacy, Texas Southern University, 3100 Cleburne St, Houston, Texas 77004, USA.

Tatsuya Morita
Faculty of Agriculture, Shizuoka University, Shizuoka 422-5829, Japan

Rita Nocerino
Food Allergy Unit, Department of Translational Medical Science, Pediatric Section, University of Naples "Federico II", Italy.

Lorella Paparo
Food Allergy Unit, Department of Translational Medical Science, Pediatric Section, University of Naples "Federico II", Italy.

Vincenza Pezzella
Food Allergy Unit, Department of Translational Medical Science, Pediatric Section, University of Naples "Federico II", Italy.

Puttur D. Prasad
Department of Biochemistry and Molecular Biology, Medical College of Georgia, Georgia Regents University, Augusta, GA 30912, USA.

Kasturi Ranganna
Department of Pharmaceutical Sciences, College of Pharmacy, Texas Southern University, 3100 Cleburne St, Houston, Texas 77004, USA.

Nagendra Singh
Department of Biochemistry and Molecular Biology, Medical College of Georgia, Georgia Regents University, Augusta, GA 30912, USA.

Muthusamy Thangaraju
Department of Biochemistry and Molecular Biology, Medical College of Georgia, Georgia Regents University, Augusta, GA 30912, USA.

David Topping
CSIRO, Preventative Health National Research Flagship, Australia;CSIRO, Animal, Food, and Health Sciences, Adelaide and North Ryde, Australia;CSIRO, Food Futures National Research Flagship, Adelaide, SA 5000, Australia.

Gianfranco Vallone
Department of Biomorphological and Functional Sciences, University of Naples "Federico II", Italy.

Xiao-Bing Zhang
Division of Regenerative Medicine MC1528B, Department of Medicine, Loma Linda University. 11234 Anderson Street, Loma Linda, California 92350, USA.

In: Butyrate: Food Sources, Functions and Health Benefits ISBN: 978-1-63117-657-9
Editor: Cong-Jun Li © 2014 Nova Science Publishers, Inc.

Chapter 1

ENHANCING BUTYRATE BIOSYNTHESIS IN THE GUT FOR HEALTH BENEFITS

Robert W. Li ***** ***and Cong-Jun Li***
USDA-ARS, Bovine Functional Genomics Laboratory,
Beltsville, Maryland, US

ABSTRACT

Butyrate is one of the major short chain fatty acids produced in the gut via microbial fermentation and a preferred energy source for gut epithelial cells. Butyrate exerts a broad range of biological effects, mainly as a potent histone deacetylase inhibitor. Butyrate also binds to its own receptors on the cell membrane. Recent RNA-seq analysis reveals that butyrate significantly alters the expression of 11,443 genes *in vitro*, representing ~65% of all genes transcribed in the epithelial transcriptome. Numerous butyrate-producing bacteria from phylogenetically diverse groups have been isolated from host-associated habitats. Luminal butyrate concentrations, which vary tremendously along the gastrointestinal tract, result from the balance between its biosynthesis, absorption, and utilization by intestinal epithelial cells, and excretion. Mounting evidence indicates that reduced butyrate production has important physiological and pathological implications. Moreover, intracellular butyrate concentrations are suggested to be a key determinant of its biological functions. Extensive research over the past decades has identified numerous butyrogenic carbohydrate substrates. The potency of these substrates in stimulating butyrate biosynthesis depends on their structural features, including polymer chain lengths. Many of these butyrogenic compounds have the potential to be prebiotics. Selected bifidogenic and butyrogenic bacterial strains, especially those hyper-butyrate producers, possess the ability to increase butyrate production. Furthermore, the capacity of butyrate biosynthesis in the gut microbiota is readily inducible. The effects of different combinations of various prebiotics or pre- and pro-biotics (synbiotics) on butyrate biosynthesis have proven to be additive or even synergistic. Alternative approaches to enhance butyrate bioavailability will also be discussed in this chapter.

---

* Phone: 301-504-5185, Email: Robert.Li@ars.usda.gov.

Keywords: Butyrate, butyrate-producing bacteria, colon, gut, histone deacetylase, hyper-butyrate producer, intestinal, inflammation, prebiotics, probiotics, synbiotics

INTRODUCTION

Butyrate is one of the major short chain fatty acids (SCFA), produced by microbial fermentation in the gut, and a preferred substrate for gut epithelial cells. In ruminants, SCFAs contribute to 70% of energy metabolism. In humans, SCFAs also play an important role in energy metabolism in the hindgut, representing 5–15% of the total energy intake [1, 2]. The percentage can be higher in individuals from developing countries where a larger amount of plant fiber is consumed. Up to 95% of the total SCFAs are either absorbed via passive diffusion or actively transported across the gut epithelium. Several butyrate transporters, such as monocarboxylate transporter 1 (MCT1) and SMCT1 (SLC5A8 or sodium-coupled monocarboxylate transporter 1), have been identified [3, 4]. The observation that reduced butyrate uptake following enteropathogenic *E. coli* infection is associated with a decreased MCT1 expression underscores the importance of MCT1 in butyrate transport [5]. At least three mechanisms contribute to overall biological functions of butyrate: 1). acting as a potent inhibitor of histone deacetylases (HDAC); 2). via its receptors: G protein-coupled receptors (free fatty acid receptor, FFAR), GPR41 (FFAR3), GPR43 (FFAR2) [6]; and 3). via direct binding to the butyrate response element in target genes [7]. Indeed, the abundant expression of GPR43 in neutrophils may represent a missing link in how butyrate regulates host immune function [8]. Butyrate receptors are also expressed in adipose cells [9]. Butyrate induces a profound change in gene expression [10], altering transcript abundance of ~65% of the genes transcribed in the epithelial transcriptome [11]. Moreover, butyrate induces numerous alternative splicing events, including 2,834 exon skipping and 13 local gene fusion or read-through events [12]. Consequently, butyrate exerts an extremely broad range of physiological and pathological effects on various functions in both the extra-intestinal (such as hemoglobinopathies, metabolic diseases, hypercholesterolemia, insulin resistance, and ischemic stroke) and the intestinal levels (such as reinforcing intestinal barrier function, regulating intestinal motility and immunity, decreasing oxidative stress, inhibiting tumorigenesis, and suppressing intestinal inflammation) [13, 14]. Butyrate is also able to inhibit the internalization of *Staphylococcus aureus* in mammary glands [15]. Furthermore, exogenous butyrate can reduce the enhanced translocation of bacteria across metabolically stressed colon epithelia [16].

SCFA concentrations in the cecum, colon, rectum, and feces of animals, range between 30 and 240 mM (typically 70 to 120 mM) [17]. The molar ratio of three major SCFAs—acetate, propionate, and butyrate—remains steady in different organs in various species—such as horses, pigs, and ruminants—and are approximately 70:20:10. The mean molar ratios of these three SCFAs are 60:20:20 in feces of normal humans fed a Western diet [17]. The butyrate concentrations in the colon and feces of animals and humans are highly variable, ranging from 5 mM to 30 mM [18]. The net luminal butyrate concentrations in the gut result from the balance between butyrate biosynthesis by the gut microbiota, absorption, and utilization primarily via β-oxidation in the mitochondria of intestinal epithelial cells, and excretion. Intraepithelial butyrate metabolism helps to maintain the concentration gradient between the cytosol and lumen, thereby facilitating absorption [19]. Upon absorption, the vast majority of the butyrate is metabolized locally, while a small amount of butyrate enters into circulation. The luminal butyrate concentration has important physiological and pathological implications. Moreover, intracellular butyrate at a low dose of up to 0.5 mM cannot act as an HDAC inhibitor, rather than serve as a stimulator of histone acetylation, and therefore affect cell proliferation [20]. At this dose, butyrate undergoes β-oxidation. At a higher dose (up to 5 mM), butyrate metabolism is saturated and excessive butyrate is accumulated to act as an HDAC inhibitor in the nucleus. These distinct dose-dependent mechanisms underscore the importance of luminal and intracellular butyrate concentrations in exerting its biological functions. Indeed, exogenous butyrate is able to rescue germfree colonocytes from deficits in mitochondrial respiration and prevent them from undergoing autophagy [21]. Butyrate concentrations vary tremendously among healthy individuals, with noted differences between healthy obese individuals following disparate carbohydrate diets [22]. Moreover, butyrate is also shown to protect against diet-induced obesity [23]. Numerous factors affect butyrate concentrations. For example, after exposure to cigarette smoke, cecal butyrate level decreases significantly in rats. Fecal butyrate concentrations are higher in infants with a cow's milk protein allergy (CMPA) than in healthy infants [24]. Butyrate is shown to have the ability to restore motility and the actin cytoskeletal network in murine colon epithelial cells with a mutated APC gene [25]. Butyrate concentrations are also correlated with intestinal pathology, such as inflammatory bowel disease (IBD). For example, ulcerative colitis (UC) patients tend to have decreased fecal SCFA, especially butyrate, resulting from the altered gut microbiota [26, 27]. Furthermore, the number of butyrate-producing bacteria is significantly reduced in patients with *Clostridium difficile* infection (CDI) and nosocomial diarrhea [28]. Anti-inflammatory and anti-neoplastic properties of butyrate have long been recognized using *in vitro* models [29, 30]. As a result, tumor targeting using butyrate-producing probiotics has been proposed [31]. Numerous studies from past decades have demonstrated that the capacity of butyrate biosynthesis by the gut microbiota is readily inducible. In this chapter, we discuss various approaches that have a potential to stimulate butyrate production in the gut for health benefits.

BUTYRATE BIOSYNTHESIS AND BUTYRATE-PRODUCING BACTERIA

Butyrate is a fermentation product synthesized by the gut microbiota. The pathways leading to the formation of butyrate include a central pathway from acetyl-CoA to butyryl-CoA and the subsequent liberation of butyrate from butyryl-CoA by two different pathways [32]. The genomic organization of the genes responsible for the central pathway is well known. A single operon, consisting of all six genes, *thl* (thiolase), *crt* (crotonase), *hbd* (β-hydroxybutyryl-CoA dehydrogenase), *bcd* (butyryl-CoA dehydrogenase), *etfB* (electron transfer flavoprotein-β), and *etfA* (ETF-α), in this order, is constitutively transcribed. This operon exists in type I strains of *Butyrivibrio fibrisolvens*. Other genomic variations include one in which five of the six form an operon and the sixth gene, either *crt* or *thl,* is located elsewhere in the genome [32, 33]. At least two pathways are known to be responsible for the liberation of butyrate from butyrate-CoA: the predominant pathway uses CoA-transferase, encoded by the *but* gene [34], while the minor pathway, with a restrained distribution, possesses phosphotransbutyrylase and butyrate kinase [35]. Indeed, only four out of the 38 anaerobic butyrate-producing bacterial strains isolated from human feces possess butyrate kinase (*buk*) activities [36].

Table 1. Selected butyrate-producing bacterial species from host-associated habitats

Species	Origin/habitat	Reference
Acetatifactor muris	Mouse intestine	[136]
Anaerofustis stercorihominis	Human feces	[137]
Anaerostipes butyraticus	Chicken cecal contents	[61]
Anaerostipes caccae	Human feces	[45]
Anaerostipes coli (SS2/1)	Human colon	[138]
Anaerostipes hadrus	Human colon	[139]
Anaerostipes rhamnosivorans	Human feces	[140]
Anaerotruncus colihominis	Human feces	[141]
Butyricicoccus pullicaecorum	Chicken cecal contents	[60]
Butyricimonas synergistica	Rat feces	[142]
Butyricimonas virosa	Rat feces	[142]
Butyrivibrio crossotus	Human gut	[143]
Butyrivibrio fibrisolvens	Rumen	[144]
Butyrivibrio hungatei	Rumen	[49]
Butyrivibrio proteoclasticus	Rumen	[145]
Christensenella minuta	Human feces	[146]
Cloacibacillus porcorum	Porcine intestine	[56]
Clostridium butyricum	Human	[147, 148]
Clostridium lactatifermentans	Chicken cecum	[149]
Coprococcus catus	Human	[39]
Coprococcus comes	Human	[39]
Coprococcus eutactus	Human	[39]
Eubacterium cylindroides	Chicken cecum	[150]
Eubacterium hallii	Human	[39]
Eubacterium ramulus	Human	[39]
Eubacterium rectale	Human	[39]
Faecalibacterium prausnitzii	Human feces	[151]
Intestinimonas butyriciproducens	Mouse intestine	[152]
Lachnoanaerobaculum orale	Human salva	[153]
Lachnoanaerobaculum umeaense	Human small intestine	[153]
Lachnobacterium bovis	Rumen	[154]
Megasphaera elsdenii	Rumen	[155]
Moryella indoligenes	Human gut	[156]
Peptostreptococcus stomatis	Human oral cavity	[157]
Porphyromonas gulae	Animal gingival sulcus	[158]
Pseudobutyrivibrio ruminis	Rumen	[159]
Pseudobutyrivibrio xylanivorans	Rumen	[49]
Roseburia cecicola	Mouse cecum	[160]
Roseburia faecis	Human	[161]
Roseburia hominis	Human	[39]
Roseburia intestinalis	Human	[59]
Roseburia inulinivorans	Human	[161]
Subdoligranulum variabile	Human feces	[162]

Hitherto, over a number of years, extensive research has been conducted to identify butyrate-producing bacteria from host-associated habitats [37-39]. As a result, an increasing number of named butyrate-producing bacterial species and novel strains and isolates have been isolated from the gut microbiome of both humans and animals (Table 1).

As a functional group, the majority of butyrate-producing bacteria belong to the phylum Firmicutes. They are widely distributed across several clostridial clusters, such as Clusters I, IV, XIVa, XIVb, XV, and XVI [38, 40]. The highest butyrate concentrations are produced by the strains from Cluster IV (family *Ruminococcaceae*) and XIVa (family Lachnospiraceae) in the chicken cecum; these two clusters are also dominant in the hindgut of humans [40, 41]. Indeed, approximately 80% of the human butyrate-producing isolates belong to Cluster XIVa [37]. The distribution of the two major butyrate producing clusters (IV and XIVa) has been examined recently [42]. A significantly higher abundance of Cluster IV is found in omnivores, while Cluster XIVa is more abundant in vegetarians and omnivores [42]. In comparison, the elderly group tends to have a lower number of bacteria in fecal samples and fewer butyrate producers than the young individuals. A decreased abundance of the Cluster XIVa population in the gut may be related to ageing [43].

The *Eubacterium rectale-Roseburia* cluster represents ~36% of isolates [37]. In another study, *E. rectale-Roseburia* accounts for approximately 6.6% and 9.5% of 16S sequences in the liquid and particle-associated fractions of fecal samples from four human donors, respectively [44]. The genus *Eubacterium*, which is the second most common genus in the human intestine, includes several known butyrate producers [45]. While the capacity for butyrate production is confirmed, selected *Eubacterium* species in this study do not appear to play a major role in butyrate production in the human intestine. Therefore, other butyrate-producing species may be responsible for fecal butyrate production in the human intestine. Indeed, *Faecalibacterium prausnitzii* and related species are highly abundant in the human colon, accounting for up to 15% of total fecal bacteria [39, 46], and can produce a large amount of butyrate, up to 40 mM. A reduction in the relative abundance of *F. prausnitzii* is associated with a higher risk of postoperative recurrence of Crohn's disease (CD) [47]. Moreover, *F. prausnitzii* also possesses anti-inflammatory properties. While species from the genera *Anaerostipes*, *Eubacterium*, *Faecalibacterium*, and *Roseburia* are highly abundant in the human colon, they are very rare in the rumen [48]. *Roseburia* species are not detected in the chicken cecum either [40].

Butyrivibrio isolates represent a large fraction (up to 30%) of culturable rumen bacteria [49]. *Butyrivibrio* is among the five most abundant genera, accounting for 1.46% of all 16S sequences in the rumen ecosystem [48]. A significant portion of these isolates is capable of fiber fermentation in the rumen, and most butyrate-producing isolates have been assigned to *B. fibrisolvens* [49]. However, differences in both substrate utilization and cell wall composition, as well as genetic *heterogeneity,* have long been recognized among these isolates, from both ruminants and humans [37]. The diversity is also reflected in genomic arrangements of genes related to the butyrate fermentation pathway [33]. As a result, two novel butyrate-producing species, *B. hungatei* and *Pseudobutyrivibrio xylanivorans*, have been proposed [49]. The latter is able to use a broad range of substrates, including polysaccharides, proteins, and nucleic acids; under various dietary conditions. They are among the predominant species in rumen butyrate-producing populations. *Butyrivibrio fibrisolvens* is abundant in the rumen of cattle and sheep. It also resides in the gut of humans, dogs, cats, rabbits, and horses [50]. The oral administration of *B. fibrisolvens* (strain MDT-1) decreases chemically induced colorectal aberrant crypt foci [51] and alleviates the symptoms of experimental enterocolitis in mice [52]. The MDT-1 strain is able to enhance intestinal butyrate production by six fold during the first seven days of oral feeding in mice [51].

Recently, a gene-targeted approach using 454 pyrosequencing and quantitative PCR has been used to survey two key genes in butyrate biosynthesis pathways, *but* and *buk*, in patients with a colectomy [53]. The results confirm the previously observed dominance of the *but* pathway in healthy individuals. The findings suggest that an abundant butyrate-producing community, representing approximately 5% to 26% of the total community, can be rapidly established following a colectomy. Approximately 75% of *but* sequences can be assigned to four species, *Roseburia intestinalis* L1-82, *R. inulinivorans* A2-194, *Acidaminococcus sp.* D21, and *E. rectale* ATCC 33656, while the same percentage of obtained *buk* sequences can be assigned to four strains, *Bacteroides species* (sp.) D2, *Bacteroides sp.* 3_2_5, *C. butyricum* 5521, and *C. perfringens* [53]. Microbial communities linked to *buk* are dominated by sequences similar to those of *C. butyricum* and *C. perfringens*, whereas sequences similar to *Acidaminococcus sp.*, *F. prausnitzii,* and *Roseburia sp.* comprise the majority of *but*-associated bacteria in both methods (i.e., 16S and target-gene approaches). However, discrepancies between phylogeny (16S) and predicted function (target-gene) approaches are observed. For example, the obtained *buk* sequences are assigned to *Bacteroides*. However, the species from this genus are currently not considered butyrate producers; and culture-based studies also confirm their inability to synthesize butyrate [54, 55].

While numerous efforts have been made to isolate butyrate-producing bacteria, many of them have yet to be identified. For example, a high percentage of mucin degraders, such as *Cloacibacillus porcorum* [56], from the porcine gut is found to be butyrogenic [57]. Fourteen of the 16 strains isolated from the chicken cecum may represent novel species [40]. Moreover, a butyrate-producing strain isolated from human feces, representing a novel genus belonging to Cluster XIVa, has yet to be named [58].

Hyper-butyrate producers, the strains capable of producing >15 mM of butyrate *in vitro*, are of interest for their potential as probiotics. In the chicken cecum, hyper-butyrate producing strains represent ~14% of all isolates. It is possible that hyper-butyrate producers dominate the butyrate biosynthesis in the gut ecosystem because these strains are abundant where the total number of butyrate producers is the lowest [40]. A similar percentage (13.5%) of hyper-butyrate producers is isolated from human fecal samples [37]. Two strains, L1-952 and A2-183, from human feces, are intriguing, as they are capable of producing >20 mM of butyrate in batch culture [37]. Several strains of hyper-butyrate producers, such as *Anaerostipes butyraticus* (strains 16-7 and 35-7), *Butyricicoccus pullicaecorum* (strains 25-3, 44-3, and 49-3), and *F. prausnitzii* (strains L2-6 and ATCC#27768), have been thoroughly studied [27, 59-63].

BUTYROGENIC SUBSTRATES AND PREBIOTICS

Butyrate is an essential nutriceutical for normal colon function. A butyrate deficit has important physiological and pathological consequences. Consequently, for decades, the means to stimulate butyrate production in the hindgut by dietary supplements have been actively sought. These research efforts have led to the identification of numerous butyrogenic components. Previous reports show that various carbohydrates, such as starch [64-66], oat bran [67], sorbitol, galacturonic and glucuronic acid [68], inulin and fructooligosaccharides [69, 70], are able to stimulate butyrate production in the gut. In the meantime, novel butyrate stimulators have continued to be discovered and characterized.

D-tagatose is a stereo-isomer of D-fructose; it has been widely used as a low-calorie sweetener to replace sucrose [71]. As an FDA-approved food additive, D-tagatose has been studied for its potential anti-diabetic and anti-obesity properties [72]. While contributing to virtually zero net energy, this compound has the potential to inhibit carbohydrase activities in the small intestine, indirectly affecting carbohydrate metabolism in the hindgut. The compound largely escapes the digestion in the stomach and small intestine in pigs, where approximately 25% of D-tagatose is digestible. However, it can be fully digested in the porcine cecum and the proximal colon [73]. In the porcine proximal colon, a 3-fold increase in butyrate production (molar composition) can be achieved, while the rate of butyrate production can be enhanced ~30 fold by D-tagatose [74]. It is estimated that approximately 10% of the total anaerobic bacteria are capable of D-tagatose degradation [74]. Moreover, a significantly higher butyrate production is achieved from D-tagatose by the bacteria of tagatose-adapted pigs than un-adapted pigs [73, 74]. In an *in vitro* model, D-tagatose results in an extremely high-level butyrate production (to 56% of the total SCFA). In human trials, while the net concentrations of butyrate as well as the total short-chain fatty acids in the feces of healthy individuals are not changed by D-tagatose, butyrate production is significantly increased after the incubation of fecal slurries with tagatose [75]. D-tagatose treatments also induce an increase in lactic acid bacteria (LAB), especially lactobacilli, without serious gastrointestinal complaints [75, 76]. When examined together, these findings suggest that D-tagatose can be used as a butyrogenic prebiotic [77].

Unlike a broad spectrum of saccharides that increase acetate production, components capable of enhancing butyrate biosynthesis in an *in vitro* human fecal incubation system are limited, including sorbitol, galacturonic, and glucuronic acids [68]. Gluconate can reach the large intestine and stimulate butyrate production, resulting in a high molar percentage, up to 26% from the normal 15% in the batch culture of pig cecal digesta [78]. Gluconate fermenters are mainly LAB. It is possible that metabolic cross-feeding between LAB and butyrate-producing bacteria, such as *Megasphaera elsdenii*, results in enhanced butyrate production. These data suggest that gluconate may be developed as a prebiotic to enhance butyrate production in the hindgut.

The health benefits of non-digestible oligosaccharides (NDO), as dietary fiber, have been studied extensively. Various forms of fructo-oligosaccharides (FOS), oligofructoses (OF), xylooligosaccharides (XOS), and galacto-oligosaccharides (GOS, reviewed by [54]) are proven to be butyrogenic. These compounds are fermented primarily by bifidobacteria, and, to a lesser extent by lactobacilli, which are not butyrate producers [79]. Nevertheless, the butyrogenic property of these compounds is well documented. FOS and GOS are not sensitive to gastric acid and do not serve as substrates for hydrolytic enzymes in the upper digestive tract [54]. Prolonged intake of FOS induces a persistent increase in cecal butyrate concentration in rats, even after its major effect, such as a short-term increase in total LAB, is abolished [70]. Similarly, higher molar proportions of fecal butyrate are observed with all diets that had been supplemented with OF in rats [80]. However, these NDO are not equally butyrogenic. Various levels of potency in stimulating butyrate production are structure-dependent; and polymer chain length is one of the important determinants. Diets containing

OF and FOS result in higher cecal butyrate concentrations in rats than diets containing XOS [81]. Similarly, FOS-containing diets yield a higher fecal butyrate production than GOS-containing diets [82]. The butyrogenicity of these compounds, which are generally recognized to be bifidogenic, may result from metabolic cross-feeding between LAB and butyrate-producing bacteria. Substrate utilization of LAB may play a key role in determining the capacity of butyrate production. For example, more clostridia strains are able to utilize FOS than XOS [82].

Arabinoxylan (AX), also known as pentosan, is a major constituent of the cell wall of cereals. Recently, AX, along with its cleaved products, arabinoxylooligosaccharides (AXOS), has received widespread interest due to its prebiotic potential. The colonic butyrate concentration in rats is significantly greater, by more than 100%, in AXOS (with an average degree of polymerization of 3 to 5) and XOS groups compared with the control group [83]. In this study, it is found that AXOS and XOS have greater potential for inducing colonic butyrate concentration than FOX and inulin. These short-chain AXOS also increase the abundance of bifidobacteria in the intestines of rats and mice. However, the prebiotic effects of these AXOS depend strongly on their structural properties [84], especially their degrees of polymerization and arabinose substitution.

Resistant starch (RS) represents the fraction of ingested starch that escapes the small intestinal digestion and enters the human large bowel [85]. Its health benefits have long been recognized [86]. Early studies show that RS intake favors butyrate production in various models. The butyrogenic potential of various RS in a porcine model is very different [87]: significantly more butyrate is produced from potato starch and RS2 than from maize starch and RS3. Moreover, the uptake of butyrate by the colonic mucosa is starch type-dependent. Among the three RS tested, only raw potato RS starch results in a significant level of butyrate in the portal blood [87]. Indeed, RS induces a significantly greater amount of cecal butyrate in dextran sulfate sodium (DSS)-induced colitis rat models (DSS rats) than control and FOS diets [88]. Using this model, it was found that RS3 improves colonic lesions, probably due to its capability to yield a higher butyrate production and an increased butyrate uptake [89]. RS protects against colonic DNA damage in rats fed a Western diet, which is inversely correlated with colonic butyrate [90]. It is generally believed that RS consumption increases the total human fecal SCFA, as well as butyrate production and excretion. Human trials involving various types of RS, such as RS2 and RS3, demonstrate that, in general, fecal butyrate concentrations can be increased significantly [86]. Nonetheless, there are a few exceptions [91]. RS intake and fecal butyrate levels are high in populations with a low risk of diet-related large bowel diseases, whereas both values are low in high-risk populations [92].

Butyrylated starch (BS), starch acrylated by butyric anhydride, has been developed recently. The cecal and distal colonic butyrate concentrations are increased by 460% and 212%, respectively, in rats fed with BS for three days, compared to the control [93]. The high potency of BS is well documented [94]. Indeed, ingestion of butyrylated high amylose maize starch (HAMSB) results in approximately 260% higher fecal butyrate concentration in healthy individuals [95]. In carcinogen-treated rats, apoptotic rates in the distal colon are increased by HAMSB and correlated with luminal butyrate concentrations [85]. Compared to low amylose maize starch (LAMS), LAMS with tributrin, and high amylose maize starch (HAMS), HAMSB is more potent in increasing butyrate concentrations, not just in the distal colon, but also in the cecum and the proximal colon, as well as in the hepatic portal system [85, 96].

Inulin is generally regarded as a mixture of naturally occurring fructose polymers with a degree of polymerization (DP) of 10 to 60. Inulin differs from FOS by polymer chain length with the DP of the latter <10. It appears that the chain length of inulin affects its fermentability, while the longe-chain inulin (DP >24) tends to yield a lower butyrate concentration [97]. Inulin is among the bifidogenic substances that have been extensively studied (see the review by [98]). Numerous studies and at least three clinical trials have been launched to exploit its therapeutic applications in blood sugar regulation and lipid management, and mineral metabolism as well as in bone remodeling [99], fatty liver disease, and gastrointestinal disorders. While the anti-tumor properties of inulin and its derivatives have been demonstrated in multiple animal experiments [100], the results from human trials on colon cancer have been mixed [101, 102]. In a recent human trial, serum butyrate is increased significantly by inulin [103]. In a batch culture, inulin stimulates butyrate production [104]. However, inulin intakes in another human trial do not seem to result in any changes in the fecal butyrate, as compared to the baseline and placebo [105].

Resistant dextrin, such as branched dextrin (NUTRIOSE), has limited absorption in the small intestine, while the majority of ingested products can reach the colon. In rats, resistant dextrin can induce a significant increase in cecal butyrate concentration in a dose-dependent manner [106].

Non-starch polysaccharides (NSP), such as cellulose, hemicellulose, pectin, and β-glucans, have important health implications for humans [107]. These compounds clearly affect the taxonomic composition and metabolic features of the fecal microbiota. Human subjects fed with a diet containing β-glucans (3g/day) for three months show an initial increase in the fecal butyrate molar ratio, compared to placebo [108]. Similarly, pectin tends to increase the cecal butyrate concentration by 100% in rats [109]. However, a significantly higher butyrate is stimulated with starch-like carbohydrates, especially RS, as compared to pectin and cellulose [66]. The relatively lower potency in inducing butyrate production has limited the use of NSP as butyrogenic prebiotics.

Enhancing Gut Butyrate Concentrations Using Probiotics and Synbiotics

Probiotics are viable microorganisms that exert beneficial health effects to the host while synbiotics are a combination of prebiotics and probiotics in which the prebiotic compound(s) selectively favors the probiotic partner [110]. In addition to being safe and efficacious, ideal probiotics should be able to colonize the gut at a desired location for a sustained period of time. There has not yet been extensive research on either the extent to which probiotics modify the native gut microbiota for a defined period of time or their ability to restore altered gut microbiota while the host is in pathological and/or critical physiological stages. Moreover, hitherto, the results from various clinical trials using probiotics to treat different manifestations of IBD have been mixed [111].

Among the numerous named butyrate-producing bacteria (Table 1) and novel strains/isolates, only a few have been tested for their potential as probiotics and even fewer have been studied with butyrate promotion as one of the major clinical objectives or the primary end point in clinical trials. Nevertheless, it is being recognized that certain probiotic and synbiotics possess the ability to enhance gut butyrate biosynthesis in both animal models and human trials. In rats fed a FOS-containing diet, an *M. elsdenii* strain of rumen origin significantly enhances cecal butyrate production (by >7 fold), while normalizing hyper-lactate production and ameliorating diarrhea resulting from lactate accumulation [112]. The oral administration of butyrate-producing *C. butyricum* strain M588 in a DSS-induced colitis rat model is shown to be able to alleviate DSS-induced colitis symptoms and increase fecal butyrate concentrations [113]. Bifidobacteria and lactobacilli account for a significant portion of the probiotics currently on the market. In rats fed *B. longum* strain IPLA E44 for 24 days, the fecal butyrate concentration is significantly increased at the end of the feeding trial, whereas the cecal butyrate concentration is significantly decreased [114], suggesting that certain probiotics may possess the ability to shift the sites of major butyrate biosynthesis in the hindgut.

Several probiotic *Lactobacillus* species and/or strains are known to increase butyrate production in both batch culture and human trials. Treatment with probiotic strain *L. acidophilus* NCFM increases butyrate production in a colon fermentation model [115]. The *L. paracasei* intake results in a significant increase of butyrate and a concomitant decrease of lactate in constipated patients [116]. Similarly, the probiotic consumption of *L. salivarius* also induced a significant increase in the fecal butyrate concentration in a six-month-old infant [117]. Butyrate enhancing abilities are also observed in patients with long-term total enteral nutrition fed with the probiotic yeast *Saccharomycin boulardii* [118]. VSL#3 is a probiotic medical food containing three *Bifidobacterium* species, four *Lactobacillus* species, and one *Streptococcus* species. Earlier clinical trials suggest that high dose probiotic VSL#3 consumption is effective in maintaining antibiotic introduced remission in patients with recurrent or refractory pouchitis [119]. Further studies demonstrate that when compared to pouchitis patients in the placebo group, probiotic therapy with VSL#3 tends to increase the total intestinal bacteria as well as the richness and diversity of the bacterial microbiota while repressing the intestinal fungal diversity [120]. Recently, VSL#3 has been shown to dramatically increase the plasma butyrate in mice fed both low- and high-fat diets in comparison to their controls ($P < 0.001$). At the same time, VSL#3 has been shown to significantly increase the abundance of *buk*-containing bacterial population in feces [121]. As a result, VSL#3 is able to ameliorate high-fat diet induced obesity and diabetes.

Strong synergistic effects in increasing butyrate production are observed in two synbiotic systems involving two strains of *L. acidophilus* in *in vitro* models [115, 122]. A synbiotic *L. acidophilus* and FOS combination increases butyrate production significantly [122]. While the *L. acidophilus* strain, NCFM, alone tends to increase butyrate production, true synergistic effects in stimulating butyrate production is documented on this strain in combination with lactitol, as a prebiotic [115]. In human trials involving patients with short bowel syndrome, fecal butyrate concentrations are significantly lower before synbiotic therapy [123], compared to healthy, age-matched children. A one-year oral consumption of synbiotics, consisting of GOS and two probiotics *B. breve* and *L. casei,* results in a significant increase in several serum immune parameters and a notable improvement in the fecal microbial profile. Both the fecal butyrate concentration and the total SCFA are increased in one of the four patients while the SCFA/total organic acid ratio is higher in the other three patients [123]. In a clinical trial comparing the efficacy of prebiotic (psyllium), probiotic (*B. longum*), and synbiotic (both) therapies to improve the quality of life in patients with UC, greater quality-of-life changes are noticed only in the synbiotic group, as reflected in a significant change in total IBD

Questionnaire (IBDQ) scores. The synergistic effects of psyllium and *B. longum* are evident; a significant reduction in C-reaction protein is observed only with the synbiotic therapy [124]. However, no fecal SCFA, including butyrate, is measured in this study. Recent results from a randomized, double-blind placebo-controlled clinical trial involving a synbiotic consisting of *B. longum* and inulin (Synergy 1) in older people have been reported [125]. While the synbiotic has no effect on bowel habits or any clinical parameters, a significant reduction in proinflammatory TNFα is detected. The synbiotic consumption leads to a significant increase in butyrate production, probably due to a significant increase in the abundance of bifidobacteria and the phylum Firmicutes, which contain numerous butyrate-producing bacteria. Overall, only a few probiotics and/or synbiotics that are able to enhance butyrate biosynthesis in the gut have been documented. Nevertheless, butyrate-producing bacteria, as novel probiotics in treating IBD, have recently received much attention [27, 126, 127]. With rapid technical progress in manufacturing and delivery, using butyrate-producing bacteria, such as *Butyricicoccus pullicaecorum*, as promising pharmabiotics will soon become a reality [63].

ALTERNATIVE APPROACHES TO INCREASE BUTYRATE BIOAVAILABILITY

Butyrate deficits have important pathological consequences. Oral butyrate administration is seemingly a logical choice. However, this approach is rarely explored because of two factors: poor palatability with an unpleasant taste and odor and low bioavailability in the hindgut. Butyrate is subject to rapid absorption in the stomach and duodenum and it is questionable if ingested butyrate can reach the desired locations in the hindgut. Nevertheless, a few published reports suggest that in healthy rats, oral butyrate administration leads to a three times increase in cecal butyrate concentrations [128], indicating that butyrate from the oral route may indeed reach the colon. In rats with experimentally induced acute UC, oral butyrate administration fails to increase cecal butyrate concentration but nevertheless improves mucosa lesions and attenuates the intestinal inflammation. This observation supports the tropic effects of butyrate on colon mucosa using rectal administration. Indeed, the efficacy of butyrate enemas in a subset of patients with distal UC, especially those with short active episodes, is documented in a double-blind, placebo controlled clinical trial [129]. Another clinical trial, involving UC patients in remission, demonstrates that rectal enemas containing 100 mM of sodium butyrate induces a minor improvement in colonic inflammation and oxidative stress [130]. Encapsulation may further improve palatability and butyrate bioavailability in the distal colon [131]. Indeed, microencapsulated sodium butyrate has been shown to reduce the frequency of abdominal pain in patients with irritable bowel syndrome [132].

Other methods to increase bioavailability and improve pharmacokinetic profiles of butyrate include emulsions, nanoparticles, and structured lipids. Structural lipids, such as butyryl triglyceride (tributyrin), present in nature, such as in milk fat and honey, is chemically stable and can be rapidly hydrolyzed by pancreatic and gastric lipases to release butyrate [18]. Tributyrin has been shown to act as a butyrate prodrug to enhance butyrate concentration over a sustained period of time with minimal toxicity [133]. Tributyrin acts on multiple anticancer cellular and molecular targets without affecting non-cancerous cells and may represent a promising anticancer agent [134]. Alternatively, compounds, such as retinoic acid, which act synergistically with butyrate so that the desired effect can be achieved at a lower butyrate concentration, have been exploited [135].

Conclusion

The butyrate concentration in the gut has important physiological and pathological implications. Reduced butyrate biosynthesis is associated with various pathological conditions. Numerous carbohydrates possess butyrogenic properties and can be developed as prebiotics. Butyrate-producing bacteria are a key component of the gut microbiome. The butyrate-producing fraction of the gut microbiota is readily inducible. Hyper-butyrate producing bacterial strains can be isolated from host-associated habitats. It is foreseeable that the synergistic effects of various prebiotics and probiotics (or synbiotics) in stimulating butyrate biosynthesis will soon be utilized for health benefits.

Acknowledgments

Mention of trade names or commercial products in this publication is solely for the purpose of providing specific information and does not imply recommendation or endorsement by the U. S. Department of Agriculture. The USDA is an equal opportunity provider and employer.

References

[1] Newmark HL, Lupton JR, Young CW. Butyrate as a differentiating agent: pharmacokinetics, analogues and current status. *Cancer letters*. 1994;78(1-3):1-5.

[2] Cummings JH. Short chain fatty acids in the human colon. *Gut*. 1981;22(9):763-79.

[3] Stein J, Zores M, Schroder O. Short-chain fatty acid (SCFA) uptake into Caco-2 cells by a pH-dependent and carrier mediated transport mechanism. *European journal of nutrition*. 2000;39(3):121-5.

[4] Miyauchi S, Gopal E, Fei YJ, Ganapathy V. Functional identification of SLC5A8, a tumor suppressor down-regulated in colon cancer, as a Na(+)-coupled transporter for short-chain fatty acids. *J. Biol. Chem*. 2004;279(14):13293-6.

[5] Borthakur A, Gill RK, Hodges K, Ramaswamy K, Hecht G, Dudeja PK. Enteropathogenic Escherichia coli inhibits butyrate uptake in Caco-2 cells by altering the apical membrane MCT1 level. *American journal of physiology Gastrointestinal and liver physiology*. 2006;290(1):G30-5.

[6] Maslowski KM, Vieira AT, Ng A, Kranich J, Sierro F, Yu D, et al. Regulation of inflammatory responses by gut microbiota and chemoattractant receptor GPR43. *Nature*. 2009;461(7268):1282-6.

[7] Haner K, Henzi T, Pfefferli M, Kunzli E, Salicio V, Schwaller B. A bipartite butyrate-responsive element in the human calretinin (CALB2) promoter acts as a repressor in colon carcinoma cells but not in mesothelioma cells. *J. Cell Biochem*. 2010;109(3):519-31.

[8] Vinolo MA, Ferguson GJ, Kulkarni S, Damoulakis G, Anderson K, Bohlooly YM, et al. SCFAs induce mouse neutrophil chemotaxis through the GPR43 receptor. *PLoS One*. 2011;6(6):e21205.

[9] Roelofsen H, Priebe MG, Vonk RJ. The interaction of short-chain fatty acids with adipose tissue: relevance for prevention of type 2 diabetes. *Beneficial microbes*. 2010;1(4):433-7.

[10] Vanhoutvin SA, Troost FJ, Hamer HM, Lindsey PJ, Koek GH, Jonkers DM, et al. Butyrate-induced transcriptional changes in human colonic mucosa. *PLoS One*. 2009;4(8):e6759.

[11] Wu S, Li RW, Li W, Li CJ. Transcriptome characterization by RNA-seq unravels the mechanisms of butyrate-induced epigenomic regulation in bovine cells. *PLoS One*. 2012;7(5):e36940.

[12] Wu S, Li C, Huang W, Li W, Li RW. Alternative splicing regulated by butyrate in bovine epithelial cells. *PLoS One*. 2012;7(6):e39182.

[13] Hamer HM, Jonkers D, Venema K, Vanhoutvin S, Troost FJ, Brummer RJ. Review article: the role of butyrate on colonic function. *Alimentary pharmacology & therapeutics*. 2008;27(2):104-19.

[14] Canani RB, Costanzo MD, Leone L, Pedata M, Meli R, Calignano A. Potential beneficial effects of butyrate in intestinal and extraintestinal diseases. *World J. Gastroenterol*. 2011;17(12):1519-28.

[15] Ochoa-Zarzosa A, Villarreal-Fernandez E, Cano-Camacho H, Lopez-Meza JE. Sodium butyrate inhibits Staphylococcus aureus internalization in bovine mammary epithelial cells and induces the expression of antimicrobial peptide genes. *Microbial pathogenesis*. 2009;47(1):1-7.

[16] Lewis K, Lutgendorff F, Phan V, Soderholm JD, Sherman PM, McKay DM. Enhanced translocation of bacteria across metabolically stressed epithelia is reduced by butyrate. *Inflammatory bowel diseases*. 2010;16(7):1138-48.

[17] Bergman EN. Energy contributions of volatile fatty acids from the gastrointestinal tract in various species. *Physiological reviews*. 1990;70(2):567-90.

[18] Wachtershauser A, Stein J. Rationale for the luminal provision of butyrate in intestinal diseases. *European journal of nutrition*. 2000;39(4):164-71.

[19] Penner GB, Steele MA, Aschenbach JR, McBride BW. Ruminant Nutrition Symposium: Molecular adaptation of ruminal epithelia to highly fermentable diets. *J. Anim. Sci*. 2011;89(4):1108-19.

[20] Bultman SJ. Molecular Pathways: Gene-environment interactions regulating dietary fiber induction of proliferation and apoptosis via butyrate for cancer prevention. *Clin. Cancer Res*. 2013.

[21] Donohoe DR, Garge N, Zhang X, Sun W, O'Connell TM, Bunger MK, et al. The microbiome and butyrate regulate energy metabolism and autophagy in the mammalian colon. *Cell metabolism*. 2011;13(5):517-26.

[22] Duncan SH, Belenguer A, Holtrop G, Johnstone AM, Flint HJ, Lobley GE. Reduced dietary intake of carbohydrates by obese subjects results in decreased concentrations of

butyrate and butyrate-producing bacteria in feces. *Applied and environmental microbiology*. 2007;73(4):1073-8.

[23] Lin HV, Frassetto A, Kowalik EJ, Jr., Nawrocki AR, Lu MM, Kosinski JR, et al. Butyrate and propionate protect against diet-induced obesity and regulate gut hormones via free fatty acid receptor 3-independent mechanisms. *PLoS One*. 2012;7(4):e35240.

[24] Thompson-Chagoyan OC, Fallani M, Maldonado J, Vieites JM, Khanna S, Edwards C, et al. Faecal microbiota and short-chain fatty acid levels in faeces from infants with cow's milk protein allergy. *International archives of allergy and immunology*. 2011;156(3):325-32.

[25] Forest V, Clement M, Pierre F, Meflah K, Menanteau J. Butyrate restores motile function and actin cytoskeletal network integrity in apc mutated mouse colon epithelial cells. *Nutrition and cancer*. 2003;45(1):84-92.

[26] Kumari R, Ahuja V, Paul J. Fluctuations in butyrate-producing bacteria in ulcerative colitis patients of North India. *World J. Gastroenterol*. 2013;19(22):3404-14.

[27] Eeckhaut V, Machiels K, Perrier C, Romero C, Maes S, Flahou B, et al. Butyricicoccus pullicaecorum in inflammatory bowel disease. *Gut*. 2013;62(12):1745-52.

[28] Antharam VC, Li EC, Ishmael A, Sharma A, Mai V, Rand KH, et al. Intestinal dysbiosis and depletion of butyrogenic bacteria in Clostridium difficile infection and nosocomial diarrhea. *Journal of clinical microbiology*. 2013;51(9):2884-92.

[29] Lupton JR. Microbial degradation products influence colon cancer risk: the butyrate controversy. *J. Nutr*. 2004;134(2):479-82.

[30] Scheppach W, Weiler F. The butyrate story: old wine in new bottles? *Current opinion in clinical nutrition and metabolic care*. 2004;7(5):563-7.

[31] Tirandaz H, Mohammadi E. Efficient tumor targeting by anaerobic butyrate-producing bacteria. *Medical hypotheses*. 2013;80(5):675-8.

[32] Louis P, McCrae SI, Charrier C, Flint HJ. Organization of butyrate synthetic genes in human colonic bacteria: phylogenetic conservation and horizontal gene transfer. *FEMS microbiology letters*. 2007;269(2):240-7.

[33] Asanuma N, Ishiwata M, Yoshii T, Kikuchi M, Nishina Y, Hino T. Characterization and transcription of the genes involved in butyrate production in Butyrivibrio fibrisolvens type I and II strains. *Current microbiology*. 2005;51(2):91-4.

[34] Charrier C, Duncan GJ, Reid MD, Rucklidge GJ, Henderson D, Young P, et al. A novel class of CoA-transferase involved in short-chain fatty acid metabolism in butyrate-producing human colonic bacteria. *Microbiology*. 2006;152(Pt 1):179-85.

[35] Walter KA, Nair RV, Cary JW, Bennett GN, Papoutsakis ET. Sequence and arrangement of two genes of the butyrate-synthesis pathway of Clostridium acetobutylicum ATCC 824. *Gene*. 1993;134(1):107-11.

[36] Louis P, Duncan SH, McCrae SI, Millar J, Jackson MS, Flint HJ. Restricted distribution of the butyrate kinase pathway among butyrate-producing bacteria from the human colon. *Journal of bacteriology*. 2004;186(7):2099-106.

[37] Barcenilla A, Pryde SE, Martin JC, Duncan SH, Stewart CS, Henderson C, et al. Phylogenetic relationships of butyrate-producing bacteria from the human gut. *Applied and environmental microbiology*. 2000;66(4):1654-61.

[38] Pryde SE, Duncan SH, Hold GL, Stewart CS, Flint HJ. The microbiology of butyrate formation in the human colon. *FEMS microbiology letters*. 2002;217(2):133-9.

[39] Louis P, Flint HJ. Diversity, metabolism and microbial ecology of butyrate-producing bacteria from the human large intestine. *FEMS microbiology letters*. 2009;294(1):1-8.

[40] Eeckhaut V, Van Immerseel F, Croubels S, De Baere S, Haesebrouck F, Ducatelle R, et al. Butyrate production in phylogenetically diverse Firmicutes isolated from the chicken caecum. *Microbial biotechnology*. 2011;4(4):503-12.

[41] Louis P, Young P, Holtrop G, Flint HJ. Diversity of human colonic butyrate-producing bacteria revealed by analysis of the butyryl-CoA:acetate CoA-transferase gene. *Environmental microbiology*. 2010;12(2):304-14.

[42] Hippe B, Zwielehner J, Liszt K, Lassl C, Unger F, Haslberger AG. Quantification of butyryl CoA:acetate CoA-transferase genes reveals different butyrate production capacity in individuals according to diet and age. *FEMS microbiology letters*. 2011;316(2):130-5.

[43] Bartosch S, Fite A, Macfarlane GT, McMurdo ME. Characterization of bacterial communities in feces from healthy elderly volunteers and hospitalized elderly patients by using real-time PCR and effects of antibiotic treatment on the fecal microbiota. *Applied and environmental microbiology*. 2004;70(6):3575-81.

[44] Walker AW, Duncan SH, Harmsen HJ, Holtrop G, Welling GW, Flint HJ. The species composition of the human intestinal microbiota differs between particle-associated and liquid phase communities. *Environmental microbiology*. 2008;10(12):3275-83.

[45] Schwiertz A, Hold GL, Duncan SH, Gruhl B, Collins MD, Lawson PA, et al. Anaerostipes caccae gen. nov., sp. nov., a new saccharolytic, acetate-utilising, butyrate-producing bacterium from human faeces. *Systematic and applied microbiology*. 2002;25(1):46-51.

[46] Suau A, Rochet V, Sghir A, Gramet G, Brewaeys S, Sutren M, et al. Fusobacterium prausnitzii and related species represent a dominant group within the human fecal flora. *Systematic and applied microbiology*. 2001;24(1):139-45.

[47] Sokol H, Pigneur B, Watterlot L, Lakhdari O, Bermudez-Humaran LG, Gratadoux JJ, et al. Faecalibacterium prausnitzii is an anti-inflammatory commensal bacterium identified by gut microbiota analysis of Crohn disease patients. *Proc. Natl. Acad. Sci. U. S. A.* 2008;105(43):16731-6.

[48] Li RW, Wu S, Baldwin RLt, Li W, Li C. Perturbation dynamics of the rumen microbiota in response to exogenous butyrate. *PLoS One*. 2012;7(1):e29392.

[49] Kopecny J, Zorec M, Mrazek J, Kobayashi Y, Marinsek-Logar R. Butyrivibrio hungatei sp. nov. and Pseudobutyrivibrio xylanivorans sp. nov., butyrate-producing bacteria from the rumen. *Int. J. Syst. Evol. Microbiol.* 2003;53(Pt 1):201-9.

[50] Rumney CJ, Duncan SH, Henderson C, Stewart CS. Isolation and characteristics of a wheatbran-degrading Butyrivibrio from human faeces. *Letters in applied microbiology*. 1995;20(4):232-6.

[51] Ohkawara S, Furuya H, Nagashima K, Asanuma N, Hino T. Oral administration of butyrivibrio fibrisolvens, a butyrate-producing bacterium, decreases the formation of aberrant crypt foci in the colon and rectum of mice. *J. Nutr.* 2005;135(12):2878-83.

[52] Ohkawara S, Furuya H, Nagashima K, Asanuma N, Hino T. Effect of oral administration of Butyrivibrio fibrisolvens MDT-1 on experimental enterocolitis in mice. *Clinical and vaccine immunology: CVI*. 2006;13(11):1231-6.

[53] Vital M, Penton CR, Wang Q, Young VB, Antonopoulos DA, Sogin ML, et al. A gene-targeted approach to investigate the intestinal butyrate-producing bacterial community. *Microbiome*. 2013;1(1):8.

[54] Macfarlane GT, Steed H, Macfarlane S. Bacterial metabolism and health-related effects of galacto-oligosaccharides and other prebiotics. *Journal of applied microbiology*. 2008;104(2):305-44.

[55] Scott DW, Longpre JM, Loo G. Upregulation of GADD153 by butyrate: involvement of MAPK. *DNA and cell biology*. 2008;27(11):607-14.

[56] Looft T, Levine UY, Stanton TB. Cloacibacillus porcorum sp. nov., a mucin-degrading bacterium from the swine intestinal tract and emended description of the genus Cloacibacillus. *Int. J. Syst. Evol. Microbiol.* 2013;63(Pt 6):1960-6.

[57] Levine UY, Looft T, Allen HK, Stanton TB. Butyrate-producing bacteria, including mucin degraders, from the swine intestinal tract. *Applied and environmental microbiology*. 2013;79(12):3879-81.

[58] Yokoyama S, Niwa T, Osawa T, Suzuki T. Characterization of an O-desmethylangolensin-producing bacterium isolated from human feces. *Archives of microbiology*. 2010;192(1):15-22.

[59] Duncan SH, Hold GL, Barcenilla A, Stewart CS, Flint HJ. Roseburia intestinalis sp. nov., a novel saccharolytic, butyrate-producing bacterium from human faeces. *Int. J. Syst. Evol. Microbiol.* 2002;52(Pt 5):1615-20.

[60] Eeckhaut V, Van Immerseel F, Teirlynck E, Pasmans F, Fievez V, Snauwaert C, et al. Butyricicoccus pullicaecorum gen. nov., sp. nov., an anaerobic, butyrate-producing bacterium isolated from the caecal content of a broiler chicken. *Int. J. Syst. Evol. Microbiol.* 2008;58(Pt 12):2799-802.

[61] Eeckhaut V, Van Immerseel F, Pasmans F, De Brandt E, Haesebrouck F, Ducatelle R, et al. Anaerostipes butyraticus sp. nov., an anaerobic, butyrate-producing bacterium from Clostridium cluster XIVa isolated from broiler chicken caecal content, and emended description of the genus Anaerostipes. *Int. J. Syst. Evol. Microbiol.* 2010; 60(Pt 5):1108-12.

[62] Geirnaert A, Steyaert A, Van den Abbeele P, Eeckhaut V, Van Immerseel F, Boon N, et al. In vitro characterization of gastrointestinal behavior of Butyricicoccus pullicaecorum, a novel butyrate producing isolate with probiotic potential to counterbalance dysbiosis in inflammatory bowel disease. *Communications in agricultural and applied biological sciences*. 2013;78(1):157-63.

[63] Eeckhaut V, Ducatelle R, Sas B, Vermeire S, Van Immerseel F. Progress towards butyrate-producing pharmabiotics: Butyricicoccus pullicaecorum capsule and efficacy in TNBS models in comparison with therapeutics. *Gut*. 2014;63(2):367.

[64] Mathers JC, Kennard J, James OF. Gastrointestinal responses to oats consumption in young adult and elderly rats: digestion, large bowel fermentation and crypt cell proliferation rates. *The British journal of nutrition*. 1993;70(2):567-84.

[65] Silvester KR, Englyst HN, Cummings JH. Ileal recovery of starch from whole diets containing resistant starch measured in vitro and fermentation of ileal effluent. *The American journal of clinical nutrition*. 1995;62(2):403-11.

[66] Weaver GA, Krause JA, Miller TL, Wolin MJ. Cornstarch fermentation by the colonic microbial community yields more butyrate than does cabbage fiber fermentation;

cornstarch fermentation rates correlate negatively with methanogenesis. *The American journal of clinical nutrition*. 1992;55(1):70-7.

[67] Knudsen KE, Jensen BB, Hansen I. Oat bran but not a beta-glucan-enriched oat fraction enhances butyrate production in the large intestine of pigs. *J. Nutr.* 1993;123(7):1235-47.

[68] Mortensen PB, Holtug K, Rasmussen HS. Short-chain fatty acid production from mono- and disaccharides in a fecal incubation system: implications for colonic fermentation of dietary fiber in humans. *J. Nutr.* 1988;118(3):321-5.

[69] Gibson GR, Wang X. Enrichment of bifidobacteria from human gut contents by oligofructose using continuous culture. *FEMS microbiology letters*. 1994;118(1-2):121-7.

[70] Le Blay G, Michel C, Blottiere HM, Cherbut C. Prolonged intake of fructo-oligosaccharides induces a short-term elevation of lactic acid-producing bacteria and a persistent increase in cecal butyrate in rats. *J. Nutr.* 1999;129(12):2231-5.

[71] Levin GV, Zehner LR, Saunders JP, Beadle JR. Sugar substitutes: their energy values, bulk characteristics, and potential health benefits. *The American journal of clinical nutrition.* 1995;62(5 Suppl):1161S-8S.

[72] Espinosa I, Fogelfeld L. Tagatose: from a sweetener to a new diabetic medication? *Expert opinion on investigational drugs*. 2010;19(2):285-94.

[73] Laerke HN, Jensen BB. D-tagatose has low small intestinal digestibility but high large intestinal fermentability in pigs. *J. Nutr.* 1999;129(5):1002-9.

[74] Laerke HN, Jensen BB, Hojsgaard S. In vitro fermentation pattern of D-tagatose is affected by adaptation of the microbiota from the gastrointestinal tract of pigs. *J. Nutr.* 2000;130(7):1772-9.

[75] Venema K, Vermunt SHF, Brink EJ. D-tagatose increase butyrate production by the colonic microbiota in healthy men and women. *Microbiol. Eco. Health Dis.* 2005; 17:47-57.

[76] Bertelsen H, Andersen H, Tvede M. Fermentation of D-tagatose by human intestinal bacteria and dairy lactic acid bacteria. *Microbiol. Eco. Health Dis*. 2001;13:87-95.

[77] Bertelsen H, Jensen BB, Buemann B. D-tagatose--a novel low-calorie bulk sweetener with prebiotic properties. *World review of nutrition and dietetics*. 1999;85:98-109.

[78] Tsukahara T, Koyama H, Okada M, Ushida K. Stimulation of butyrate production by gluconic acid in batch culture of pig cecal digesta and identification of butyrate-producing bacteria. *J. Nutr.* 2002;132(8):2229-34.

[79] Kolida S, Tuohy K, Gibson GR. Prebiotic effects of inulin and oligofructose. *The British journal of nutrition.* 2002;87 Suppl 2:S193-7.

[80] Kleessen B, Hartmann L, Blaut M. Oligofructose and long-chain inulin: influence on the gut microbial ecology of rats associated with a human faecal flora. *The British journal of nutrition.* 2001;86(2):291-300.

[81] Campbell JM, Fahey GC, Jr., Wolf BW. Selected indigestible oligosaccharides affect large bowel mass, cecal and fecal short-chain fatty acids, pH and microflora in rats. *J. Nutr*. 1997;127(1):130-6.

[82] Djouzi Z, Andrieux C. Compared effects of three oligosaccharides on metabolism of intestinal microflora in rats inoculated with a human faecal flora. *The British journal of nutrition*. 1997;78(2):313-24.

[83] Van Craeyveld V, Swennen K, Dornez E, Van de Wiele T, Marzorati M, Verstraete W, et al. Structurally different wheat-derived arabinoxylooligosaccharides have different prebiotic and fermentation properties in rats. *J. Nutr.* 2008;138(12):2348-55.

[84] Damen B, Verspreet J, Pollet A, Broekaert WF, Delcour JA, Courtin CM. Prebiotic effects and intestinal fermentation of cereal arabinoxylans and arabinoxylan oligosaccharides in rats depend strongly on their structural properties and joint presence. *Molecular nutrition & food research.* 2011;55(12):1862-74.

[85] Clarke JM, Young GP, Topping DL, Bird AR, Cobiac L, Scherer BL, et al. Butyrate delivered by butyrylated starch increases distal colonic epithelial apoptosis in carcinogen-treated rats. *Carcinogenesis.* 2012;33(1):197-202.

[86] Topping DL, Clifton PM. Short-chain fatty acids and human colonic function: roles of resistant starch and nonstarch polysaccharides. *Physiological reviews.* 2001;81(3):1031-64.

[87] Martin LJ, Dumon HJ, Lecannu G, Champ MM. Potato and high-amylose maize starches are not equivalent producers of butyrate for the colonic mucosa. *The British journal of nutrition.* 2000;84(5):689-96.

[88] Moreau NM, Martin LJ, Toquet CS, Laboisse CL, Nguyen PG, Siliart BS, et al. Restoration of the integrity of rat caeco-colonic mucosa by resistant starch, but not by fructo-oligosaccharides, in dextran sulfate sodium-induced experimental colitis. *The British journal of nutrition.* 2003;90(1):75-85.

[89] Moreau NM, Champ MM, Goupry SM, Le Bizec BJ, Krempf M, Nguyen PG, et al. Resistant starch modulates in vivo colonic butyrate uptake and its oxidation in rats with dextran sulfate sodium-induced colitis. *J. Nutr.* 2004;134(3):493-500.

[90] Conlon MA, Kerr CA, McSweeney CS, Dunne RA, Shaw JM, Kang S, et al. Resistant starches protect against colonic DNA damage and alter microbiota and gene expression in rats fed a Western diet. *J. Nutr.* 2012;142(5):832-40.

[91] Holt PR, Atillasoy E, Lindenbaum J, Ho SB, Lupton JR, McMahon D, et al. Effects of acarbose on fecal nutrients, colonic pH, and short-chain fatty acids and rectal proliferative indices. *Metabolism: clinical and experimental.* 1996;45(9):1179-87.

[92] Bird AR, Conlon MA, Christophersen CT, Topping DL. Resistant starch, large bowel fermentation and a broader perspective of prebiotics and probiotics. *Beneficial microbes.* 2010;1(4):423-31.

[93] Annison G, Illman RJ, Topping DL. Acetylated, propionylated or butyrylated starches raise large bowel short-chain fatty acids preferentially when fed to rats. *J. Nutr.* 2003; 133(11):3523-8.

[94] Bajka BH, Topping DL, Cobiac L, Clarke JM. Butyrylated starch is less susceptible to enzymic hydrolysis and increases large-bowel butyrate more than high-amylose maize starch in the rat. *The British journal of nutrition.* 2006;96(2):276-82.

[95] West NP, Christophersen CT, Pyne DB, Cripps AW, Conlon MA, Topping DL, et al. Butyrylated starch increases colonic butyrate concentration but has limited effects on immunity in healthy physically active individuals. *Exercise immunology review.* 2013; 19:102-19.

[96] Clarke JM, Topping DL, Christophersen CT, Bird AR, Lange K, Saunders I, et al. Butyrate esterified to starch is released in the human gastrointestinal tract. *The American journal of clinical nutrition.* 2011;94(5):1276-83.

[97] Stewart ML, Timm DA, Slavin JL. Fructooligosaccharides exhibit more rapid fermentation than long-chain inulin in an in vitro fermentation system. *Nutrition research*. 2008;28(5):329-34.

[98] Kelly G. Inulin-type prebiotics--a review: part 1. *Alternative medicine review: a journal of clinical therapeutic*. 2008;13(4):315-29.

[99] Scholz-Ahrens KE, Schrezenmeir J. Inulin and oligofructose and mineral metabolism: the evidence from animal trials. *J. Nutr*. 2007;137(11 Suppl):2513S-23S.

[100] Roberfroid MB. Introducing inulin-type fructans. *The British journal of nutrition*. 2005;93 Suppl 1:S13-25.

[101] Boutron-Ruault MC, Marteau P, Lavergne-Slove A, Myara A, Gerhardt MF, Franchisseur C, et al. Effects of a 3-mo consumption of short-chain fructo-oligosaccharides on parameters of colorectal carcinogenesis in patients with or without small or large colorectal adenomas. *Nutrition and cancer*. 2005;53(2):160-8.

[102] Pool-Zobel BL. Inulin-type fructans and reduction in colon cancer risk: review of experimental and human data. *The British journal of nutrition*. 2005;93 Suppl 1:S73-90.

[103] Tarini J, Wolever TM. The fermentable fibre inulin increases postprandial serum short-chain fatty acids and reduces free-fatty acids and ghrelin in healthy subjects. *Applied physiology, nutrition, and metabolism = Physiologie appliquee, nutrition et metabolisme*. 2010;35(1):9-16.

[104] Nazzaro F, Fratianni F, Orlando P, Coppola R. Biochemical Traits, Survival and Biological Properties of the Probiotic Lactobacillus plantarum Grown in the Presence of Prebiotic Inulin and Pectin as Energy Source. *Pharmaceuticals*. 2012;5(5):481-92.

[105] Petry N, Egli I, Chassard C, Lacroix C, Hurrell R. Inulin modifies the bifidobacteria population, fecal lactate concentration, and fecal pH but does not influence iron absorption in women with low iron status. *The American journal of clinical nutrition*. 2012;96(2):325-31.

[106] Guerin-Deremaux L, Ringard F, Desailly F, Wils D. Effects of a soluble dietary fibre NUTRIOSE(R) on colonic fermentation and excretion rates in rats. *Nutrition research and practice*. 2010;4(6):470-6.

[107] Kumar V, Sinha AK, Makkar HP, de Boeck G, Becker K. Dietary roles of non-starch polysaccharides in human nutrition: a review. *Critical reviews in food science and nutrition*. 2012;52(10):899-935.

[108] Turunen K, Tsouvelakidou E, Nomikos T, Mountzouris KC, Karamanolis D, Triantafillidis J, et al. Impact of beta-glucan on the faecal microbiota of polypectomized patients: a pilot study. *Anaerobe*. 2011;17(6):403-6.

[109] Licht TR, Hansen M, Bergstrom A, Poulsen M, Krath BN, Markowski J, et al. Effects of apples and specific apple components on the cecal environment of conventional rats: role of apple pectin. *BMC microbiology*. 2010;10:13.

[110] Schrezenmeir J, de Vrese M. Probiotics, prebiotics, and synbiotics--approaching a definition. *The American journal of clinical nutrition*. 2001;73(2 Suppl):361S-4S.

[111] Hedin C, Whelan K, Lindsay JO. Evidence for the use of probiotics and prebiotics in inflammatory bowel disease: a review of clinical trials. *The Proceedings of the Nutrition Society*. 2007;66(3):307-15.

[112] Hashizume K, Tsukahara T, Yamada K, Koyama H, Ushida K. Megasphaera elsdenii JCM1772T normalizes hyperlactate production in the large intestine of

fructooligosaccharide-fed rats by stimulating butyrate production. *J. Nutr.* 2003; 133(10):3187-90.

[113] Okamoto T, Sasaki M, Tsujikawa T, Fujiyama Y, Bamba T, Kusunoki M. Preventive efficacy of butyrate enemas and oral administration of Clostridium butyricum M588 in dextran sodium sulfate-induced colitis in rats. *Journal of gastroenterology.* 2000;35(5):341-6.

[114] Salazar N, Binetti A, Gueimonde M, Alonso A, Garrido P, Gonzalez del Rey C, et al. Safety and intestinal microbiota modulation by the exopolysaccharide-producing strains Bifidobacterium animalis IPLA R1 and Bifidobacterium longum IPLA E44 orally administered to Wistar rats. *International journal of food microbiology.* 2011;144(3):342-51.

[115] Makivuokko H, Forssten S, Saarinen M, Ouwehand A, Rautonen N. Synbiotic effects of lactitol and Lactobacillus acidophilus NCFM in a semi-continuous colon fermentation model. *Beneficial microbes.* 2010;1(2):131-7.

[116] Valerio F, Russo F, de Candia S, Riezzo G, Orlando A, Lonigro SL, et al. Effects of probiotic Lactobacillus paracasei-enriched artichokes on constipated patients: a pilot study. *Journal of clinical gastroenterology.* 2010;44 Suppl 1:S49-53.

[117] Maldonado J, Lara-Villoslada F, Sierra S, Sempere L, Gomez M, Rodriguez JM, et al. Safety and tolerance of the human milk probiotic strain Lactobacillus salivarius CECT5713 in 6-month-old children. Nutrition. 2010;26(11-12):1082-7.

[118] Schneider SM, Girard-Pipau F, Filippi J, Hebuterne X, Moyse D, Hinojosa GC, et al. Effects of Saccharomyces boulardii on fecal short-chain fatty acids and microflora in patients on long-term total enteral nutrition. *World J. Gastroenterol.* 2005;11(39):6165-9.

[119] Mimura T, Rizzello F, Helwig U, Poggioli G, Schreiber S, Talbot IC, et al. Once daily high dose probiotic therapy (VSL#3) for maintaining remission in recurrent or refractory pouchitis. *Gut.* 2004;53(1):108-14.

[120] Kuhbacher T, Ott SJ, Helwig U, Mimura T, Rizzello F, Kleessen B, et al. Bacterial and fungal microbiota in relation to probiotic therapy (VSL#3) in pouchitis. *Gut.* 2006;55(6):833-41.

[121] Yadav H, Lee JH, Lloyd J, Walter P, Rane SG. Beneficial metabolic effects of a probiotic via butyrate-induced GLP-1 hormone secretion. *J. Biol. Chem.* 2013;288(35): 25088-97.

[122] Gmeiner M, Kneifel W, Kulbe KD, Wouters R, De Boever P, Nollet L, et al. Influence of a synbiotic mixture consisting of Lactobacillus acidophilus 74-2 and a fructooligosaccharide preparation on the microbial ecology sustained in a simulation of the human intestinal microbial ecosystem (SHIME reactor). *Applied microbiology and biotechnology.* 2000;53(2):219-23.

[123] Uchida K, Takahashi T, Inoue M, Morotomi M, Otake K, Nakazawa M, et al. Immunonutritional effects during synbiotics therapy in pediatric patients with short bowel syndrome. *Pediatric surgery international.* 2007;23(3):243-8.

[124] Fujimori S, Gudis K, Mitsui K, Seo T, Yonezawa M, Tanaka S, et al. A randomized controlled trial on the efficacy of synbiotic versus probiotic or prebiotic treatment to improve the quality of life in patients with ulcerative colitis. *Nutrition.* 2009;25(5):520-5.

[125] Macfarlane S, Cleary S, Bahrami B, Reynolds N, Macfarlane GT. Synbiotic consumption changes the metabolism and composition of the gut microbiota in older people and modifies inflammatory processes: a randomised, double-blind, placebo-controlled crossover study. *Alimentary pharmacology & therapeutics*. 2013;38(7):804-16.

[126] Van Immerseel F, Ducatelle R, De Vos M, Boon N, Van De Wiele T, Verbeke K, et al. Butyric acid-producing anaerobic bacteria as a novel probiotic treatment approach for inflammatory bowel disease. *Journal of medical microbiology*. 2010;59(Pt 2):141-3.

[127] Marteau P, Guyonnet D, Lafaye de Micheaux P, Gelu S. A randomized, double-blind, controlled study and pooled analysis of two identical trials of fermented milk containing probiotic Bifidobacterium lactis CNCM I-2494 in healthy women reporting minor digestive symptoms. *Neurogastroenterology and motility: the official journal of the European Gastrointestinal Motility Society*. 2013;25(4):331-e252.

[128] Vieira EL, Leonel AJ, Sad AP, Beltrao NR, Costa TF, Ferreira TM, et al. Oral administration of sodium butyrate attenuates inflammation and mucosal lesion in experimental acute ulcerative colitis. *J. Nutr. Biochem*. 2012;23(5):430-6.

[129] Breuer RI, Soergel KH, Lashner BA, Christ ML, Hanauer SB, Vanagunas A, et al. Short chain fatty acid rectal irrigation for left-sided ulcerative colitis: a randomised, placebo controlled trial. *Gut*. 1997;40(4):485-91.

[130] Hamer HM, Jonkers DM, Vanhoutvin SA, Troost FJ, Rijkers G, de Bruine A, et al. Effect of butyrate enemas on inflammation and antioxidant status in the colonic mucosa of patients with ulcerative colitis in remission. *Clinical nutrition*. 2010;29(6):738-44.

[131] Roda A, Simoni P, Magliulo M, Nanni P, Baraldini M, Roda G, et al. A new oral formulation for the release of sodium butyrate in the ileo-cecal region and colon. *World J. Gastroenterol*. 2007;13(7):1079-84.

[132] Banasiewicz T, Krokowicz L, Stojcev Z, Kaczmarek BF, Kaczmarek E, Maik J, et al. Microencapsulated sodium butyrate reduces the frequency of abdominal pain in patients with irritable bowel syndrome. *Colorectal disease: the official journal of the Association of Coloproctology of Great Britain and Ireland*. 2013;15(2):204-9.

[133] Chen ZX, Breitman TR. Tributyrin: a prodrug of butyric acid for potential clinical application in differentiation therapy. *Cancer Res*. 1994;54(13):3494-9.

[134] Heidor R, Ortega JF, de Conti A, Ong TP, Moreno FS. Anticarcinogenic actions of tributyrin, a butyric acid prodrug. *Current drug targets*. 2012;13(14):1720-9.

[135] Breitman TR, He RY. Combinations of retinoic acid with either sodium butyrate, dimethyl sulfoxide, or hexamethylene bisacetamide synergistically induce differentiation of the human myeloid leukemia cell line HL60. *Cancer Res*. 1990; 50(19):6268-73.

[136] Pfeiffer N, Desmarchelier C, Blaut M, Daniel H, Haller D, Clavel T. Acetatifactor muris gen. nov., sp. nov., a novel bacterium isolated from the intestine of an obese mouse. *Archives of microbiology*. 2012;194(11):901-7.

[137] Finegold SM, Lawson PA, Vaisanen ML, Molitoris DR, Song Y, Liu C, et al. Anaerofustis stercorihominis gen. nov., sp. nov., from human feces. *Anaerobe*. 2004;10(1):41-5.

[138] Munoz-Tamayo R, Laroche B, Walter E, Dore J, Duncan SH, Flint HJ, et al. Kinetic modelling of lactate utilization and butyrate production by key human colonic bacterial species. *FEMS microbiology ecology*. 2011;76(3):615-24.

[139] Allen-Vercoe E, Daigneault M, White A, Panaccione R, Duncan SH, Flint HJ, et al. Anaerostipes hadrus comb. nov., a dominant species within the human colonic microbiota; reclassification of Eubacterium hadrum Moore et al. 1976. *Anaerobe.* 2012;18(5):523-9.

[140] Bui TP, de Vos W, Plugge CM. Anaerostipes rhamnosivorans sp. nov., a human intestinal butyrate forming bacterium. *Int. J. Syst. Evol. Microbiol.* 2013.

[141] Lawson PA, Song Y, Liu C, Molitoris DR, Vaisanen ML, Collins MD, et al. Anaerotruncus colihominis gen. nov., sp. nov., from human faeces. *Int. J. Syst. Evol. Microbiol.* 2004;54(Pt 2):413-7.

[142] Sakamoto M, Takagaki A, Matsumoto K, Kato Y, Goto K, Benno Y. Butyricimonas synergistica gen. nov., sp. nov. and Butyricimonas virosa sp. nov., butyric acid-producing bacteria in the family 'Porphyromonadaceae' isolated from rat faeces. *Int. J. Syst. Evol. Microbiol.* 2009;59(Pt 7):1748-53.

[143] Ben-Amor K, Heilig H, Smidt H, Vaughan EE, Abee T, de Vos WM. Genetic diversity of viable, injured, and dead fecal bacteria assessed by fluorescence-activated cell sorting and 16S rRNA gene analysis. *Applied and environmental microbiology.* 2005;71(8):4679-89.

[144] Kalmokoff ML, Teather RM. Isolation and characterization of a bacteriocin (Butyrivibriocin AR10) from the ruminal anaerobe Butyrivibrio fibrisolvens AR10: evidence in support of the widespread occurrence of bacteriocin-like activity among ruminal isolates of B. fibrisolvens. *Applied and environmental microbiology.* 1997;63(2):394-402.

[145] Moon CD, Pacheco DM, Kelly WJ, Leahy SC, Li D, Kopecny J, et al. Reclassification of Clostridium proteoclasticum as Butyrivibrio proteoclasticus comb. nov., a butyrate-producing ruminal bacterium. *Int. J. Syst. Evol. Microbiol.* 2008;58(Pt 9):2041-5.

[146] Morotomi M, Nagai F, Watanabe Y. Description of Christensenella minuta gen. nov., sp. nov., isolated from human faeces, which forms a distinct branch in the order Clostridiales, and proposal of Christensenellaceae fam. nov. *Int. J. Syst. Evol. Microbiol.* 2012;62(Pt 1):144-9.

[147] Abbad-Andaloussi S, Durr C, Raval G, Petitdemange. Carbon and electron flow in Clostridium butyricum grown in chemostat culture on glycerol and on glucose. *Microbiol.* 1996;142:1149-1158.

[148] Seki H, Shiohara M, Matsumura T, Miyagawa N, Tanaka M, Komiyama A, Kurata S. 2003. Prevention of antibiotic-associated diarrhea in children by Clostridium butyricum MIYAIRI. *Pediatr. Int.* 2003;45:86–90.

[149] van der Wielen PW, Rovers GM, Scheepens JM, Biesterveld S. Clostridium lactatifermen tans sp. nov., a lactate-fermenting anaerobe isolated from the caeca of a chicken. *Int. J. Syst. Evol. Microbiol.* 2002;52(Pt 3):921-5.

[150] Schwiertz A, Le Blay G, Blaut M. Quantification of different Eubacterium spp. in human fecal samples with species-specific 16S rRNA-targeted oligonucleotide probes. *Applied and environmental microbiology.* 2000;66(1):375-82.

[151] Duncan SH, Hold GL, Harmsen HJ, Stewart CS, Flint HJ. Growth requirements and fermentation products of Fusobacterium prausnitzii, and a proposal to reclassify it as Faecalibacterium prausnitzii gen. nov., comb. nov. *Int. J. Syst. Evol. Microbiol.* 2002;52(Pt 6):2141-6.

[152] Klaring K, Hanske L, Bui N, Charrier C, Blaut M, Haller D, et al. Intestinimonas butyriciproducens gen. nov., sp. nov., a butyrate-producing bacterium from the mouse intestine. *Int. J. Syst. Evol. Microbiol.* 2013;63(Pt 12):4606-12.

[153] Hedberg ME, Moore ER, Svensson-Stadler L, Horstedt P, Baranov V, Hernell O, et al. Lachnoanaerobaculum gen. nov., a new genus in the Lachnospiraceae: characterization of Lachnoanaerobaculum umeaense gen. nov., sp. nov., isolated from the human small intestine, and Lachnoanaerobaculum orale sp. nov., isolated from saliva, and reclassification of Eubacterium saburreum (Prevot 1966) Holdeman and Moore 1970 as Lachnoanaerobaculum saburreum comb. nov. *Int. J. Syst. Evol. Microbiol.* 2012;62(Pt 11):2685-90.

[154] Whitford MF, Yanke LJ, Forster RJ, Teather RM. Lachnobacterium bovis gen. nov., sp. nov., a novel bacterium isolated from the rumen and faeces of cattle. *Int. J. Syst. Evol. Microbiol.* 2001;51(Pt 6):1977-81.

[155] Weimer PJ, Moen GN. Quantitative analysis of growth and volatile fatty acid production by the anaerobic ruminal bacterium Megasphaera elsdenii T81. *Applied microbiology and biotechnology*. 2013;97(9):4075-81.

[156] Carlier JP, K'Ouas G, Han XY. Moryella indoligenes gen. nov., sp. nov., an anaerobic bacterium isolated from clinical specimens. *Int. J. Syst. Evol. Microbiol.* 2007;57(Pt 4):725-9.

[157] Downes J, Wade WG. Peptostreptococcus stomatis sp. nov., isolated from the human oral cavity. *Int. J. Syst. Evol. Microbiol.* 2006;56(Pt 4):751-4.

[158] Fournier D, Mouton C, Lapierre P, Kato T, Okuda K, Menard C. Porphyromonas gulae sp. nov., an anaerobic, gram-negative coccobacillus from the gingival sulcus of various animal hosts. *Int. J. Syst. Evol. Microbiol.* 2001;51(Pt 3):1179-89.

[159] van Gylswyk NO, Hippe H, Rainey FA. Pseudobutyrivibrio ruminis gen. nov., sp. nov., a Butyrate-Producing Bacterium from the Rumen That Closely Resembles Butyrivibrio fibrisolvens in Phenotype. *International journal of systematic bacteriology*. 1996; 46(2):559-63.

[160] Stanton TB, Savage DC. Colonization of gnotobiotic mice by Roseburia cecicola, a motile, obligately anaerobic bacterium from murine ceca. *Applied and environmental microbiology*. 1983;45(5):1677-84.

[161] Duncan SH, Aminov RI, Scott KP, Louis P, Stanton TB, Flint HJ. Proposal of Roseburia faecis sp. nov., Roseburia hominis sp. nov. and Roseburia inulinivorans sp. nov., based on isolates from human faeces. *Int. J. Syst. Evol. Microbiol.* 2006;56(Pt 10):2437-41.

[162] Holmstrom K, Collins MD, Moller T, Falsen E, Lawson PA. Subdoligranulum variabile gen. nov., sp. nov. from human feces. *Anaerobe*. 2004;10(3):197-203.

In: Butyrate: Food Sources, Functions and Health Benefits ISBN: 978-1-63117-657-9
Editor: Cong-Jun Li © 2014 Nova Science Publishers, Inc.

Chapter 2

BUTYRATE AND INTESTINAL FUNCTION

Jacqueline I. Alvarez-Leite* and Edenil Costa Aguilar

Department of Biochemistry and Immunology,
Federal University of Minas Gerais,
Belo Horizonte, Brazil

ABSTRACT

Butyrate is a 4-carbon fatty acid that is physiologically produced by the microbial fermentation of dietary fibers and other carbohydrates that escaped of enzymatic digestion. Food sources of butyrate comprise mainly milk and dairy products.

The important role that butyrate plays in maintaining intestinal homeostasis is now uncontestable. Butyrate is the main fuel to colonocytes and almost all of the butyrate is oxidized in the colonocytes to produce ATP, accelerating cell proliferation and mucosa recovery. Butyrate is also able to regulate intestinal barrier and intestinal motility and to reduce oxidative stress. All these actions make butyrate a promisor adjuvant on the treatment and prevention of several intestinal disorders including short bowel syndrome, mucositis, Crohn's disease and ulcerative colitis.

Several of the butyrate actions are linked to its capacity to inhibit the enzyme histone deacetylase which is crucial for the chromatin organization and activation of specific genes. As immunomodulator, butyrate enhances anti-inflammatory responses and reduces pro-inflammatory cytokines secretion. The mechanism of those actions involve the lower expression and activation of the nuclear factor kappa B (NF-κB) which controls the expression of proinflammatory cytokines, chemokines, adhesion molecules, growth factors, heat shock proteins and immune receptors, among others.

In vivo and *in vitro* studies showed that butyrate induces cell differentiation and apoptosis of malignant cells in models of colorectal cancer (CTC). The apparent paradoxical effect of butyrate in malignant colonocytes (inducing apoptosis) compared to normal colonocytes (inducing proliferation) is due to its different intracellular fates. Differently of normal colonocytes, in malignant ones butyrate is poorly oxidized and will be available to translocate to the nucleus and, through the inhibition of histone deacetylases, regulates several genes including those involved in apoptosis and cell differentiation.

* Corresponding author: Alvarez-Leite, J.I.(jalvarezleite@gmail.com).

The effects of butyrate on the small intestine and colon occurs when it is administered as an enema and also when it is given orally as demonstrated by the improvement of ulcerative colitis and mucositis after oral supplementation of butyrate or tributyrin. These actions make butyrate an important factor for the maintenance of gut health and potential adjuvant on the treatment of intestinal disorders.

PHYSIOLOGICAL CHARACTERISTICS AND FUNCTIONS OF BUTYRATE

Short chain fatty acids (SCFAs), acetate, propionate, and butyrate, are organic acids produced through the bacterial fermentation of dietary fiber in the lumen of the colon. Fermentation rescues unabsorbed energy from food in the small intestine, contributing 5 to 15% of the total caloric requirement in humans [66, 93]. The concentration of SCFA, produced in the human intestine, varies according to the site of fermentation (proximal or distal colon), type of nutrients (fiber, undigested starch or amino acids), and microbiota composition [13, 66, 162]. Acetate, propionate and butyrate are present in the colon at a relative proportion of about 60:25:15 and contribute to the colon integrity, improving colonic musculature, vasculature and metabolism [57, 162].

Absorption: The absorption of short chain fatty acids occurs through different mechanisms [91, 105, 155]. The protonated form is absorbed through diffusion and the ionic (dissociated) form is absorbed through ionic exchanges. Monocarboxylate transporter-1 (MCT1) has been described as a significant transporter of monocarboxylate molecules across the plasma membrane, catalyzing the cell influx of pyruvate, lactate, ketone bodies and SCFAs, including butyrate [61, 63]. Butyrate, in turn, is able to increase the MCT1 in a concentration and time-dependent manner, resulting in the enhanced uptake of itself, dependently of the NF-κB activation [16, 17, 33].

After absorption, butyrate is retained in colonocytes and used as substrate for oxidation and ATP formation in aerobic conditions. Butyrate is the preferential fuel for colonic epithelium compared with glucose or glutamine [29, 62, 161]. This important role in colon metabolism makes butyrate a key component in colon health and trophism as evidenced in studies with germ-free mice. In these mice, the absence of microbiota and, consequently, the absence of colonic production of short-chain fatty acids have been associated with exacerbated inflammation after dextran sodium sulfate (DSS)-induced colitis [74, 105].

Butyrate is important not only as an intracellular energy source but also for other functions associated with cell homeostasis and gene regulation (Figure 1).

The effects of butyrate on cell proliferation, differentiation and apoptosis are essential for tissue protection against cancer and other diseases [34, 36]. Although normal colonocytes use butyrate as the primary energy source, colorectal cancer (CRC) cells shift their fuel preference to glucose. Oxidation of butyrate in malignant colonocytes is inhibited through the Warburg effect, causing butyrate accumulation [44]. The Warburg effect is related to high rate of glycolysis, even in the presence of oxygen (aerobic glycolysis) in malignant cells leading to increased lactic acid concentrations and faster depletion of glucose.

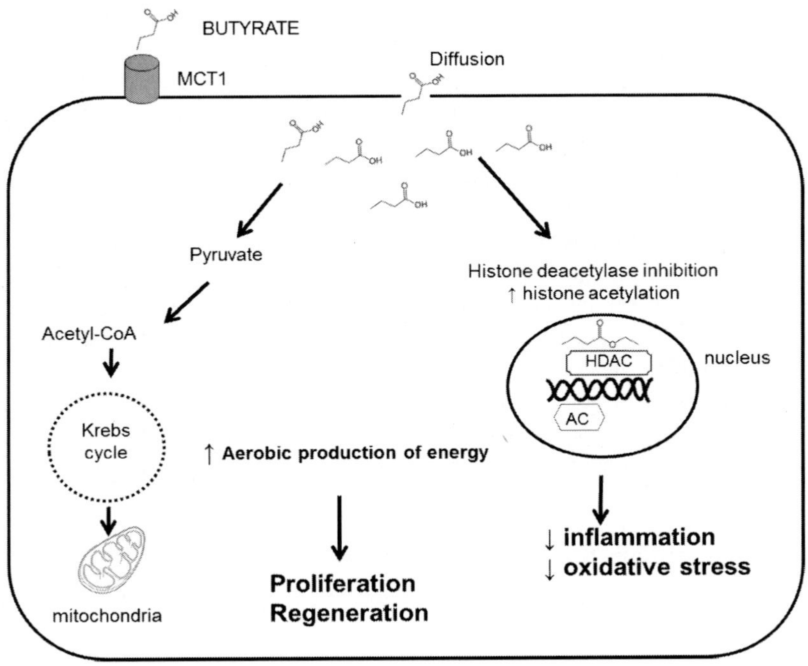

A

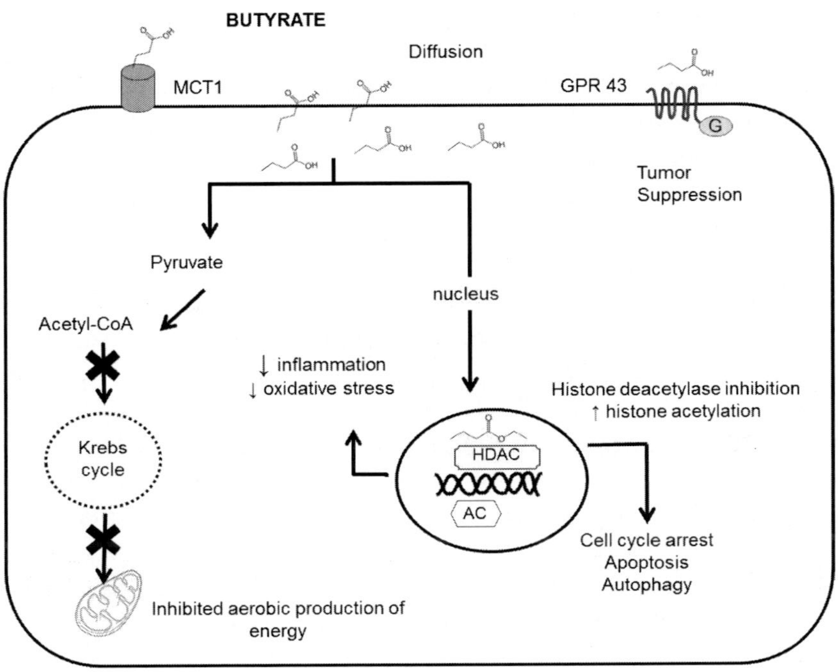

B

A- *Normal colonocytes*: The absorption of butyrate occurs through different mechanisms. The protonated form is absorbed through diffusion and the ionic form is absorbed through ionic exchanges. Monocarboxylate transporter 1 (MCT1) has been described as a significant transporter of monocarboxylate molecules across the plasma membrane. G protein-coupled receptors GPR41 (FFA3) and GPR43 (FFA2) are associated to butyrate and its actions in several cells. Butyrate preferentially binds to G protein-coupled receptors GPR41 (FFA3), but can also associate with GRP3 (FFA2). (Continued on next page)

After absorption, butyrate is retained in colonocyte used as substrate for oxidation and ATP formation in aerobic conditions. Butyrate is the preferential fuel for colonic epithelium compared with glucose or glutamine. This important role in colon metabolism makes butyrate a key component in colon health and trophism. Butyrate inhibits the activity of histone deacetylases (HDAC). This enzyme regulates gene transcription through the modification of chromatin structure by deacetylating histone proteins. Histone hyperacetylation alters the expression of genes that interfere in several processes, including inhibition of nuclear factor kappa B (NF-κB), involved in pro-inflammatory cytokines and iNOS synthesis.

B- *Malignant colonocytes:* Due to the metabolic reprogramming in cancer cells given to anaerobic glycolysis the priority in the energy production, butyrate is oxidized to a lesser extent, crossing the nucleus membrane. In the nucleus of these cells, butyrate acts as HDAC inhibitor to epigenetically regulate gene expression. Butyrate can also induce cell death in malignant or inflamed cells through a mechanism dependent on caspase-3 activation (apoptosis) or in a caspase 3 independent manner (autophagy).

Figure 1. Butyrate metabolism in normal and malignant colonocytes.

In CRC cells, the difficulty of aerobic oxidation leads to the higher availability of butyrate in the intracellular milieu, directing it to other functions such as HDAC inhibition.

GPR-mediated effects of butyrate: G protein-coupled receptors (GPR, or free fat acid receptor - FFA), particularly GPR41 (FFA3) and GPR43 (FFA2) are associated to butyrate and its actions in several cells such as colonocytes, adipocytes, bone marrow cells and immune cells [19, 79, 80, 160, 166]. Butyrate preferentially binds to GPR41, but can also be associated with GRP3. GPR43 is present in high levels in polymorphonuclear cells (PMBCs), mainly in neutrophils, while GPR41 is widely expressed in the spleen, lymph node, bone marrow, and PBMCs [91]. *In vitro* studies have suggested that butyrate activates neutrophil migration in a mechanism dependent on GPR43 [144]. Moreover, GPR43 deficient mice (Gpr43-/-), develop diseases such as colitis, arthritis and asthma, exhibiting intense inflammation, with the increased production of inflammatory mediators and recruitment of leukocytes. It has been shown that signaling via p38 mitogen-activated protein kinases (MAPK) and the phosphorylation of p38 MAPK mediated through butyrate is dependent on GPR43 [112, 137].

Inhibition of histone deacetylase: Butyrate influences cell metabolism through several mechanisms, including reducing inflammation and nitric oxide production; inducing apoptosis and increasing the cell antioxidant potential [7, 134]. These activities are primarily associated with the ability of butyrate to inhibit the activity of histone deacetylases (HDAC) [93, 122, 169]. This enzyme regulates gene transcription through the modification of chromatin structure by deacetylating histone proteins. Histone deacetylases and histone acetyltransferases are enzymes that synergistically remove or add acetyl moieties on histones, respectively. The histone acetyltransferase-mediated addition of one acetyl moiety relaxes chromatin structure and facilitates the access of transcription factors to target gene promoters [122, 169]. Thus, hyperacetylation through HDAC inhibitors, such as butyrate, is associated with the transcriptional activation of several genes. Histone hyperacetylation through butyrate alters the expression of genes that interfere with the inflammatory process, decreasing pro-inflammatory cytokines and/or increasing anti-inflammatory cytokines [7, 54, 111, 152]. The inhibitory effect of butyrate on HDAC also affects genes associated with apoptosis through the regulation of the expression of components of the BcL-2 family, caspase activation and anexin-1 externalization [4, 109, 113, 155, 176].

Inhibition of Nitric Oxide Synthase: The nitric oxide (NO) is an important cell-signaling molecule, which acts as a potent vasodilator. In addition, physiological concentrations of NO inhibit leukocyte adhesion, platelet aggregation and endothelial permeability. The diminution of NO synthesis or viability impairs endothelium-dependent vasodilatation, leading to endothelial dysfunction [30, 90, 141]. On the other hand, the exacerbated production of NO occurs under inflammatory conditions, increasing oxidative stress and causing damage on endothelium [53, 148].

NO is produced by one of the 3 isoforms of nitric oxide synthase (NOS). Neuronal nitric oxide synthase (nNOS) and endothelial nitric oxide synthase (eNOS) are essential for NO synthesis under physiological conditions, and the inducible nitric oxide synthase (iNOS) is induced through inflammation [3, 35, 55]. Although NO acts as a cytotoxic agent for cancer cells or infectious agents, the increased production of this molecule through iNOS presents adverse effects on vessels [83, 148]. The increased production of NO through iNOS has been associated with peroxynitrite formation, which induces protein peroxidation (nitrotyrosine formation) and contributes oxidative stress [77].

Several studies have shown that butyrate reduces the *in vivo* and *in vitro* production of NO through iNOS in macrophage under inflammatory stimulation [24, 99, 128]. In LPS-stimulated RAW264.7 cells, SCFAs (acetate, propionate, and butyrate) reduced the production of proinflammatory factors, including NO, and inhibited the iNOS [99]. Butyrate prevents the activation of NF-κB through the stabilization of IκB-α and IκB-β. Butyrate did not affect the phosphorylation of mitogen-activated protein (MAP) kinases by LPS [24]. Those results suggest that butyrate down-regulated LPS-induced NO production in RAW cells through preventing the expression of iNOS, and that it was due to the inhibitory action of butyrate on the activation of NF-κB.

Anti-inflammatory effects: Butyrate may exert anti-inflammatory activity by several mechanisms, including reduction of endothelium activation, adhesion and transmigration of leukocyte, secretion of pro-inflammatory cytokine and induction of apoptosis in activated immune cell [93, 107, 134, 169, 170].

The endothelium is critical for the production of regulatory molecules, actively regulating vascular tone and permeability, coagulation, platelet aggregation, proliferation of smooth muscle cells (SMC) and leukocyte adhesion and extravasation [42, 139]. Vascular inflammation causes endothelial cell activation, resulting in the secretion of chemokines, cytokines and adhesion molecules which interact with circulating leukocytes [42, 115].

The reduction in leukocyte recruitment caused by butyrate has been described and results from its ability to reduce the chemotaxis and adhesion [107, 169]. The chemotaxis of leukocytes to the site of inflammation depends on the actions of chemotactic proteins, such as CCL2 (MCP1 - monocyte chemotaxis protein -1), produced by endothelial cells [43]. Butyrate has been shown to effectively reduce the expression and secretion of CCL2 under various *in vitro* experimental conditions of inflammation [32, 107, 114, 135, 169], suggesting that butyrate could decrease the activation of endothelial cells through the reduction of chemotactic molecule secretion and inflammatory cell migration, thereby preventing the development or exacerbation of vascular inflammation.

Firm adhesion is induced through the expression of vascular adhesion molecules, such as vascular cell adhesion molecule (VCAM) and intercellular adhesion molecule (ICAM), which are respectively associated with the integrins very late antigen-4 (VLA–4) and present leukocyte function-associated antigen-1 (LFA–1) in leukocytes. The leukocyte transmigration is mediated through other adhesion molecules such as platelet endothelial cell adhesion molecule-1 (PECAM-1), which is also expressed in endothelial cells, particularly at intercellular junctions [9, 56, 145]. Studies using endothelial cells stimulated with TNF-α and IL-1β showed that the expression and concentration of VCAM-1 and ICAM-1 were reduced after incubation with butyrate [108, 175]. This effect is associated with a reduction in the activity of NF-kB, and an increase in the activity of peroxisome proliferator-activated receptor α (PPAR-α). NF-kB is responsible for the expression of genes that encode proinflammatory cytokines and other molecules such as adhesion molecules, growth factors, heat shock proteins and immune receptors [93]. Butyrate is able to inhibit NF-κB in different cell types, including cancer cell lines, cells from colon lamina propria, macrophages and neutrophils. In addition, butyrate also inhibits the secretion of the inflammatory cytokines TNF-α, IL-1β and IL-16, and induces the anti-inflammatory cytokine IL-10 in macrophages [32, 99, 106].

Neutrophils play an important role in innate immunity, particularly in the response against invading pathogens, and their rapid recruitment is essential for the body's defense. Activated neutrophils release reactive oxygen species and toxic granules for bacteria in order to protect the host against infection. The excess of proinflammatory agents can lead to host tissues damage [4, 85]. Neutrophils have a key role in the development of ulcerative colitis in humans and in DSS-induced colitis animal models [82, 110] and reduced apoptosis of these cells may maintain the local inflammation or generate a systemic inflammation. The apoptosis of neutrophils occurs naturally, but inflammatory stimuli such as pro-inflammatory cytokines and bacterial products extend the lifespan of these cells.

Induction of apoptosis and cell death: Apoptotic cell death is executed by caspases. There are two well characterized mammalian caspase activation pathways, the death receptor pathway and the mitochondria/cytochrome c-mediated pathway. In the first pathway, binding of agonists to the death receptors induce activation caspase-8, which in turn activates the effector caspase, caspase-3. In the cytochrome c-mediated (internal) pathway, the main event is cytochrome c release from mitochondria to cytoplasm, an event regulated by the Bcl-2 family of proteins. Released cytochrome c induces the key mediator Apaf-1 to form a multimeric protein complex, the apoptosome that induces the activation of caspase-9, which activates the executioner caspases [142].

Autophagic cell death is characterized by massive degradation of cellular contents, including essential organelles such as mitochondria. Caspases are not required for and Bcl-2 and Bcl-XL are not inhibitors of autophagic cell death in a mammary epithelial morphogenesis model [142]. However, both processes are involved in tumorigenesis.

The role of butyrate in authophagic cell death has been studied [46, 142, 153, 163]. Tang and colleagues [154] have shown that the treatment of CRC cells with 1-3 mM of butyrate and propionate did not induce overt apoptosis but rather induced extensive morphological alterations characteristics of autophagy. Shao et al. [142] showed that autophagic cell death can be induced by histone deacetylase inhibitors. The authors showed that high concentrations of Z-VAD-FMK, a potent cell-permeable caspase did not block the cell death induced by butyrate in either wild-type or Apaf-1-knockout mouse embryonic fibroblasts. Moreover, in HeLa cell line stably transfected with Bcl-XL, the cell death induced by butyrate was not blocked by overexpression of Bcl-XL [142].

The action of butyrate as an apoptotic agent has been more extensively explored and is mainly related to its ability to inhibit HDAC inhibitor [1, 4, 5, 22, 26, 102, 103, 113, 116, 128, 149, 176]. Apoptosis is regulated by a cascade of signal carried by a family of cysteine proteases called caspases [51]. The mechanisms apparently diverge among the tested cells and tissues. In some cell lines such as HT-29 cell line [28], macrophage [127] and 2C4 human fibrosarcoma cells [125], the mechanism of apoptosis is dependent on caspase 3 activation. In other cells, however, apoptosis induced by butyrate can occur in a caspase-3 independent manner [67, 68].

In intestinal diseases such UC or CRC, the induction of apoptosis in inflammatory or malignant cells will favor the control of the disease. Butyrate induces apoptosis in most of inflammatory cells, including neutrophils, monocytes and lymphocytes [1, 4, 127, 128]. Butyrate is able to induce apoptosis in both non-activated or LPS (or TNF) activated neutrophils. This effect is dependent on the activity of caspase-8 and caspase-9 and also dependent on HDAC inhibition [4].

The pro-apoptotic effect of butyrate has also been shown in macrophages. Ramos and colleagues [127, 128] evaluated the effect of butyrate on murine macrophages and showed that butyrate induces apoptosis in a dose dependent manner. The effect was more accentuated in presence of an inflammatory stimulus (LPS) and mediated via caspase-3. This butyrate action was also later confirmed by other authors [7, 113].

Butyrate also induced apoptosis of T cells in models of ulcerative colitis [106] and inhibits IFN-γ trough inhibition of STAT1 signaling regulation in T cells through inhibition of HDAC [176]. The increased Fas expression results in T cell apoptosis, eliminating the source of colonic mucosa inflammation. These data suggest that butyrate is not only able to reduce IFN-γ pro-inflammatory signaling, but also promotes apoptosis in lymphocytes, that is critical in the secretion of this cytokine, especially in colonic tissue. This finding confirms the key role of butyrate to inhibit HDAC and highlights an important mode of anti-inflammatory action of butyrate in intestinal inflammation.

It has been described that the incubation of mouse macrophages with several HDAC inhibitors, including butyrate, caused the externalization of anexin A1 (AnxA), with the concomitant, but independent, inhibition of cytokine gene expression and secretion [109]. In a murine model of acute inflammation, butyrate treatment at the peak of the disease, accelerated resolution processes in wild-type mice, but a much more modest resolution was observed in AnxA1 null mice. On the other hand, butyrate maintained the inhibition of cytokine secretion even in AnxA1 null macrophage [109]. The authors propose non-genomic modulation of AnxA1 in immune cells as a novel mechanism of action for HDAC inhibitors, which may underlie their reported efficacy in models of chronic inflammatory pathologies.

Anticancer property: The Warburg effect is responsible for changes in metabolic fate of butyrate in colorectal cancer cells. Due to the metabolic reprogramming in cancer cells given to anaerobic glycolysis the priority in the energy production, butyrate is oxidized to a lesser extent, goes through nucleus membrane and accumulates in the nucleus of cancerous colonocytes. There, it acts as HDAC inhibitor to epigenetically regulate gene expression [21, 44].

In a recent review, Bultman [21] presented two distinct mechanisms in which butyrate maintains histone acetylated; inhibiting HDAC or stimulating histone acetyltransferases (HAT). The first one is the classic and well recognized mechanism that occurs as a consequence of the increased concentration of non-oxidized butyrate in the nucleus (due to

Warburg effect), inhibiting the deacetylation of histones. However, even in cancer cells, this mechanism is seen only with high intracellular concentrations of butyrate. The HDAC inhibition mechanism is only seen at butyrate concentrations of 2mM and it is more relevant at 5mM. In these concentrations, butyrate is not metabolized in the mitochondria and accumulates as HDAC inhibitors in the nucleus [45]. However, a different mechanism HDAC –independent occurs in lower concentrations of butyrate (0.5mM), resulting in histone hyperacetylation [70]. In such low dose, butyrate undergoes β-oxidation in the mitochondria, and is driven to Krebs cycle, forming citrate. Citrate can exit the mitochondria and be converted into acetyl-CoA in the cytosol and nucleus, via ATP citrate lyase activity. In the nucleus, acetyl-CoA serves as the acetyl group donor for histone acetyltransferases. Since the aerobic metabolism is repressed in malignant cells, butyrate derived acetylCoA will serve as substrate for histone acetyltransferases inducing histone hyperacetylation [172].

Antioxidant effect: Oxidative stress is the result of the imbalance between the generation of reactive oxygen species (ROS) and antioxidant defenses. The antioxidant defense includes enzymes, such as glutathione-S-transferase (GST) and glutathione peroxidase (GPX), and non-enzymatic antioxidant, such as glutathione (GSH) and uric acid. Increased oxidative stress in the intestinal epithelium has been shown to disrupt mucosal barrier function, resulting in increased permeability [64].

Several *in vitro* and experimental models have shown that butyrate may reduce oxidative stress induced by colon inflammation that is related to the disruption of the intestinal barrier and cancer induction [2, 94, 95, 98, 100, 110, 131, 134, 138]. Physiological concentrations of butyrate reduced H_2O_2-induced DNA damage, increased the expression of catalase and reduced the expression of cyclooxygenase- 2 in human colonocytes [138]. In rats, sodium butyrate was able to attenuate inflammatory responses, neutrophil infiltration, and oxidative stress in the lungs, and protects against acute lung injury induced by severe burn. This effect was associated with inhibition of the high-mobility group box 1 protein (HMGB1) expression, a ubiquitous nuclear protein that drives proinflammatory responses when released extracellularly [98]. In DSS induced colitis models, administration of tributyrin - the triacylglycerol containing 3 molecules of butyrate - reduced eosinophil peroxidase and hydroperoxide levels and increased SOD and catalase activities compared to mice receiving placebo solution [94]. The involvement of the glutathione/glutathione S-transferase (GST) antioxidant system was evaluated in vascular smooth muscle cells (VSMC) [129]. The treatment of proliferating VSMCs with butyrate induced GST, increased glutathione content, and reduced reactive oxygen species [129].

Although those studies showed beneficial effects of butyrate, clinical studies addressed to the antioxidant effect of butyrate are still scarce. A cross-over study compared colon mucosa biopsies obtained from healthy volunteers [64] treated daily with butyrate enema or saline for 2 weeks. The results showed a significantly higher expression and concentration of the antioxidant glutathione (GSH) and a lower expression and concentration of uric acid after butyrate enemas compared to saline ones. However, in a similar experimental protocol using biopsies of patients with ulcerative colitis in remission, butyrate enemas induced minor effects on colonic inflammation and oxidative stress [65]. Only a significant increase of the colonic interleukin (IL)-10/IL-12 ratio was found within butyrate-treated patients. Colonic concentrations of chemokine (C–C motif) ligand 5 (CCL5, also known as RANTES) were also increased after butyrate compared to placebo treatment. The results suggest that the effects of butyrate enemas on total colonic glutathione appeared to be dependent on the level of inflammation. The authors concluded that, although UC patients in remission were characterized by low-grade oxidative stress and inflammation, rectal butyrate enemas showed only minor effects on inflammatory and oxidative stress parameters [65].

EFFECT OF BUTYRATE IN INTESTINAL DISEASES

Butyrate and Colorectal Cancer: The incidence of CRC is increasing in the whole world. This increase in the risk of CRC has been attributed to industrialization and modifiable factors such as tabagism, sedentarism, alcohol consumption, obesity, low fiber diet. Although some authors have not confirmed the beneficial effects of butyrate on CRC prevention [140, 143, 164], most *in vitro* studies reported the beneficial effects of butyrate on the control of CRC cells [27, 28, 47]. The main action of butyrate in CRC cells is the induction of apoptosis and cell cycle arrest as a consequence of the cell proliferation inhibition as demonstrated in several studies with different CRC cell lines [7, 27, 69, 75, 84, 117, 118]. Butyrate is reported to activate the intrinsic (cytochrome c release) pathway of apoptosis, to sensitize cancer cells to apoptosis mediated by the extrinsic pathway (via death receptors) and, more recently, to induce autophagic cell death [84, 93]. Several of the anticancer mechanisms result from either the direct butyrate action or from its HDAC inhibitor activity. The main actions of butyrate inducing apoptosis include the up regulation the death receptor pathway, $p21^{WAF1}$ and BAK; and the down regulation of Bcl-xL and cyclin D1, Neuropilin-1 (NRP-1). Butyrate also inhibits DNA methylation and modulates the canonical Wnt signaling, a pathway constitutively activated in the majority of CRC. In HT-29 and FHC (non-transformed) cells butyrate induced cycle arrest in the G0/G1, while in HCT-116 cells it induced cell cycle arrest in the G2/M phase [52, 93].

The ability to prevent or repair DNA damage caused by dietary carcinogens contributes to the reduction of the risk of cancer. A favorable balance of biotransformation enzymes, which include phase II enzymes such as glutathione S-transferases (GST), UDP-glucuronosyl transferases, might protect tumor target cells from accumulating additional mutations. This mechanism is related to inhibition of cell cancer growth or induction of apoptosis [123]. Butyrate transcriptionally up regulates detoxifying enzymes that protect cells from genotoxic carcinogens [27, 123] as showed in HT29 adenocarcinoma cell line. In those cells butyrate induced up regulation of GST (GSTA2, GSTT2) that are known to be involved in the defense against oxidative stress [123]. In addition, in primary invasive CRC cells butyrate was able to inhibit cellular migration by reducing $\alpha 2\beta 1$ integrin levels and inhibiting of cell adhesion to basement membrane [20].

Butyrate and chemotherapy induced mucositis: Additionally to its anti-proliferative and apoptotic effect in CRC cells, butyrate has shown improve chemotherapy related mucositis in several studies [54] and potentiates the effect of anticancer drug therapy, such as ARA-C, 5-fluorouracil (5FU), vincristine, celecoxib, cisplatin and etoposide [25, 58, 76, 78, 86, 104, 119, 124, 126, 127, 171]. Studies in 5FU treated mice confirm that the beneficial effect of butyrate is due to the increase mucosa proliferation, reduction of inflammatory infiltration and of the oxidative stress. These studies show that enterocytes that do not use butyrate as preferential fuel for metabolism is also beneficiated by oral supplementation of this fatty acid. This effect is due in part to a local action of butyrate. Although butyrate concentration in physiological conditions is low in small intestine, the oral administration of butyrate exposes the stomach and small intestinal mucosa to higher concentrations, increasing its absorption and intracellular concentration in enterocytes. Moreover, oral administration promotes higher butyrate absorption and concentrations in the liver [59]. In that organ, butyrate can be metabolized into glutamate and acetoacetate, which are important fuels for enterocytes, and glutamine, a well-known trophic agent for enterocytes. Butyrate also increases pancreatic secretion and jejunal brush-border enzymatic activity [54, 60], which increases nutrient availability that is necessary for enterocyte regeneration and stimulates GLP-2, a pleiotropic intestinotrophic hormone that enhances bowel digestive and absorptive capacity [71].

Butyrate also reduces the alteration in intestinal permeability that is typically seen in 5FU treated mice [54, 132, 133, 174]. The mechanism of this effect can be linked to gene expression of tight junction proteins, since butyrate and trichostatin A, an inhibitor of histone acetylase, decreased tight junction permeability in Caco-2 cells via lipoxynase activation [126]. All these components propitiate the mucosa integrity protecting cells from 5FU damage, including the increase of intestinal permeability. As a consequence, the bacterial translocation is reduced minimizing the inflammation. For these reason, butyrate is a promising adjuvant in cancer chemotherapy, since butyrate could induce apoptosis of malignant cells [37, 132] and reduce inflammatory damage in non-malignant enterocytes [54].

Inflammatory Bowel Disease: Inflammatory bowel disease (IBD) is a chronic multifactorial inflammatory disorder that attacks the gastrointestinal tract and includes Crohn's disease (CD) and ulcerative colitis (UC). Although the knowledge of the etiology of IBD has been improved in the least years, it is not still totally understood. IBD is the result of genetic susceptibility, environmental influences (tabagism etc.), microbiota characteristics, triggering an abnormal immune response in genetically susceptible individuals [81, 92, 136, 173]. One of the characteristics of IBD is a vast mucosa inflammation of small or/and large intestine. IBD patients experience diverse symptoms and lesions ranging from weight loss, abdominal pain, diarrhea and intestinal obstruction to ulceration and perforation of the gastrointestinal tract.

Butyrate has been involved with both etiology and treatment of IBD, mainly of UC. UC is a disease that affects the mucous layer, altering periods of activity and remission. It affects the rectum and extends continuously to the colon in a continuous pattern [14, 15, 173]. Initially, the immune response in ulcerative colitis exhibits characteristics of a Th2 profile response, but with normal levels of IL-4 and IFN-γ. With the progression of the disease, occurs the subsequent involvement of other cytokines such as IL -6, TNF and IL- 1β [10, 150]. The conventional treatment, consists of aminosalicylates, corticosteroids, immunomodulators and antitumor necrosis factor α (TNFα) to counteract inflammation [101].

Several studies have reported the association of defective colonic epithelial oxidation of butyrate with the pathogenesis of mucosal damage and inflammation in UC [39, 97, 161]. It has been described that the activity of two mitochondrial enzymes related to butyrate oxidation, the acetoacetyl CoA thiolase and 3-hydroxy-3- methylglutaryl CoA synthase 2, which are responsible for butyrate oxidation and butyrate ketogenesis are reduced in the colons of UC patients [96]. Moreover, decreased mucosal sulfide detoxification related to impaired butyrate oxidation [38] as well as reduced absorption caused by MCT1 transporter down-regulation are also described in those patients [41, 161]. Moreover, the concomitant glucose transporter GLUT1 induction suggests that inflammation could induce a metabolic switch from butyrate to glucose oxidation [161].

Experimental studies using dextran sulphate sodium induced colitis in mice showed that butyrate is responsible for a faster mucosa recovery rather than reduce mucosal damage [168], probably due to its trophic effects. Biopsies from IBD patients show an improvement in inflammation symptoms following butyrate irrigation. However, high concentrations of butyrate are required in IBD patients to inhibit the release of the proinflammatory cytokines. Moreover, rectal butyrate enemas have only minor effects on inflammatory and oxidative stress parameters in ulcerative colitis patients in remission that present with low-grade of oxidative stress and inflammation [65]. Ulcerative colitis treatment results concerning the association of butyrate and conventional drugs, such as mesalazine, have presented conflicting results, and until now, there is no formal indication for such an association [31].

It is now believed that UC patients present alterations in the normal intestinal microbiota or dysbiosis [49]. The most abundant butyrate producers appear to be *Faecalibacterium prausnitzii*, belonging to clostridial cluster IV, and *Eubacterium rectale*, which belong to clostridial cluster XIVa [50]. It has been described a reduced biodiversity in the intestine of UC patients compared with healthy individuals, specially lower counts of bacteria belonging to the clostridial clusters IV and XIVa. These finding could explain the reduction of butyrate in intestinal content of UC patients and also highlight the possibility of prebiotic therapy. These results are stimulating the studies addressed to the use of different prebiotics in the treatment of experimental colitis [49]. However, although butyrate or prebiotic intakes show positive effects in experimental studies of UC [49, 93, 95, 101], clinical studies show conflicting results [40].

Butyrate and Intestinal Barrier: The intestinal barrier is dependent on several factors, including the mucus barrier and the apical junctional complex. The mucus layer, is a major factor in the protection of the intestinal epithelium and mainly consists of mucin glycoproteins (such as MUC2), trefoil factor 3 (TFF3) and secretory IgA. Most mucosal surfaces are covered by a hydrated gel formed by mucins. Mucins are secreted by specialized epithelial cells, such as intestinal goblet cells, and create a barrier that prevents large particles, including most bacteria, from directly contacting the epithelial cell layer [165]. Defective mucus production has been reported in cystic fibrosis and in spontaneous colitis models [165].

There are no consensus about the effect of butyrate on those components of the intestinal barrier. Experimental studies show that both MUC2 synthesis and tff3, the gene responsible for synthesis of trefoils factors, are stimulated by butyrate incubation [6, 73, 146]. However, these results could not be confirmed in one clinical study that did not find differences in the colonic MUC2 and TFF3 expression levels of UC patients after butyrate enemas [65].

The apical junctional complex is also important to the intestinal barrier. It is composed of the tight junction (TJ) and subjacent adherens junction (AJ). Both tight and adherens junctions are supported by a dense peri-junctional ring of actin and myosin that can regulate barrier function. Tight junctions (TJ) are a protein complex which connects the adjacent cells and function as filters with selective paracellular passage to ions, water, larger molecules and even cells. Dysfunction of this barrier will result in disorders such as inflammatory bowel disease and diarrhea among others. TJ is composed by transmembrane, cytoplasmic and cytoskeletal proteins. The main transmembrane proteins are claudins and occludin, whose extracellular elements are thought to directly control the intercellular space flux, and select the diffusion of different kinds of ions and molecules [72, 165]. Zonula occludens-1,-2,-3 (ZO-1,2,3) are scaffolding proteins that interact with claudins and occludin. The ZO proteins can recruit a large amount of proteins to the site of TJs and play a crucial role in the assembly of TJs [72]

There are two routes of transport through the tight junction proteins that appear to be regulated independently. The first allows the paracellular transport of large solutes, including the limited flow of proteins and lipopolysaccharide (LPS). The second form of transport is characterized by small pores, associated with proteins claudins and feature selectivity charge and exclude molecules larger than 4A [165].

The effect of butyrate on the intestinal barrier has been demonstrated in the Caco-2 cell monolayer model and occurs, at least in part, by facilitating the assembly of tight junctions. Specifically, butyrate accelerates the relocation of ZO-1 and occludin to the tight junctions during calcium switch-induced tight junction assembly, which enhances the barrier function. This dynamic process is mediated by AMP-activated protein kinase (AMPK) activation [120, 121]. Butyrate also reduces bacterial translocation in animal models of inflammatory disease [97] associated with the decreased expression of steA, which is a virulence effector associated with *Salmonella enterica* translocation [23].

Effects on the enteric nervous system: The enteric nervous system (ENS) is a neuronal network organized in myenteric and submucosal plexus. Myenteric neurons control gastrointestinal motility and peristalsis. Excitatory myenteric motor neurons contain acetylcholine and substance P that induce smooth muscle contraction, whereas inhibitory motor neurons contain nitric oxide (NO) and vasointestinal peptide, which induce muscle relaxation [151].

The effects of butyrate on the ENS were studied in colons of adult and newborn rats [147, 151]. In adult rats, effects of butyrate were studied in colons of rats given a resistant starch containing diet or intracecal perfusion of short chain fatty acids as well as in primary cultures of ENS incubated with butyrate [147]. Resistant starch diet and butyrate significantly increased the proportion of choline acetyltransferase (ChAT) immunoreactive neurons. The induction of a cholinergic phenotype by butyrate involves the monocarboxylate co-transporter-2 (MCT2), which was specifically detected in enteric neurons. This effect of butyrate on acetyltransferase expression is involved in the Src-kinase signaling pathway and in the acetylation of histone H3, which suggests that butyrate could play an important role in controlling neuromediator gene expression in the enteric nervous system and, consequently, on the intestinal motility [147]. In newborn rats, butyrate enemas (2.5mM) induced a significant increase in both nitrergic and cholinergic components of the neuromuscular transmission and also increased distal colonic transit time compared with control rats. These findings suggest that butyrate enemas induce neuroplastic changes in myenteric and submucosal neurons, leading to changes in gastrointestinal functions and support a potential use of butyrate in preterm infants with delayed maturation of the ENS [151].

Studies using experimental models of colitis have suggested that, besides the beneficial effects, butyrate instillation could increase visceral sensitivity [18, 159]. Nevertheless, in a study with healthy volunteers, daily self-administration of butyrate enemas caused a dose-dependent reduction of pain, urge and discomfort compared with placebo (saline) enemas. These results suggest that colonic administration of butyrate, at physiologically relevant concentrations, dose-dependently decreases visceral sensitivity in healthy volunteers [167]. The reduction in visceral perception could be caused by directly modulating

5-hydroxytryptamine (5-HT or serotonin) release and activating transient receptor potential vanilloid 1 (TRPV1) receptors in the colonic mucosa, which in turn may indirectly lead to the release of 5-HT in the gut to alter the perception of pain and alternatively attenuate visceral perception via histone deacetylase inhibition [167]. Although healthy humans present reduction in pain sensitivity, is not clear if in situations of intestinal inflammation butyrate treatment will act in the same sense that in healthy humans or, if it will follow the pattern of colonic hypersensitivity seen in experimental models of colitis.

Other effects of butyrate on the small intestine: The effects of butyrate in the gastrointestinal tract extend beyond the colon by influencing the integrity and immune defenses of the small intestine. Experimental studies indicate that oral butyrate administration improves the structural and functional indexes of adaptation in short bowel syndrome [156]. Butyrate also exerts pro-absorptive/anti-secretory effects due its characteristics of inducing ion and water absorption. SCFA are absorbed by colonic epithelial cells and stimulate Na-dependent fluid absorption via a cyclic AMP–independent process involving apical membrane Na-H, SCFA-HCO_3, and Cl-SCFA exchanges [11]. Butyrate inhibits Cl^- secretion induced by prostaglandin E2, cholera toxin, and phosphocholine [89]. This effect is due to reduced production of intracellular cyclic AMP (cAMP) secondary to the expression and regulation of adenylate cyclase [12]. For these reasons, butyrate and SCFA solutions are potentially useful in diarrhea linked disorders such as antibiotic and osmolarity-associated diarrhea; diversion colitis and short bowel syndrome [11].

Total parenteral nutrition (TPN) reduces the mass of the remaining intestinal mucosa, whereas adaptation to small bowel resection is associated with increased mucosal mass. Experimental studies has presented that the addition of short chain fatty acids (SCFA) to TPN has been shown to prevent the hypotrophy related to prolonged TPN and to enhance structural markers of adaptation to small-bowel resection [87, 88]. Adult rats underwent an 80% small bowel resection receiving TPN showed significant loss of jejunal mucosal weight, after small bowel resection, whereas animals receiving SCFA-supplemented TPN showed no significant change in the jejunal mucosal parameters and a significant increase in ileal mucosal protein. These data demonstrated that SCFA-supplemented TPN reduces the mucosal atrophy associated with TPN after massive bowel resection and may facilitate adaptation to small bowel resection [88]. It has been shown that systemic SCFA is able to increase GLUT2 expression following intestinal resection [157, 158], suggesting a potential effect of these fatty acids in modulating gene expression and transport capacity of glucose and other hexoses. The concept that SCFAs can be provided intravenously to prepare the intestinal brush border for effective digestion and absorption of enteral nutrients is particularly attractive for patients with intestinal failure [156]. The mechanism of this effect of butyrate is not totally understood but could be at least partially due to increases on sodium-glucose co-transporter 1 (SGLT-1) activity and GLP-2 concentrations [8].

Use of Butyrate in the clinical practice of intestinal diseases: Despite its positive effects pointed out in this chapter, the current use of butyrate as a functional food or pharmacological agent is still limited due to several factors. Besides the controversies of some of its clinical effects, rectal enemas are the most common and studied via of administration. However, they impose low acceptability by the patients and require several daily applications. The oral supplementation sodium butyrate is also limited by its short half-life (about 4 h), its fast metabolism and excretion and some side-effects observed such as unpleasant odor, nauseas, and headache. Alternatives for these common routes of administration such as coated tablets and micro and nanoparticles that contain butyrate or butyrate producing prebiotics and probiotics have been tested with promising results [27, 78, 130, 144]. Tributyrin (TBT) is an oily (liquid) triglyceride that contains three butyrate moieties esterified with glycerol. TBT can be delivered orally and releases butyrate when metabolized by intestinal enzymes. TBT (150 to 200mg/kg three times daily) was already tested in 20 patients with solid tumors [48]. The results showed that blood concentration of TBT presented considerable interpatient variability, with median butyrate concentration of 52μM. This concentration is a lower effective concentration related to butyrate effects on differentiation and apoptosis. However, no toxic effects were registered and no objective responses were seen, although four patients presented prolonged disease stabilization and two patients with chemotherapy-refractory non-small-cell lung cancer had survived for >1 year without evidence of progression.

Conclusion

Butyrate presents a vast beneficial effect in the gastrointestinal tract that could be associated to the improvement and prevention of various disorders of the colon and also of the small intestine. These effects can be obtained using different routes of administration: in situ (enema), oral or even parenteral administration.

Although the effects of butyrate are being studied for over 20 years, few clinical studies have been conducted until now. For this reason, its use in intestinal diseases, particularly CRC and UC, although promising, requires further investigation.

References

[1] K. Abe, 'Butyric Acid Induces Apoptosis in Both Human Monocytes and Lymphocytes Equivalently', *J Oral Sci,* 54 (2012), 7-14.

[2] S. L. Abrahamse, B. L. Pool-Zobel, and G. Rechkemmer, 'Potential of Short Chain Fatty Acids to Modulate the Induction of Dna Damage and Changes in the Intracellular Calcium Concentration by Oxidative Stress in Isolated Rat Distal Colon Cells', *Carcinogenesis,* 20 (1999), 629-34.

[3] W. K. Alderton, C. E. Cooper, and R. G. Knowles, 'Nitric Oxide Synthases: Structure, Function and Inhibition', *Biochem J,* 357 (2001), 593-615.

[4] M. Aoyama, J. Kotani, and M. Usami, 'Butyrate and Propionate Induced Activated or Non-Activated Neutrophil Apoptosis Via Hdac Inhibitor Activity but without Activating Gpr-41/Gpr-43 Pathways', *Nutrition,* 26 (2010), 653-61.

[5] V. R. Babaev, J. D. Chew, L. Ding, S. Davis, M. D. Breyer, R. M. Breyer, J. A. Oates, S. Fazio, and M. F. Linton, 'Macrophage Ep4 Deficiency Increases Apoptosis and Suppresses Early Atherosclerosis', *Cell Metab,* 8 (2008), 492-501.

[6] Z. Bai, Z. Zhang, Y. Ye, and S. Wang, 'Sodium Butyrate Induces Differentiation of Gastric Cancer Cells to Intestinal Cells Via the Pten/Phosphoinositide 3-Kinase Pathway', *Cell Biol Int,* 34 (2010), 1141-5.

[7] E. Bailón, M. Cueto-Sola, P. Utrilla, M. E. Rodriguez-Cabezas, N. Garrido-Mesa, A. Zarzuelo, J. Xaus, J. Galvez, and M. Comalada, 'Butyrate in Vitro Immune-Modulatory

Effects Might Be Mediated through a Proliferation-Related Induction of Apoptosis', *Immunobiology,* 215 (2010), 863-73.

[8] A. L. Bartholome, D. M. Albin, D. H. Baker, J. J. Holst, and K. A. Tappenden, 'Supplementation of Total Parenteral Nutrition with Butyrate Acutely Increases Structural Aspects of Intestinal Adaptation after an 80% Jejunoileal Resection in Neonatal Piglets', *JPEN J Parenter Enteral Nutr,* 28 (2004), 210-22; discussion 22-3.

[9] D. Behrendt and P. Ganz, 'Endothelial Function. From Vascular Biology to Clinical Applications', *Am J Cardiol,* 90 (2002), 40L-48L.

[10] J. Bilski, A. I. Mazur-Bialy, M. Wierdak, and T. Brzozowski, 'The Impact of Physical Activity and Nutrition on Inflammatory Bowel Disease: The Potential Role of Cross Talk between Adipose Tissue and Skeletal Muscle', *J Physiol Pharmacol,* 64 (2013), 143-55.

[11] H. J. Binder, 'Role of Colonic Short-Chain Fatty Acid Transport in Diarrhea', *Annu Rev Physiol,* 72 (2010), 297-313.

[12] H. J. Binder and P. Mehta, 'Short-Chain Fatty Acids Stimulate Active Sodium and Chloride Absorption in Vitro in the Rat Distal Colon', *Gastroenterology,* 96 (1989), 989-96.

[13] M. Blaut and T. Clavel, 'Metabolic Diversity of the Intestinal Microbiota: Implications for Health and Disease', *J Nutr,* 137 (2007), 751S-5S.

[14] R. S. Blumberg, L. J. Saubermann, and W. Strober, 'Animal Models of Mucosal Inflammation and Their Relation to Human Inflammatory Bowel Disease', *Curr Opin Immunol,* 11 (1999), 648-56.

[15] R. S. Blumberg and W. Strober, 'Prospects for Research in Inflammatory Bowel Disease', *JAMA,* 285 (2001), 643-7.

[16] A. Borthakur, R. K. Gill, K. Hodges, K. Ramaswamy, G. Hecht, and P. K. Dudeja, 'Enteropathogenic Escherichia Coli Inhibits Butyrate Uptake in Caco-2 Cells by Altering the Apical Membrane Mct1 Level', *Am J Physiol Gastrointest Liver Physiol,* 290 (2006), G30-5.

[17] A. Borthakur, S. Saksena, R. K. Gill, W. A. Alrefai, K. Ramaswamy, and P. K. Dudeja, 'Regulation of Monocarboxylate Transporter 1 (Mct1) Promoter by Butyrate in Human Intestinal Epithelial Cells: Involvement of Nf-Kappab Pathway', *J Cell Biochem,* 103 (2008), 1452-63.

[18] S. Bourdu, M. Dapoigny, E. Chapuy, F. Artigue, M. P. Vasson, P. Dechelotte, G. Bommelaer, A. Eschalier, and D. Ardid, 'Rectal Instillation of Butyrate Provides a Novel Clinically Relevant Model of Noninflammatory Colonic Hypersensitivity in Rats', *Gastroenterology,* 128 (2005), 1996-2008.

[19] A. J. Brown, S. M. Goldsworthy, A. A. Barnes, M. M. Eilert, L. Tcheang, D. Daniels, A. I. Muir, M. J. Wigglesworth, I. Kinghorn, N. J. Fraser, N. B. Pike, J. C. Strum, K. M. Steplewski, P. R. Murdock, J. C. Holder, F. H. Marshall, P. G. Szekeres, S. Wilson, D. M. Ignar, S. M. Foord, A. Wise, and S. J. Dowell, 'The Orphan G Protein-Coupled Receptors Gpr41 and Gpr43 Are Activated by Propionate and Other Short Chain Carboxylic Acids', *J Biol Chem,* 278 (2003), 11312-9.

[20] A. Buda, D. Qualtrough, M. A. Jepson, D. Martines, C. Paraskeva, and M. Pignatelli, 'Butyrate Downregulates Alpha2beta1 Integrin: A Possible Role in the Induction of Apoptosis in Colorectal Cancer Cell Lines', *Gut,* 52 (2003), 729-34.

[21] S. J. Bultman, 'Molecular Pathways: Gene-Environment Interactions Regulating Dietary Fiber Induction of Proliferation and Apoptosis Via Butyrate for Cancer Prevention', *Clin Cancer Res* (2013).

[22] X. X. Cao, I. Mohuiddin, F. Ece, D. J. McConkey, and W. R. Smythe, 'Histone Deacetylase Inhibitor Downregulation of Bcl-Xl Gene Expression Leads to Apoptotic Cell Death in Mesothelioma', *Am J Respir Cell Mol Biol,* 25 (2001), 562-8.

[23] E. Cardenal-Muñoz and F. Ramos-Morales, 'Analysis of the Expression, Secretion and Translocation of the Salmonella Enterica Type Iii Secretion System Effector Stea', *PLoS One,* 6 (2011), e26930.

[24] D. Chakravortty, N. Koide, Y. Kato, T. Sugiyama, M. M. Mu, T. Yoshida, and T. Yokochi, 'The Inhibitory Action of Butyrate on Lipopolysaccharide-Induced Nitric Oxide Production in Raw 264.7 Murine Macrophage Cells', *J Endotoxin Res,* 6 (2000), 243-7.

[25] W. Chen, F. Wei, J. Xu, Y. Wang, L. Chen, J. Wang, and X. Guan, 'Trastuzumab Enhances the Anti-Tumor Effects of the Histone Deacetylase Inhibitor Sodium Butyrate on a Her2-Overexpressing Breast Cancer Cell Line', *Int J Mol Med,* 28 (2011), 985-91.

[26] D. H. Chung, F. Zhang, F. Chen, W. P. McLaughlin, and M. Ljungman, 'Butyrate Attenuates Bclx(L) Expression in Human Fibroblasts and Acts in Synergy with Ionizing Radiation to Induce Apoptosis', *Radiat Res,* 149 (1998), 187-94.

[27] J. M. Clarke, G. P. Young, D. L. Topping, A. R. Bird, L. Cobiac, B. L. Scherer, J. G. Winkler, and T. J. Lockett, 'Butyrate Delivered by Butyrylated Starch Increases Distal Colonic Epithelial Apoptosis in Carcinogen-Treated Rats', *Carcinogenesis,* 33 (2012), 197-202.

[28] K. O. Clarke, R. Feinman, and L. E. Harrison, 'Tributyrin, an Oral Butyrate Analogue, Induces Apoptosis through the Activation of Caspase-3', *Cancer Lett,* 171 (2001), 57-65.

[29] M. R. Clausen and P. B. Mortensen, 'Kinetic Studies on Colonocyte Metabolism of Short Chain Fatty Acids and Glucose in Ulcerative Colitis', *Gut,* 37 (1995), 684-9.

[30] J. P. Cooke, 'The Pivotal Role of Nitric Oxide for Vascular Health', *Can J Cardiol,* 20 Suppl B (2004), 7B-15B.

[31] M. Cottone, S. Renna, I. Modesto, and A. Orlando, 'Is 5-Asa Still the Treatment of Choice for Ulcerative Colitis?', *Curr Drug Targets,* 12 (2011), 1396-405.

[32] M. A. Cox, J. Jackson, M. Stanton, A. Rojas-Triana, L. Bober, M. Laverty, X. Yang, F. Zhu, J. Liu, S. Wang, F. Monsma, G. Vassileva, M. Maguire, E. Gustafson, M. Bayne, C. C. Chou, D. Lundell, and C. H. Jenh, 'Short-Chain Fatty Acids Act as Antiinflammatory Mediators by Regulating Prostaglandin E(2) and Cytokines', *World J Gastroenterol,* 15 (2009), 5549-57.

[33] M. A. Cuff, D. W. Lambert, and S. P. Shirazi-Beechey, 'Substrate-Induced Regulation of the Human Colonic Monocarboxylate Transporter, Mct1', *J Physiol,* 539 (2002), 361-71.

[34] M. A. Cuff and S. P. Shirazi-Beechey, 'The Importance of Butyrate Transport to the Regulation of Gene Expression in the Colonic Epithelium', *Biochem Soc Trans,* 32 (2004), 1100-2.

[35] S. Daff, 'No Synthase: Structures and Mechanisms', *Nitric Oxide,* 23 (2010), 1-11.

[36] K. Daly, M. A. Cuff, F. Fung, and S. P. Shirazi-Beechey, 'The Importance of Colonic Butyrate Transport to the Regulation of Genes Associated with Colonic Tissue Homoeostasis', *Biochem Soc Trans,* 33 (2005), 733-5.

[37] M. C. Daroqui and L. H. Augenlicht, 'Transcriptional Attenuation in Colon Carcinoma Cells in Response to Butyrate', *Cancer Prev Res (Phila),* 3 (2010), 1292-302.

[38] V. De Preter, I. Arijs, K. Windey, W. Vanhove, S. Vermeire, F. Schuit, P. Rutgeerts, and K. Verbeke, 'Decreased Mucosal Sulfide Detoxification Is Related to an Impaired Butyrate Oxidation in Ulcerative Colitis', *Inflamm Bowel Dis,* 18 (2012), 2371-80.

[39] ———, 'Impaired Butyrate Oxidation in Ulcerative Colitis Is Due to Decreased Butyrate Uptake and a Defect in the Oxidation Pathway', *Inflamm Bowel Dis,* 18 (2012), 1127-36.

[40] V. De Preter, V. Bulteel, P. Suenaert, K. P. Geboes, G. De Hertogh, A. Luypaerts, K. Geboes, K. Verbeke, and P. Rutgeerts, 'Pouchitis, Similar to Active Ulcerative Colitis, Is Associated with Impaired Butyrate Oxidation by Intestinal Mucosa', *Inflamm Bowel Dis,* 15 (2009), 335-40.

[41] V. De Preter, K. P. Geboes, V. Bulteel, G. Vandermeulen, P. Suenaert, P. Rutgeerts, and K. Verbeke, 'Kinetics of Butyrate Metabolism in the Normal Colon and in Ulcerative Colitis: The Effects of Substrate Concentration and Carnitine on the Β-Oxidation Pathway', *Aliment Pharmacol Ther,* 34 (2011), 526-32.

[42] J. E. Deanfield, J. P. Halcox, and T. J. Rabelink, 'Endothelial Function and Dysfunction: Testing and Clinical Relevance', *Circulation,* 115 (2007), 1285-95.

[43] S. L. Deshmane, S. Kremlev, S. Amini, and B. E. Sawaya, 'Monocyte Chemoattractant Protein-1 (Mcp-1): An Overview', *J Interferon Cytokine Res,* 29 (2009), 313-26.

[44] D. R. Donohoe, L. B. Collins, A. Wali, R. Bigler, W. Sun, and S. J. Bultman, 'The Warburg Effect Dictates the Mechanism of Butyrate-Mediated Histone Acetylation and Cell Proliferation', *Mol Cell,* 48 (2012), 612-26.

[45] D. R. Donohoe, K. P. Curry, and S. J. Bultman, 'Microbial Oncotarget: Bacterial-Produced Butyrate, Chemoprevention and Warburg Effect', *Oncotarget,* 4 (2013), 182-3.

[46] D. R. Donohoe, N. Garge, X. Zhang, W. Sun, T. M. O'Connell, M. K. Bunger, and S. J. Bultman, 'The Microbiome and Butyrate Regulate Energy Metabolism and Autophagy in the Mammalian Colon', *Cell Metab,* 13 (2011), 517-26.

[47] M. P. dos Santos, G. Schwartsmann, R. Roesler, A. L. Brunetto, and A. L. Abujamra, 'Sodium Butyrate Enhances the Cytotoxic Effect of Antineoplastic Drugs in Human Lymphoblastic T-Cells', *Leuk Res,* 33 (2009), 218-21.

[48] M. J. Edelman, K. Bauer, S. Khanwani, N. Tait, J. Trepel, J. Karp, N. Nemieboka, E. J. Chung, and D. Van Echo, 'Clinical and Pharmacologic Study of Tributyrin: An Oral Butyrate Prodrug', *Cancer Chemother Pharmacol,* 51 (2003), 439-44.

[49] V. Eeckhaut, R. Ducatelle, B. Sas, S. Vermeire, and F. Van Immerseel, 'Progress Towards Butyrate-Producing Pharmabiotics: Butyricicoccus Pullicaecorum Capsule and Efficacy in Tnbs Models in Comparison with Therapeutics', *Gut,* 63 (2014), 367.

[50] V. Eeckhaut, K. Machiels, C. Perrier, C. Romero, S. Maes, B. Flahou, M. Steppe, F. Haesebrouck, B. Sas, R. Ducatelle, S. Vermeire, and F. Van Immerseel, 'Butyricicoccus Pullicaecorum in Inflammatory Bowel Disease', *Gut,* 62 (2013), 1745-52.

[51] T. J. Fan, L. H. Han, R. S. Cong, and J. Liang, 'Caspase Family Proteases and Apoptosis', *Acta Biochim Biophys Sin (Shanghai),* 37 (2005), 719-27.

[52] J. K. Fauser, L. D. Prisciandaro, A. G. Cummins, and G. S. Howarth, 'Fatty Acids as Potential Adjunctive Colorectal Chemotherapeutic Agents', *Cancer Biol Ther,* 11 (2011), 724-31.

[53] Q. Feng, X. Lu, D. L. Jones, J. Shen, and J. M. Arnold, 'Increased Inducible Nitric Oxide Synthase Expression Contributes to Myocardial Dysfunction and Higher Mortality after Myocardial Infarction in Mice', *Circulation,* 104 (2001), 700-4.

[54] T. M. Ferreira, A. J. Leonel, M. A. Melo, R. R. Santos, D. C. Cara, V. N. Cardoso, M. I. Correia, and J. I. Alvarez-Leite, 'Oral Supplementation of Butyrate Reduces Mucositis and Intestinal Permeability Associated with 5-Fluorouracil Administration', *Lipids,* 47 (2012), 669-78.

[55] U. Forstermann and T. Munzel, 'Endothelial Nitric Oxide Synthase in Vascular Disease: From Marvel to Menace', *Circulation,* 113 (2006), 1708-14.

[56] E. Galkina and K. Ley, 'Vascular Adhesion Molecules in Atherosclerosis', *Arterioscler Thromb Vasc Biol,* 27 (2007), 2292-301.

[57] R. K. Gill and P. K. Dudeja, 'A Novel Facet to Consider for the Effects of Butyrate on Its Target Cells. Focus On "The Short-Chain Fatty Acid Butyrate Is a Substrate of Breast Cancer Resistance Protein"', *Am J Physiol Cell Physiol,* 301 (2011), C977-9.

[58] A. Gospodinov, S. Popova, I. Vassileva, and B. Anachkova, 'The Inhibitor of Histone Deacetylases Sodium Butyrate Enhances the Cytotoxicity of Mitomycin C', *Mol Cancer Ther,* 11 (2012), 2116-26.

[59] P. Guilloteau, L. Martin, V. Eeckhaut, R. Ducatelle, R. Zabielski, and F. Van Immerseel, 'From the Gut to the Peripheral Tissues: The Multiple Effects of Butyrate', *Nutr Res Rev,* 23 (2010), 366-84.

[60] P. Guilloteau, G. Savary, Y. Jaguelin-Peyrault, V. Rome, L. Le Normand, and R. Zabielski, 'Dietary Sodium Butyrate Supplementation Increases Digestibility and Pancreatic Secretion in Young Milk-Fed Calves', *J Dairy Sci,* 93 (2010), 5842-50.

[61] C. Hadjiagapiou, L. Schmidt, P. K. Dudeja, T. J. Layden, and K. Ramaswamy, 'Mechanism(S) of Butyrate Transport in Caco-2 Cells: Role of Monocarboxylate Transporter 1', *Am J Physiol Gastrointest Liver Physiol,* 279 (2000), G775-80.

[62] A. Hague, A. J. Butt, and C. Paraskeva, 'The Role of Butyrate in Human Colonic Epithelial Cells: An Energy Source or Inducer of Differentiation and Apoptosis?', *Proc Nutr Soc,* 55 (1996), 937-43.

[63] A. P. Halestrap, 'The Monocarboxylate Transporter Family--Structure and Functional Characterization', *IUBMB Life,* 64 (2012), 1-9.

[64] H. M. Hamer, D. M. Jonkers, A. Bast, S. A. Vanhoutvin, M. A. Fischer, A. Kodde, F. J. Troost, K. Venema, and R. J. Brummer, 'Butyrate Modulates Oxidative Stress in the Colonic Mucosa of Healthy Humans', *Clin Nutr,* 28 (2009), 88-93.

[65] H. M. Hamer, D. M. Jonkers, S. A. Vanhoutvin, F. J. Troost, G. Rijkers, A. de Bruïne, A. Bast, K. Venema, and R. J. Brummer, 'Effect of Butyrate Enemas on Inflammation and Antioxidant Status in the Colonic Mucosa of Patients with Ulcerative Colitis in Remission', *Clin Nutr,* 29 (2010), 738-44.

[66] H. M. Hamer, D. Jonkers, K. Venema, S. Vanhoutvin, F. J. Troost, and R. J. Brummer, 'Review Article: The Role of Butyrate on Colonic Function', *Aliment Pharmacol Ther,* 27 (2008), 104-19.

[67] B. G. Heerdt, M. A. Houston, G. M. Anthony, and L. H. Augenlicht, 'Initiation of Growth Arrest and Apoptosis of Mcf-7 Mammary Carcinoma Cells by Tributyrin, a

Triglyceride Analogue of the Short-Chain Fatty Acid Butyrate, Is Associated with Mitochondrial Activity', *Cancer Res,* 59 (1999), 1584-91.
[68] R. Heidor, J. F. Ortega, A. de Conti, T. P. Ong, and F. S. Moreno, 'Anticarcinogenic Actions of Tributyrin, a Butyric Acid Prodrug', *Curr Drug Targets,* 13 (2012), 1720-9.
[69] A. Hernandez, R. Thomas, F. Smith, J. Sandberg, S. Kim, D. H. Chung, and B. M. Evers, 'Butyrate Sensitizes Human Colon Cancer Cells to Trail-Mediated Apoptosis', *Surgery,* 130 (2001), 265-72.
[70] B. F. Hinnebusch, S. Meng, J. T. Wu, S. Y. Archer, and R. A. Hodin, 'The Effects of Short-Chain Fatty Acids on Human Colon Cancer Cell Phenotype Are Associated with Histone Hyperacetylation', *J Nutr,* 132 (2002), 1012-7.
[71] P. J. Hornby and B. A. Moore, 'The Therapeutic Potential of Targeting the Glucagon-Like Peptide-2 Receptor in Gastrointestinal Disease', *Expert Opin Ther Targets,* 15 (2011), 637-46.
[72] Y. J. Hu, Y. D. Wang, F. Q. Tan, and W. X. Yang, 'Regulation of Paracellular Permeability: Factors and Mechanisms', *Mol Biol Rep,* 40 (2013), 6123-42.
[73] T. Hudcovic, J. Kolinska, J. Klepetar, R. Stepankova, T. Rezanka, D. Srutkova, M. Schwarzer, V. Erban, Z. Du, J. M. Wells, T. Hrncir, H. Tlaskalova-Hogenova, and H. Kozakova, 'Protective Effect of Clostridium Tyrobutyricum in Acute Dextran Sodium Sulphate-Induced Colitis: Differential Regulation of Tumour Necrosis Factor-A and Interleukin-18 in Balb/C and Severe Combined Immunodeficiency Mice', *Clin Exp Immunol,* 167 (2012), 356-65.
[74] T. Høverstad and T. Midtvedt, 'Short-Chain Fatty Acids in Germfree Mice and Rats', *J Nutr,* 116 (1986), 1772-6.
[75] H. Inoue, K. Shiraki, S. Ohmori, T. Sakai, M. Deguchi, T. Yamanaka, H. Okano, and T. Nakano, 'Histone Deacetylase Inhibitors Sensitize Human Colonic Adenocarcinoma Cell Lines to Tnf-Related Apoptosis Inducing Ligand-Mediated Apoptosis', *Int J Mol Med,* 9 (2002), 521-5.
[76] R. Joachimiak, A. Kaźnica, and T. Drewa, 'Influence of Sodium Butyrate on Hepatocellular Carcinoma (Hepg2) and Glioblastoma (C6) Cell Lines in Vitro', *Acta Pol Pharm,* 64 (2007), 561-3.
[77] M. Kajita, T. Murata, K. Horiguchi, M. Iizuka, M. Hori, and H. Ozaki, 'Inos Expression in Vascular Resident Macrophages Contributes to Circulatory Dysfunction of Splanchnic Vascular Smooth Muscle Contractions in Portal Hypertensive Rats', *Am J Physiol Heart Circ Physiol,* 300 (2011), H1021-31.
[78] S. N. Kang, S. S. Hong, M. K. Lee, and S. J. Lim, 'Dual Function of Tributyrin Emulsion: Solubilization and Enhancement of Anticancer Effect of Celecoxib', *Int J Pharm,* 428 (2012), 76-81.
[79] S. Karaki, R. Mitsui, H. Hayashi, I. Kato, H. Sugiya, T. Iwanaga, J. B. Furness, and A. Kuwahara, 'Short-Chain Fatty Acid Receptor, Gpr43, Is Expressed by Enteroendocrine Cells and Mucosal Mast Cells in Rat Intestine', *Cell Tissue Res,* 324 (2006), 353-60.
[80] S. Karaki, H. Tazoe, H. Hayashi, H. Kashiwabara, K. Tooyama, Y. Suzuki, and A. Kuwahara, 'Expression of the Short-Chain Fatty Acid Receptor, Gpr43, in the Human Colon', *J Mol Histol,* 39 (2008), 135-42.
[81] H. Kayahan, I. Sari, N. Cullu, F. Yuksel, S. Demir, M. Akarsu, Y. Goktay, B. Unsal, and H. Akpinar, 'Evaluation of Early Atherosclerosis in Patients with Inflammatory Bowel Disease', *Dig Dis Sci,* 57 (2012), 2137-43.

[82] S. Kayo, Y. Ikura, T. Suekane, N. Shirai, Y. Sugama, M. Ohsawa, K. Adachi, K. Watanabe, S. Nakamura, Y. Fujiwara, N. Oshitani, K. Higuchi, K. Maeda, K. Hirakawa, T. Arakawa, and M. Ueda, 'Close Association between Activated Platelets and Neutrophils in the Active Phase of Ulcerative Colitis in Humans', *Inflamm Bowel Dis,* 12 (2006), 727-35.

[83] M. Kibbe, T. Billiar, and E. Tzeng, 'Inducible Nitric Oxide Synthase and Vascular Injury', *Cardiovasc Res,* 43 (1999), 650-7.

[84] Y. H. Kim, J. W. Park, J. Y. Lee, and T. K. Kwon, 'Sodium Butyrate Sensitizes Trail-Mediated Apoptosis by Induction of Transcription from the Dr5 Gene Promoter through Sp1 Sites in Colon Cancer Cells', *Carcinogenesis,* 25 (2004), 1813-20.

[85] S. D. Kobayashi and F. R. DeLeo, 'Towards a Comprehensive Understanding of the Role of Neutrophils in Innate Immunity: A Systems Biology-Level Approach', *Wiley Interdiscip Rev Syst Biol Med,* 1 (2009), 309-33.

[86] M. Koprinarova, P. Botev, and G. Russev, 'Histone Deacetylase Inhibitor Sodium Butyrate Enhances Cellular Radiosensitivity by Inhibiting Both Dna Nonhomologous End Joining and Homologous Recombination', *DNA Repair (Amst),* 10 (2011), 970-7.

[87] M. J. Koruda, R. H. Rolandelli, D. Z. Bliss, J. Hastings, J. L. Rombeau, and R. G. Settle, 'Parenteral Nutrition Supplemented with Short-Chain Fatty Acids: Effect on the Small-Bowel Mucosa in Normal Rats', *Am J Clin Nutr,* 51 (1990), 685-9.

[88] M. J. Koruda, R. H. Rolandelli, R. G. Settle, D. M. Zimmaro, and J. L. Rombeau, 'Effect of Parenteral Nutrition Supplemented with Short-Chain Fatty Acids on Adaptation to Massive Small Bowel Resection', *Gastroenterology,* 95 (1988), 715-20.

[89] S. Krishnan, B. S. Ramakrishna, and H. J. Binder, 'Stimulation of Sodium Chloride Absorption from Secreting Rat Colon by Short-Chain Fatty Acids', *Dig Dis Sci,* 44 (1999), 1924-30.

[90] D. W. Laight, J. Matz, B. Caesar, M. J. Carrier, and E. E. Anggard, 'Investigation of Endogenous Nitric Oxide Vascular Function in the Carotid Artery of Cholesterol-Fed Rabbits', *Br J Pharmacol,* 117 (1996), 1471-4.

[91] E. Le Poul, C. Loison, S. Struyf, J. Y. Springael, V. Lannoy, M. E. Decobecq, S. Brezillon, V. Dupriez, G. Vassart, J. Van Damme, M. Parmentier, and M. Detheux, 'Functional Characterization of Human Receptors for Short Chain Fatty Acids and Their Role in Polymorphonuclear Cell Activation', *J Biol Chem,* 278 (2003), 25481-9.

[92] V. Leone, E. B. Chang, and S. Devkota, 'Diet, Microbes, and Host Genetics: The Perfect Storm in Inflammatory Bowel Diseases', *J Gastroenterol,* 48 (2013), 315-21.

[93] A. J. Leonel and J. I. Alvarez-Leite, 'Butyrate: Implications for Intestinal Function', *Curr Opin Clin Nutr Metab Care,* 15 (2013), 474-9.

[94] A. J. Leonel, L. G. Teixeira, R. P. Oliveira, A. F. Santiago, N. V. Batista, T. R. Ferreira, R. C. Santos, V. N. Cardoso, D. C. Cara, A. M. Faria, and J. Alvarez-Leite, 'Antioxidative and Immunomodulatory Effects of Tributyrin Supplementation on Experimental Colitis', *Br J Nutr,* 109 (2012), 1396-407.

[95] ———, 'Antioxidative and Immunomodulatory Effects of Tributyrin Supplementation on Experimental Colitis', *Br J Nutr,* 109 (2013), 1396-407.

[96] P. Lepage, R. Häsler, M. E. Spehlmann, A. Rehman, A. Zvirbliene, A. Begun, S. Ott, L. Kupcinskas, J. Doré, A. Raedler, and S. Schreiber, 'Twin Study Indicates Loss of Interaction between Microbiota and Mucosa of Patients with Ulcerative Colitis', *Gastroenterology,* 141 (2011), 227-36.

[97] K. Lewis, F. Lutgendorff, V. Phan, J. D. Söderholm, P. M. Sherman, and D. M. McKay, 'Enhanced Translocation of Bacteria across Metabolically Stressed Epithelia Is Reduced by Butyrate', *Inflamm Bowel Dis,* 16 (2010), 1138-48.

[98] X. Liang, R. S. Wang, F. Wang, S. Liu, F. Guo, L. Sun, Y. J. Wang, Y. X. Sun, and X. L. Chen, 'Sodium Butyrate Protects against Severe Burn-Induced Remote Acute Lung Injury in Rats', *PLoS One,* 8 (2013), e68786.

[99] T. Liu, J. Li, Y. Liu, N. Xiao, H. Suo, K. Xie, C. Yang, and C. Wu, 'Short-Chain Fatty Acids Suppress Lipopolysaccharide-Induced Production of Nitric Oxide and Proinflammatory Cytokines through Inhibition of Nf-Kappab Pathway in Raw264.7 Cells', *Inflammation,* 35 (2012), 1676-84.

[100] R. A. Machado, S. Constantino Lde, C. D. Tomasi, H. A. Rojas, F. S. Vuolo, M. F. Vitto, P. A. Cesconetto, C. T. de Souza, C. Ritter, and F. Dal-Pizzol, 'Sodium Butyrate Decreases the Activation of Nf-Kappab Reducing Inflammation and Oxidative Damage in the Kidney of Rats Subjected to Contrast-Induced Nephropathy', *Nephrol Dial Transplant,* 27 (2012), 3136-40.

[101] K. Machiels, M. Joossens, J. Sabino, V. De Preter, I. Arijs, V. Eeckhaut, V. Ballet, K. Claes, F. Van Immerseel, K. Verbeke, M. Ferrante, J. Verhaegen, P. Rutgeerts, and S. Vermeire, 'A Decrease of the Butyrate-Producing Species Roseburia Hominis and Faecalibacterium Prausnitzii Defines Dysbiosis in Patients with Ulcerative Colitis', *Gut* (2013).

[102] M. Mandal, L. Adam, J. Mendelsohn, and R. Kumar, 'Nuclear Targeting of Bax During Apoptosis in Human Colorectal Cancer Cells', *Oncogene,* 17 (1998), 999-1007.

[103] M. Mandal, D. J. Olson, T. Sharma, R. K. Vadlamudi, and R. Kumar, 'Butyric Acid Induces Apoptosis by up-Regulating Bax Expression Via Stimulation of the C-Jun N-Terminal Kinase/Activation Protein-1 Pathway in Human Colon Cancer Cells', *Gastroenterology,* 120 (2001), 71-8.

[104] T. Maruyama, S. Yamamoto, J. Qiu, Y. Ueda, T. Suzuki, M. Nojima, and H. Shima, 'Apoptosis of Bladder Cancer by Sodium Butyrate and Cisplatin', *J Infect Chemother,* 18 (2012), 288-95.

[105] K. M. Maslowski, A. T. Vieira, A. Ng, J. Kranich, F. Sierro, D. Yu, H. C. Schilter, M. S. Rolph, F. Mackay, D. Artis, R. J. Xavier, M. M. Teixeira, and C. R. Mackay, 'Regulation of Inflammatory Responses by Gut Microbiota and Chemoattractant Receptor Gpr43', *Nature,* 461 (2009), 1282-6.

[106] H. Masuda, S. Iwai, T. Tanaka, and S. Hayakawa, 'Expression of Il-8, Tnf-Alpha and Ifn-Gamma M-Rna in Ulcerative Colitis, Particularly in Patients with Inactive Phase', *J Clin Lab Immunol,* 46 (1995), 111-23.

[107] K. Meijer, P. de Vos, and M. G. Priebe, 'Butyrate and Other Short-Chain Fatty Acids as Modulators of Immunity: What Relevance for Health?', *Curr Opin Clin Nutr Metab Care,* 13 (2010), 715-21.

[108] T. Menzel, H. Luhrs, S. Zirlik, J. Schauber, T. Kudlich, T. Gerke, A. Gostner, M. Neumann, R. Melcher, and W. Scheppach, 'Butyrate Inhibits Leukocyte Adhesion to Endothelial Cells Via Modulation of Vcam-1', *Inflamm Bowel Dis,* 10 (2004), 122-8.

[109] T. Montero-Melendez, J. Dalli, and M. Perretti, 'Gene Expression Signature-Based Approach Identifies a Pro-Resolving Mechanism of Action for Histone Deacetylase Inhibitors', *Cell Death Differ,* 20 (2013), 567-75.

[110] Y. Naito, T. Takagi, and T. Yoshikawa, 'Neutrophil-Dependent Oxidative Stress in Ulcerative Colitis', *J Clin Biochem Nutr,* 41 (2007), 18-26.

[111] Y. F. Ni, J. Wang, X. L. Yan, F. Tian, J. B. Zhao, Y. J. Wang, and T. Jiang, 'Histone Deacetylase Inhibitor, Butyrate, Attenuates Lipopolysaccharide-Induced Acute Lung Injury in Mice', *Respir Res,* 11 (2010), 33.

[112] J. A. Nick, N. J. Avdi, S. K. Young, L. A. Lehman, P. P. McDonald, S. C. Frasch, M. A. Billstrom, P. M. Henson, G. L. Johnson, and G. S. Worthen, 'Selective Activation and Functional Significance of P38alpha Mitogen-Activated Protein Kinase in Lipopolysaccharide-Stimulated Neutrophils', *J Clin Invest,* 103 (1999), 851-8.

[113] K. Nohara, Y. Yokoyama, and K. Kano, 'The Important Role of Caspase-10 in Sodium Butyrate-Induced Apoptosis', *Kobe J Med Sci,* 53 (2007), 265-73.

[114] H. Ohira, Y. Fujioka, C. Katagiri, R. Mamoto, M. Aoyama-Ishikawa, K. Amako, Y. Izumi, S. Nishiumi, M. Yoshida, M. Usami, and M. Ikeda, 'Butyrate Attenuates Inflammation and Lipolysis Generated by the Interaction of Adipocytes and Macrophages', *J Atheroscler Thromb,* 20 (2013), 425-42.

[115] D. Onat, D. Brillon, P. C. Colombo, and A. M. Schmidt, 'Human Vascular Endothelial Cells: A Model System for Studying Vascular Inflammation in Diabetes and Atherosclerosis', *Curr Diab Rep,* 11 (2011), 193-202.

[116] R. G. Pacheco, C. C. Esposito, L. C. Müller, M. T. Castelo-Branco, L. P. Quintella, V. L. Chagas, H. S. de Souza, and A. Schanaider, 'Use of Butyrate or Glutamine in Enema Solution Reduces Inflammation and Fibrosis in Experimental Diversion Colitis', *World J Gastroenterol,* 18 (2012), 4278-87.

[117] B. Pajak, B. Gajkowska, and A. Orzechowski, 'Sodium Butyrate Sensitizes Human Colon Adenocarcinoma Colo 205 Cells to Both Intrinsic and Tnf-Alpha-Dependent Extrinsic Apoptosis', *Apoptosis,* 14 (2009), 203-17.

[118] B. Pajak and A. Orzechowski, 'Sodium Butyrate-Dependent Sensitization of Human Colon Adenocarcinoma Colo 205 Cells to Tnf-Alpha-Induced Apoptosis', *J Physiol Pharmacol,* 58 Suppl 3 (2007), 163-76.

[119] C. D. Palani, J. F. Beck, and J. Sonnemann, 'Histone Deacetylase Inhibitors Enhance the Anticancer Activity of Nutlin-3 and Induce P53 Hyperacetylation and Downregulation of Mdm2 and Mdm4 Gene Expression', *Invest New Drugs,* 30 (2012), 25-36.

[120] L. Peng, Z. He, W. Chen, I. R. Holzman, and J. Lin, 'Effects of Butyrate on Intestinal Barrier Function in a Caco-2 Cell Monolayer Model of Intestinal Barrier', *Pediatr Res,* 61 (2007), 37-41.

[121] L. Peng, Z. R. Li, R. S. Green, I. R. Holzman, and J. Lin, 'Butyrate Enhances the Intestinal Barrier by Facilitating Tight Junction Assembly Via Activation of Amp-Activated Protein Kinase in Caco-2 Cell Monolayers', *J Nutr,* 139 (2009), 1619-25.

[122] T. X. Pham and J. Lee, 'Dietary Regulation of Histone Acetylases and Deacetylases for the Prevention of Metabolic Diseases', *Nutrients,* 4 (2013), 1868-86.

[123] B. L. Pool-Zobel, V. Selvaraju, J. Sauer, T. Kautenburger, J. Kiefer, K. K. Richter, M. Soom, and S. Wölfl, 'Butyrate May Enhance Toxicological Defence in Primary, Adenoma and Tumor Human Colon Cells by Favourably Modulating Expression of Glutathione S-Transferases Genes, an Approach in Nutrigenomics', *Carcinogenesis,* 26 (2005), 1064-76.

[124] O. Queirós, A. Preto, A. Pacheco, C. Pinheiro, J. Azevedo-Silva, R. Moreira, M. Pedro, Y. H. Ko, P. L. Pedersen, F. Baltazar, and M. Casal, 'Butyrate Activates the Monocarboxylate Transporter Mct4 Expression in Breast Cancer Cells and Enhances the Antitumor Activity of 3-Bromopyruvate', *J Bioenerg Biomembr,* 44 (2012), 141-53.

[125] F. L. Rabelo, M. G. Ramos, G. Brumatti, G. P. Amarante-Mendes, C. Ropert, C. A. Bonjardim, and J. I. Alvarez-Leite, 'Apoptosis Induced by Butyrate Is Independent of Jak/Stat Signaling in a Fibrosarcoma Cell Line', *Biochem Biophys Res Commun,* 301 (2003), 968-73.

[126] M. G. Ramos, E. A. Bambirra, D. C. Cara, E. C. Vieira, and J. I. Alvarez-Leite, 'Oral Administration of Short-Chain Fatty Acids Reduces the Intestinal Mucositis Caused by Treatment with Ara-C in Mice Fed Commercial or Elemental Diets', *Nutr Cancer,* 28 (1997), 212-7.

[127] M. G. Ramos, F. L. Rabelo, G. Brumatti, A. E. Bueno-da-Silva, G. P. Amarante-Mendes, and J. I. Alvarez-Leite, 'Butyrate Increases Apoptosis Induced by Different Antineoplastic Drugs in Monocytic Leukemia Cells', *Chemotherapy,* 50 (2004), 221-8.

[128] M. G. Ramos, F. L. Rabelo, T. Duarte, R. T. Gazzinelli, and J. I. Alvarez-Leite, 'Butyrate Induces Apoptosis in Murine Macrophages Via Caspase-3, but Independent of Autocrine Synthesis of Tumor Necrosis Factor and Nitric Oxide', *Braz J Med Biol Res,* 35 (2002), 161-73.

[129] K. Ranganna, O. P. Mathew, F. M. Yatsu, Z. Yousefipour, B. E. Hayes, and S. G. Milton, 'Involvement of Glutathione/Glutathione S-Transferase Antioxidant System in Butyrate-Inhibited Vascular Smooth Muscle Cell Proliferation', *FEBS J,* 274 (2007), 5962-78.

[130] A. Roda, P. Simoni, M. Magliulo, P. Nanni, M. Baraldini, G. Roda, and E. Roda, 'A New Oral Formulation for the Release of Sodium Butyrate in the Ileo-Cecal Region and Colon', *World J Gastroenterol,* 13 (2007), 1079-84.

[131] P. Rosignoli, R. Fabiani, A. De Bartolomeo, F. Spinozzi, E. Agea, M. A. Pelli, and G. Morozzi, 'Protective Activity of Butyrate on Hydrogen Peroxide-Induced Dna Damage in Isolated Human Colonocytes and Ht29 Tumour Cells', *Carcinogenesis,* 22 (2001), 1675-80.

[132] M. E. Rothenberg, 'Eosinophilic Gastrointestinal Disorders (Egid)', *J Allergy Clin Immunol,* 113 (2004), 11-28; quiz 29.

[133] M. E. Rothenberg, A. Mishra, E. B. Brandt, and S. P. Hogan, 'Gastrointestinal Eosinophils', *Immunol Rev,* 179 (2001), 139-55.

[134] I. Russo, A. Luciani, P. De Cicco, E. Troncone, and C. Ciacci, 'Butyrate Attenuates Lipopolysaccharide-Induced Inflammation in Intestinal Cells and Crohn's Mucosa through Modulation of Antioxidant Defense Machinery', *PLoS One,* 7 (2012), e32841.

[135] S. Saegusa, M. Totsuka, S. Kaminogawa, and T. Hosoi, 'Cytokine Responses of Intestinal Epithelial-Like Caco-2 Cells to Non-Pathogenic and Opportunistic Pathogenic Yeasts in the Presence of Butyric Acid', *Biosci Biotechnol Biochem,* 71 (2007), 2428-34.

[136] A. R. Safarpour, S. V. Hosseini, and D. Mehrabani, 'Epidemiology of Inflammatory Bowel Diseases in Iran and Asia; a Mini Review', *Iran J Med Sci,* 38 (2013), 140-49.

[137] S. Saika, Y. Okada, T. Miyamoto, O. Yamanaka, Y. Ohnishi, A. Ooshima, C. Y. Liu, D. Weng, and W. W. Kao, 'Role of P38 Map Kinase in Regulation of Cell Migration

and Proliferation in Healing Corneal Epithelium', *Invest Ophthalmol Vis Sci,* 45 (2004), 100-9.

[138] J. Sauer, K. K. Richter, and B. L. Pool-Zobel, 'Physiological Concentrations of Butyrate Favorably Modulate Genes of Oxidative and Metabolic Stress in Primary Human Colon Cells', *J Nutr Biochem,* 18 (2007), 736-45.

[139] C. G. Schalkwijk and C. D. Stehouwer, 'Vascular Complications in Diabetes Mellitus: The Role of Endothelial Dysfunction', *Clin Sci (Lond),* 109 (2005), 143-59.

[140] J. Serpa, F. Caiado, T. Carvalho, C. Torre, L. G. Gonçalves, C. Casalou, P. Lamosa, M. Rodrigues, Z. Zhu, E. W. Lam, and S. Dias, 'Butyrate-Rich Colonic Microenvironment Is a Relevant Selection Factor for Metabolically Adapted Tumor Cells', *J Biol Chem,* 285 (2010), 39211-23.

[141] A. M. Shah, 'Inducible Nitric Oxide Synthase and Cardiovascular Disease', *Cardiovasc Res,* 45 (2000), 148-55.

[142] Y. Shao, Z. Gao, P. A. Marks, and X. Jiang, 'Apoptotic and Autophagic Cell Death Induced by Histone Deacetylase Inhibitors', *Proc Natl Acad Sci U S A,* 101 (2004), 18030-5.

[143] F. G. Silva, L. C. Penido, F. X. Valente, M. C. Mendes, D. D. Rosa, M. B. Glória, and M.o C Peluzio, 'Sodium Butyrate Does Not Decrease the Evolution of Precancerous Lesions in Rats', *Acta Cir Bras,* 25 (2010), 507-12.

[144] C. Sina, O. Gavrilova, M. Forster, A. Till, S. Derer, F. Hildebrand, B. Raabe, A. Chalaris, J. Scheller, A. Rehmann, A. Franke, S. Ott, R. Hasler, S. Nikolaus, U. R. Folsch, S. Rose-John, H. P. Jiang, J. Li, S. Schreiber, and P. Rosenstiel, 'G Protein-Coupled Receptor 43 Is Essential for Neutrophil Recruitment During Intestinal Inflammation', *J Immunol,* 183 (2009), 7514-22.

[145] C. W. Smith, '3. Adhesion Molecules and Receptors', *J Allergy Clin Immunol,* 121 (2008), S375-9; quiz S414.

[146] M. Song, B. Xia, and J. Li, 'Effects of Topical Treatment of Sodium Butyrate and 5-Aminosalicylic Acid on Expression of Trefoil Factor 3, Interleukin 1beta, and Nuclear Factor Kappab in Trinitrobenzene Sulphonic Acid Induced Colitis in Rats', *Postgrad Med J,* 82 (2006), 130-5.

[147] R. Soret, J. Chevalier, P. De Coppet, G. Poupeau, P. Derkinderen, J. P. Segain, and M. Neunlist, 'Short-Chain Fatty Acids Regulate the Enteric Neurons and Control Gastrointestinal Motility in Rats', *Gastroenterology,* 138 (2010), 1772-82.

[148] P. B. Stathopulos, X. Lu, J. Shen, J. A. Scott, J. R. Hammond, D. G. McCormack, J. M. Arnold, and Q. Feng, 'Increased L-Arginine Uptake and Inducible Nitric Oxide Synthase Activity in Aortas of Rats with Heart Failure', *Am J Physiol Heart Circ Physiol,* 280 (2001), H859-67.

[149] N. H. Stollman and A. I. Rogers, 'Butyrate and Colonocytes: Bax to the Front', *Am J Gastroenterol,* 92 (1997), 1573-4.

[150] W. Strober, I. Fuss, and P. Mannon, 'The Fundamental Basis of Inflammatory Bowel Disease', *J Clin Invest,* 117 (2007), 514-21.

[151] E. Suply, P. de Vries, R. Soret, F. Cossais, and M. Neunlist, 'Butyrate Enemas Enhance Both Cholinergic and Nitrergic Phenotype of Myenteric Neurons and Neuromuscular Transmission in Newborn Rat Colon', *Am J Physiol Gastrointest Liver Physiol,* 302 (2012), G1373-80.

[152] M. D. Säemann, G. A. Bohmig, C. H. Osterreicher, H. Burtscher, O. Parolini, C. Diakos, J. Stockl, W. H. Horl, and G. J. Zlabinger, 'Anti-Inflammatory Effects of Sodium Butyrate on Human Monocytes: Potent Inhibition of Il-12 and up-Regulation of Il-10 Production', *FASEB J,* 14 (2000), 2380-2.

[153] Y. Tang, Y. Chen, H. Jiang, and D. Nie, 'Short-Chain Fatty Acids Induced Autophagy Serves as an Adaptive Strategy for Retarding Mitochondria-Mediated Apoptotic Cell Death', *Cell Death Differ,* 18 (2011), 602-18.

[154] ———, 'The Role of Short-Chain Fatty Acids in Orchestrating Two Types of Programmed Cell Death in Colon Cancer', *Autophagy,* 7 (2011), 235-7.

[155] Y. Tang, Y. Chen, H. Jiang, G. T. Robbins, and D. Nie, 'G-Protein-Coupled Receptor for Short-Chain Fatty Acids Suppresses Colon Cancer', *Int J Cancer,* 128 (2011), 847-56.

[156] K. A. Tappenden, 'Emerging Therapies for Intestinal Failure', *Arch Surg,* 145 (2010), 528-32.

[157] K. A. Tappenden, L. A. Drozdowski, A. B. Thomson, and M. I. McBurney, 'Short-Chain Fatty Acid-Supplemented Total Parenteral Nutrition Alters Intestinal Structure, Glucose Transporter 2 (Glut2) Mrna and Protein, and Proglucagon Mrna Abundance in Normal Rats', *Am J Clin Nutr,* 68 (1998), 118-25.

[158] K. A. Tappenden and M. I. McBurney, 'Systemic Short-Chain Fatty Acids Rapidly Alter Gastrointestinal Structure, Function, and Expression of Early Response Genes', *Dig Dis Sci,* 43 (1998), 1526-36.

[159] A. L. Tarrerias, M. Millecamps, A. Alloui, C. Beaughard, J. L. Kemeny, S. Bourdu, G. Bommelaer, A. Eschalier, M. Dapoigny, and D. Ardid, 'Short-Chain Fatty Acid Enemas Fail to Decrease Colonic Hypersensitivity and Inflammation in Tnbs-Induced Colonic Inflammation in Rats', *Pain,* 100 (2002), 91-7.

[160] H. Tazoe, Y. Otomo, S. Karaki, I. Kato, Y. Fukami, M. Terasaki, and A. Kuwahara, 'Expression of Short-Chain Fatty Acid Receptor Gpr41 in the Human Colon', *Biomed Res,* 30 (2009), 149-56.

[161] R. Thibault, F. Blachier, B. Darcy-Vrillon, P. de Coppet, A. Bourreille, and J. P. Segain, 'Butyrate Utilization by the Colonic Mucosa in Inflammatory Bowel Diseases: A Transport Deficiency', *Inflamm Bowel Dis,* 16 (2010), 684-95.

[162] D. L. Topping and P. M. Clifton, 'Short-Chain Fatty Acids and Human Colonic Function: Roles of Resistant Starch and Nonstarch Polysaccharides', *Physiol Rev,* 81 (2001), 1031-64.

[163] H. Tsuda, K. Ochiai, N. Suzuki, and K. Otsuka, 'Butyrate, a Bacterial Metabolite, Induces Apoptosis and Autophagic Cell Death in Gingival Epithelial Cells', *J Periodontal Res,* 45 (2010), 626-34.

[164] H. F. Turk, S. S. Kolar, Y. Y. Fan, C. A. Cozby, J. R. Lupton, and R. S. Chapkin, 'Linoleic Acid and Butyrate Synergize to Increase Bcl-2 Levels in Colonocytes', *Int J Cancer,* 128 (2011), 63-71.

[165] J. R. Turner, 'Intestinal Mucosal Barrier Function in Health and Disease', *Nat Rev Immunol,* 9 (2009), 799-809.

[166] T. Ulven, 'Short-Chain Free Fatty Acid Receptors Ffa2/Gpr43 and Ffa3/Gpr41 as New Potential Therapeutic Targets', *Front Endocrinol (Lausanne),* 3 (2012), 111.

[167] S. A. Vanhoutvin, F. J. Troost, T. O. Kilkens, P. J. Lindsey, H. M. Hamer, D. M. Jonkers, K. Venema, and R. J. Brummer, 'The Effects of Butyrate Enemas on Visceral Perception in Healthy Volunteers', *Neurogastroenterol Motil,* 21 (2009), 952-e76.

[168] E. L. Vieira, A. J. Leonel, A. P. Sad, N. R. Beltrão, T. F. Costa, T. M. Ferreira, A. C. Gomes-Santos, A. M. Faria, M. C. Peluzio, D. C. Cara, and J. I. Alvarez-Leite, 'Oral Administration of Sodium Butyrate Attenuates Inflammation and Mucosal Lesion in Experimental Acute Ulcerative Colitis', *J Nutr Biochem,* 23 (2012), 430-6.

[169] M. A. Vinolo, H. G. Rodrigues, R. T. Nachbar, and R. Curi, 'Regulation of Inflammation by Short Chain Fatty Acids', *Nutrients,* 3 (2011), 858-76.

[170] C. Voltolini, S. Battersby, S. L. Etherington, F. Petraglia, J. E. Norman, and H. N. Jabbour, 'A Novel Antiinflammatory Role for the Short-Chain Fatty Acids in Human Labor', *Endocrinology,* 153 (2012), 395-403.

[171] D. Wang, Z. Wang, B. Tian, X. Li, S. Li, and Y. Tian, 'Two Hour Exposure to Sodium Butyrate Sensitizes Bladder Cancer to Anticancer Drugs', *Int J Urol,* 15 (2008), 435-41.

[172] K. E. Wellen, G. Hatzivassiliou, U. M. Sachdeva, T. V. Bui, J. R. Cross, and C. B. Thompson, 'Atp-Citrate Lyase Links Cellular Metabolism to Histone Acetylation', *Science,* 324 (2009), 1076-80.

[173] H. R. Williams, J. D. Willsmore, I. J. Cox, D. G. Walker, J. F. Cobbold, S. D. Taylor-Robinson, and T. R. Orchard, 'Serum Metabolic Profiling in Inflammatory Bowel Disease', *Dig Dis Sci,* 57 (2012), 2157-65.

[174] R. J. Xavier and D. K. Podolsky, 'Unravelling the Pathogenesis of Inflammatory Bowel Disease', *Nature,* 448 (2007), 427-34.

[175] D. Zapolska-Downar, A. Siennicka, M. Kaczmarczyk, B. Kolodziej, and M. Naruszewicz, 'Butyrate Inhibits Cytokine-Induced Vcam-1 and Icam-1 Expression in Cultured Endothelial Cells: The Role of Nf-Kappab and Pparalpha', *J Nutr Biochem,* 15 (2004), 220-8.

[176] M. A. Zimmerman, N. Singh, P. M. Martin, M. Thangaraju, V. Ganapathy, J. L. Waller, H. Shi, K. D. Robertson, D. H. Munn, and K. Liu, 'Butyrate Suppresses Colonic Inflammation through Hdac1-Dependent Fas Upregulation and Fas-Mediated Apoptosis of T Cells', *Am J Physiol Gastrointest Liver Physiol,* 302 (2012), G1405-15.

In: Butyrate: Food Sources, Functions and Health Benefits ISBN: 978-1-63117-657-9
Editor: Cong-Jun Li © 2014 Nova Science Publishers, Inc.

Chapter 3

LARGE BOWEL SHORT CHAIN FATTY ACID PRODUCTION, IMMUNE STATUS AND IMMUNE CELL FUNCTION: IMPLICATIONS FOR CHRONIC INFLAMMATORY DISEASE

Kim Y. C. Fung[1,2,*], Leah Cosgrove[1,2], Julie Clarke[1,2], Trevor Lockett[1,2], Tatsuya Morita[3], Koji Hase[4,5,6] and David Topping[1,2,7]

[1]CSIRO, Preventative Health National Research Flagship, Australia
[2]CSIRO, Animal, Food, and Health Sciences, Adelaide and North Ryde, Australia
[3]Faculty of Agriculture, Shizuoka University, Shizuoka, Japan
[4]RIKEN Centre for Integrative Medical Sciences, Kanagawa, Japan
[5]The Institute for Medical Sciences, University of Tokyo, Tokyo, Japan
[6]PRESTO, Japan Science and Technology Agency, Saitama, Japan
[7]CSIRO, Food Futures National Research Flagship, Adelaide, SA, Australia

ABSTRACT

It is thought that short chain fatty acids (SCFA) formed by the fermentation of dietary fibre carbohydrates by the large bowel microbiota play a key role in lowering the risk of serious diseases including colorectal cancer and inflammatory bowel disease.

---

* Correspondence: Kim Fung, Ph. D., CSIRO Preventative Health National Research Flagship, Life Sciences Centre, Riverside Corporate Park, 11 Julius Ave, North Ryde NSW, 2113. (T) +61 2 9490 8710, (E) kim.fung@csiro.au.

Recent data indicate that the major SCFA (butyrate, propionate and acetate) may have a wider role in maintaining human health where they contribute to intestinal homeostasis by regulating immune cell function and inflammatory processes. These effects are thought to occur via activation of G-protein coupled receptors (GPRs) such as GPR43 and GPR41 by SCFA which results in regulation of T cell function and production of anti-inflammatory cytokines. GPR43/41-SCFA interactions in the colon also result in secretion of gut hormones that regulate gut motility and nutrient absorption, appetite and satiety and there is emerging evidence to indicate that these interactions may influence lipolysis and adipogenesis in the periphery. This chapter outlines current evidence from in vivo and in vitro studies supporting the potential role of SCFA in inflammation, including the importance of the mode and route of delivery of SCFA and their effects on immune status. These experimental factors, when considered in combination with a systems biology approach, will delineate how SCFA exert their effects to prevent chronic inflammatory diseases.

Keywords: Short chain fatty acids, butyrate, inflammation, immune system

INTRODUCTION

Dietary fibre consists largely of carbohydrates of plant origin which resist digestion in the human small intestine and pass into the large bowel. The main components of fibre are non-starch polysaccharides (NSP), starch which resist small intestinal amylolysis (resistant starch, RS) and oligosaccharides. The health benefits of dietary fibre are well established with population studies showing that greater consumption improves gastrointestinal health and reduces risk of non-communicable conditions such as cardiovascular diseases (CVD), colorectal cancer (CRC) and obesity [1, 2]. Despite the known health benefits, daily intakes of dietary fibre in countries such as the US remains below recommended levels [3], which may contribute to their relatively high rates of diet-related disease. However, the situation is not entirely simple and anomalies exist. One of these is the Australian paradox which is the persistence of high rates of disease such as CRC despite comparatively high intakes of fibre, largely as cereal NSP. It is becoming clear that interest in fibre should be directed at the components which are fermented by the colonic microbiota, especially RS [4]. Dietary intakes of RS are low in countries where diet-related disease rates are high making for the attractive hypothesis that they reflect a deficiency of fermentable fibre. More accurately, it could be said that the deficiency is actually of the products of fermentation, mainly (but not only) the short chain fatty acids (SCFA). This brings the role of the colonic microbiome to the fore. The colonic microbiota consists of at least 1000 different bacterial species which contribute to the maintenance of host homeostasis and energy metabolism [4], and the composition of the microbiome appears to vary between individuals and be affected by diet [5-7]. Specific species of the colonic microbiota are responsible for fermentation of RS to produce SCFA [7-10]. The three primary SCFA are acetate, propionate and butyrate with physiological levels ranging from 70 mM to 130 mM [11]. In humans they are produced in molar ratios of approximately 60:30:10 with acetate being the most abundant acid produced, followed by propionate and butyrate [12, 13]. These SCFA play an important role in maintaining homeostasis in the colon by regulating gut barrier function, immune cell function and inflammatory processes and they are also implicated in reducing the risk of developing serious diseases [14]. Although the beneficial health effects of SCFA in humans are well known, the underlying mechanisms involved are poorly understood. Furthermore, recent data has identified a new potential role for SCFA in appetite regulation and satiety, implying that dietary fibre production may also have a role in prevention of obesity and metabolic syndrome through the products of fermentation [15, 16].

Of the major acids, butyrate has been studied most extensively with a primary focus on its ability to prevent CRC (reviewed in [17-19]). In the normal colon, butyrate is the main energy source for colonocytes and is essential for their maturation and function [20]. Physiologically, butyrate promotes gut barrier function, modulates colonic motility, regulates cell growth and differentiation and reduces inflammation [14]. At the cellular level, in vitro studies have shown that butyrate induces apoptosis and inhibits proliferation and the cell cycle in colorectal and other cancer cell types. Butyrate is believed to exert these effects primarily by inhibition of histone deacetylase (HDAC) activity, although additional mechanisms such as autophagy and involvement of the intrinsic and extrinsic apoptotic pathways have been identified [21-24].

SCFA are recognised for their ability to maintain or enhance the host immune response in the colon although the exact mechanisms are not understood. In vitro studies have identified G-protein coupled receptors (GPR) with specificity for the SCFA as playing essential roles in mediating these effects. The cell surface receptors GPR41, GPR43 and GPR109A are thought to be critical. They are expressed most highly on immune cells (e.g., peripheral blood mononuclear cell (PBMC), monocytes, neutrophils, lymphocytes) and GPR41 and GPR43 are also highly expressed on adipocytes with lower expression reported on intestinal enteroendocrine and epithelial cells [25-27]. Loss of expression of GPR43 and GPR109A has been shown to occur in CRC cells that support a role for these receptors in maintaining normal colonic function and tumour suppression [28, 29]. In vivo studies have also shown release of peptide YY (PYY) and glucagon-like peptide-1 (GLP1) from colonic enteroendocrine cells following activation of GPR41 and GPR43, implying a critical role for regulation of satiety by influencing blood glucose and insulin levels [15, 30-35]. In the periphery, activation of these receptors on adipocytes appears to regulate fatty acid metabolism, thus affecting lipolysis, and provides further evidence for their role in preventing the consequences of obesity [36]. In this review, we focus on the interaction between SCFA and GPR, in particular GPR41 and GPR43, and how inflammatory processes that underlie human diseases such as inflammatory bowel disease (IBD), obesity and metabolic syndrome are potentially regulated. We also discuss the inconsistencies regarding hypothesised mechanisms of action and interpretation of experimental data. Although in vitro studies have been used to study potential mechanisms of action, whether comparable (millimolar) concentrations of SCFA are reached in vivo, especially in the peripheral circulation, are not known. Furthermore, interpretation of results from animal studies have been dependent on the mode of delivery of SCFA, i.e., the type of fibre consumed as a dietary supplement versus administration of individual or mixtures SCFA in drinking water or as an enema, and the contribution of dietary fibre to some of the observed physiological effects cannot be conclusively determined. Together, these factors have potentially confounded results of human trials involving dietary supplementation with fibre or RS. The use of novel tools, such as delivery of individual SCFA preferentially to the large colon with acylated high amylose starches [37], will provide better understanding of the influence of these metabolites on the immune and inflammatory response to provide additional insight into the role of dietary fibre in maintaining optimal human health and will provide a basis for developing novel strategies for delivery of SCFA to manage and support personal nutrition.

SCFA AND REGULATION OF COLONIC INFLAMMATION

There are numerous reports supporting the link between the gut microbiota, fermentation and inflammatory conditions such as ulcerative colitis (UC). Recent reports describe an intimate relationship between the gut microbiota and the immune response where commensal bacterial species (e.g., *Bacteroides fragilis*, *Clostridium* spp.) are able to influence the development of pro- and anti-inflammatory pathways, in particular by inducing the maturation of a subset of T regulatory cells (Treg cells) resident in the lamina propia of the colon [38-40]. Colonic Treg cells are characterised by expression of the transcription factor FOXP3 and modulate the intestinal immune and inflammatory response by producing and secreting the pleiotrophic inflammatory cytokine, IL10, which is essential for intestinal immune homeostasis [40, 41]. Both forms of IBD (Crohn's disease and UC) are characterised by chronic inflammation of the gut mucosa and aberrant T cell function has been identified as the primary factor mediating the severity of their symptoms [42]. SCFA, in particular butyrate, have shown promise for reducing inflammation in experimental colitis in animal models [43, 44]. However the results of human studies have not been as conclusive in showing that butyrate administration, e.g., via enema, is effective in alleviating the severity of the disease [45-48]. To understand these observations, transcriptional profiling of colonic mucosa in humans, rats and pigs following consumption of dietary fibre or RS, or butyrate administration have revealed involvement of specific pathways mediating the cellular effects of SCFA [49-52]. These include activation of metabolic pathways, and inhibition of immune and inflammatory pathways. Importantly, it was reported recently that, in pigs, raising large bowel SCFA by feeding RS altered the profile of colonocyte gene expression from an immune pattern and led to increased expression of genes responsible for fatty acid oxidation and the tricarboxylic acid cycle [53]. This is consistent with an increased energy supply for the mucosa and also greater O_2 supply [54]. Transcriptional and proteomic profiling data from in vitro experiments where colorectal adenocarcinoma cell lines were treated with butyrate corroborate these findings [55-59]. Although global transcriptional and proteomic analysis have provided some insight into the biological pathways involved with the effects of SCFA, in particular butyrate, at the physiological and cellular level, the specific mechanisms are still understood poorly.

The effects of SCFA on immune cells are well described and involve chemotaxis, production of reactive oxygen species (ROS) and modulation of both pro- and anti-inflammatory cytokine expression, most likely via suppression of nuclear factor kappa beta (NFkB) activity and inhibition of HDAC activity. SCFA also appear to have both pro- and anti-inflammatory effects depending on the cell type being studied [60, 61]. These opposing effects provide a potential explanation for the inconclusive results seen in human trials mentioned above for butyrate enemas [45-48]. For example, Usami et al. demonstrated a pro-inflammatory effect by measuring TNF-α release in isolated human peripheral blood mononuclear cells (PMBC) stimulated with lipopolysaccharide (LPS) [60]. Both butyrate and acetate were equally effective at stimulating TNF-α secretion but propionate was less potent.

Furthermore, while butyrate and propionate both suppressed NFkB activity, acetate appeared to be acting via a different mechanism and this was not investigated as part of this study. Vinolo et al. performed similar experiments on LPS-activated neutrophils and demonstrated an anti-inflammatory effect where butyrate and propionate both inhibited TNF-α production but acetate had no effect [61]. It was concluded that these effects were due to attenuation of NFkB activity. While the authors of both studies indicated that HDAC inhibition by butyrate and propionate was linked to and likely preceded the effects on NFkB activity, this was not demonstrated definitively.

In addition to the widely reported effect on HDAC inhibition and NFkB activity, various reports have identified a link between SCFA and activation of GPR43 and GPR41 in the induction of an inflammatory response in the colon [62-65]. For example, administration of individual or a mixture SCFA to germ free (GF) and specific pathogen free (SPF) mice (150 mM SCFA in the drinking water) increased the number of colonic Treg cells specifically [65]. Treg cells of the spleen, mesenteric lymph node or thymus were not increased, nor were colonic T helper cells (Th1 or Th17). In the same study, treatment of isolated colonic Treg cells in vitro with propionate increased the expression of FOXP3 and IL10. The authors also demonstrated that increases in colonic Treg cell numbers and their anti-inflammatory function were dependent on GPR43 expression. However, the relevance of these effects to the effects of SCFA produced by large bowel fermentation remains uncertain.

An in vivo study utilising GPR43 and GPR41 knockout mice has demonstrated that these receptors are essential for mounting an acute inflammatory response following immunological challenges to the colon [62]. Reduced leukocyte infiltration and expression of inflammatory cytokines, chemokines and metalloproteinases were observed in the knockout mice when compared with wildtype mice following treatment with agents such as ethanol and 4,6-trinitrobenzene sulfonic acid (TNBS), or infection with a bacterial pathogen (*Citrobacter rodentium*). Furthermore, Kim et al. demonstrated that either acetate or propionate could enhance the immune response in wildtype mice and that this effect was mediated by GPR43- and GPR41-dependent activation of ERK signalling [62]. Further support for the involvement of GPR43 was demonstrated by Maslowski et al. [63]. In a mouse model of colitis, the authors showed that GPR43-acetate interaction was important in the resolution of symptoms of inflammation [63]. GPR43 knockout mice exhibited a greater inflammatory response than wildtype mice following administration of DSS in the drinking water. These effects were ameliorated by the addition of 200 mM acetate in the water supply. The authors were also able to show that acetate reduced inflammation in other mouse models of systemic inflammation, in particular arthritis and allergic airway inflammation, indicating that SCFA may possibly have similar effects in the peripheral organs.

Again, the relevance of oral administration of SCFA is open to question, given the relatively short half-life of the acids in the circulation. While these studies have attempted to draw a link between SCFA generated by the colonic microbiota and effects on the immune system, the relevance of oral SCFA administration to dietary effects is questionable. Production of SCFA through large bowel fermentation is a sustained process and the absorbed acids are transported via the portal vein to the liver. Animal studies have shown that the three major acids (acetate, propionate and butyrate) are present in the portal circulation in rough proportion to their concentrations in large bowel digesta. However, the concentration of butyrate is disproportionately low, presumably reflecting preferential utilisation by cells of the mucosa. Further, while significant concentrations of SCFA (up to the millimolar range) are present in the hepatic portal vein, only micromolar concentrations have been reported in the peripheral circulation due to visceral uptake [12, 66]. The situation is quite different for SCFA administered orally. Pomare and colleagues showed a very rapid, transient rise in mixed venous concentrations when volunteers consumed drinks containing acetate [67].

Studies in pigs administered propionate orally have shown a similar very rapid and relatively brief rise in circulating concentrations (including the hepatic portal vein), consistent with absorption in the upper intestine. In vitro studies indicate that GPR43 and GPR41 are both activated by millimolar concentrations of SCFA [25, 26], i.e., circulating levels of SCFA are likely not sufficiently high enough to activate these receptors in peripheral tissues. Although high levels of SCFA have been reported at sites of bacterial infection [68], it is more likely that alternate and additional mechanisms are involved with the peripheral effects of SCFA, especially in the maintenance and promotion of health. A recent study by Arpaia et al. has demonstrated that administration of butyrate via the drinking water to microbiota deficient mice treated with antibiotics resulted in undetectable levels of butyrate in faeces [69]. Although an increase in peripheral Treg cells numbers was noted, the number of Treg cells derived from the thymus or colon was unchanged. The authors concluded that these observed effects were due to increased systemic levels of butyrate that occurred due to butyrate absorption in the upper gastrointestinal tract. However, when butyrate was either delivered by enema or when mice were fed butyrylated starch, an increase in colonic Treg cell numbers was observed. To delineate the possible mechanisms of action, in vitro studies also demonstrated that butyrate, and to a lesser extent propionate, increased extrathymic Treg cell numbers and induced differentiation of FOXP3 expressing dendritic cells, whereas acetate had no effect. Cells pretreated with pertussis toxin, a GPR inhibitor, showed no change in FOXP3 expression but when cells were exposed to known HDAC inhibitors (trichostatin A, valproate and phenylbutyrate), FOXP3 expression was induced, leading the authors to conclude that the observed peripheral effects were most likely mediated by HDAC inhibition rather than GPR activation. This conclusion was further consolidated by a microarray study that showed similar changes in the gene expression profile of butyrate and trichostatin A treated dendritic cells.

The study by Arpaia et al. [69] highlights the importance of the mode of SCFA delivery in in vivo studies that attempt to establish a direct link between the fermentation of dietary fibre by the colonic microbiota and potential health benefits and determination of the underlying mechanisms involved. While SCFA have been associated strongly with induction of an inflammatory and immune response in the colon, Furusawa et al. have established a direct link between the fermentative production of SCFA and induction of an inflammatory response [70]. GF mice that were inoculated with chloroform-resistant bacteria consisting primarily of Clostridia and fed a high fibre diet showed higher levels of colonic Treg cell induction than mice fed a low fibre diet. This effect was attributed particularly to butyrate, with propionate showing only a moderate increase while acetate was ineffective. This finding was corroborated by delivery of individual SCFA as acylated high amylose starches. These starches bypass small intestinal digestion and enter the large bowel where the esterified acids are released by large bowel bacterial enzymes [37]. Using acetylated, propionylated and butyrylated starch to increase the luminal concentrations of the respective acid in SPF mice [37, 70] it was shown butyrate was specifically responsible for increased Treg numbers in SPF mice but not GF mice. This gives further support for the essential role of the commensal bacteria in Treg cell induction. Because GPR43 and GPR41 have higher affinity for acetate and propionate and lowest affinity for butyrate, it was hypothesised that additional mechanisms were involved in the induction of the inflammatory response to SCFA.

In another study by Fukuda et al., a combined metabolomic and transcriptomic approach was used to investigate the mechanisms involved with the protective effects of Bifidobacteria in a mouse model of enterohaemorrhagic *Escherichia coli* (O157 H7) infection, a known source of food borne disease that can result in severe diarrhoea [71]. Inoculation of mice with a protective Bifidobacteria strain which was followed by infection with an infectious *E. coli* strain led to dysregulated expression of several inflammation-associated genes in the distal colonic epithelium. These effects were evident prior to any microscopic evidence of inflammation and were linked to induction of apoptosis in the epithelial cells. Metabolomic analysis of faecal material from mice inoculated with different preventive and non-preventive Bifidobacteria strains indicated that efficient metabolism of carbohydrate and production of acetate was likely responsible for the protective effects against the infectious *E. coli*. This effect was further validated by feeding mice infected with *E. Coli* and a non-preventive Bifidobacteria strain a diet supplemented with a modified starch that specifically releases acetate following digestion in the colon [37].

In vitro studies and experiments with animal models fed diets supplemented with dietary fibres, including RS, have identified common mechanisms involved with immune and anti-inflammatory action of SCFA action. These have concentrated primarily on GPR activation and induction of MAPK signalling but more work is required to understand the role of each specific SCFA properly in vivo, especially in the peripheral organs and tissues. These have shown clearly a link between the health benefits of dietary fibre and the specific metabolites produced by its large bowel fermentation in the colon, and acylated starch enhanced the power of mechanistic studies considerably [70, 71]. The use of probes such as these facilitates the segregation of local (i.e., colonic) effects of SCFA and those which occur when SCFA are administered by more general routes such as intravenously or via the diet or drinking water. Coupled with powerful systems biology tools, there may be an opportunity to identify the particular mechanisms which can be directly attributed to dietary fibre consumption.

Regulation of Satiety and Appetite

Consumption of diets high in fibre has been linked to a lower propensity for developing obesity, insulin resistance and CVD [15, 16]. Numerous animal and human studies have shown that dietary fibre reduces plasma lipid levels, reduces fat deposition and improves insulin sensitivity and SCFA are believed to mediate some of these effects [72-80]. SCFA have been reported to suppress cholesterol biosynthesis in the liver leading to lower plasma lipid levels with the effect being particularly strong for propionate [81]. Butyrate (5 mM) has been shown to downregulate genes essential to the intestinal cholesterol biosynthetic pathway in the CACO-2/TC-7 enterocyte cell line but 2 mM propionate was equally effective [82]. However, it is unlikely that this action occurs in vivo. The proposal that propionate mediated the lipid-lowering effects of fibre came from both in vitro studies with cell lines and also from feeding trials in which animals were fed propionate-supplemented diets. As noted, the time course of the entry of oral SCFA is quite different to that of the same acids formed in the large bowel. Further, measurement of hepatic cholesterol synthesis in a physiologically relevant perfusion system showed that inhibition by propionate did not occur at concentrations likely to be encountered in the portal vein in vivo [83].

SCFA have also been shown to regulate the expression of satiety related hormones such as GLP-1 and PYY in the colon [33, 35, 84]. Release of both PYY and GLP-1 following food intake slows gastric emptying and its effects on satiety and food intake behaviour appear to be regulated in the hypothalamic region of the central nervous system [85-91]. Human studies have shown reduced plasma levels of both peptides in obese individuals when compared to lean individuals, and treatment of overweight or obese individuals with either GLP-1 or PYY has been shown to reduce appetite, possibly contributing to weight loss in these individuals [88, 91-97].

Animal studies have been used to investigate the effects of butyrate in adiposity and insulin sensitivity. Vinolo et al. utilised tributyrin (i.e., glyceryl tributyrate) as the source of butyrate for dietary supplementation in a mouse feeding experiment [98]. Tributyrin sustains circulating butyrate levels in plasma following oral administration and overcomes the short half life associated with its rapid metabolism when given orally or intravenously [99, 100]. In their study, mice were fed either a high fat diet alone or a high fat diet supplemented with tributyrin and physiological indicators of obesity (e.g., weight gain, insulin sensitivity) and circulating levels of cytokines and adipokines were measured. Mice fed the high fat diet supplemented with tributyrin demonstrated reduced body weight and fat accumulation (adiposity) than mice fed the high fat diet only, and overall displayed improved insulin sensitivity. Tributyrin fed mice also had lower levels of proinflammatory cytokines in adipose tissue and liver, and reduced macrophage infiltration of adipose tissue was observed. This opens up the important question of whether the effects of the oral administration of butyrate differ from the butyrate produced in the colon solely because of the very short half life of the former. In this regard, a diet supplemented with 28% RS as a high amylose cornstarch was more effective than sodium butyrate supplementation (3.2%) or combined RS/butyrate supplementation at increasing levels of serum GLP-1 and PYY in rats fed an energy controlled diet [75]. In contrast, supplementation with sodium butyrate alone did not increase the levels of either peptide hormone when compared to the control group, and the rats fed a combined RS/butyrate supplemented diet demonstrated lower GLP-1 and PYY serum concentrations than the RS alone. These effects correlated with caecal butyrate concentrations but the authors did not report on the levels of acetate or propionate or investigate the potential role of either of the GPR. All three experimental groups showed reduced body fat when compared to the control group fed the energy controlled diet only.

In the colon, enteroendocrine cells that express and secrete GLP-1 and PYY also express the GPR43 and GPR41 receptors and SCFA have been shown to stimulate release of these hormones, most likely via receptor activation [31, 33, 84, 101], although this is still inconclusive [34, 35, 75, 79, 102]. While these studies show that activation of GPR43 or GPR41 may have a role in appetite control, energy expenditure and adiposity, the exact mechanisms involved have yet to be elucidated. Only one study has attempted to determine the role of GPR-SCFA interaction in mediating these effects [34]. Lin et al. have shown that dietary supplementation with butyrate (5% w/w) or propionate (4.3% w/w) as sodium salts completely blocked diet-induced obesity in lean C57BL/6N mice fed a high fat diet over a 4 week period [34]. Dietary supplementation with the sodium salt of acetate (3.7%) had only a moderate effect (suppressed excessive weight gain by 40%). Improved insulin sensitivity was seen with each of the three SCFA. Furthermore, butyrate- and propionate- fed mice showed a reduction in cumulative food intake (22% and 9%, respectively) whereas mice fed an acetate supplemented diet did not (food intake increased by 23%). Plasma levels of GLP-1 and PYY were increased significantly with butyrate administration but not with administration of propionate or acetate, indicating that different mechanisms are responsible for the effects observed with each SCFA. The authors also showed that GLP-1 and PYY stimulation by butyrate was, in part, mediated by GPR41 activation, but that the reduction in food intake and suppressed weight gain as a result of butyrate or propionate supplementation was not. Again, it is unclear whether these effects are relevant to those of colonic-produced SCFA.

SCFA are also hypothesised to reduce the risk of CVD and symptoms of metabolic syndrome by modulating leptin expression and secretion in visceral adipose tissue and adipocytes in culture. Leptin is an adipokine, or hormone released by adipocytes, that suppresses food intake and increases energy expenditure [103, 104]. Experiments with cultured mouse adipocytes and animal studies have shown contradictory results concerning the activation of GPR41 and GPR43 by SCFA in leptin production and secretion [105-107]. For example, Hong et al. showed that micromolar concentrations of acetate and propionate increased the expression of GPR43 on 3T3-L1 cells and subsequent activation of the receptor resulted in accumulation of lipids and inhibition of lipolysis [105]. These results were supported by Ge et al. who also determined that acetate was able to reduce plasma free fatty acid levels in mice [36]. Intraperitoneal injection of acetate equating to 0.23-1.05 mM in plasma resulted in a significant reduction in circulating free fatty acid levels in wildtype and *ob/ob* obese mice, but not in GPR43 knockout mice, indicating that this effect was, in part, mediated by activation of this receptor. Butyrate was not investigated in either of these studies. Using GPR41 knockout mice, Zaibi et al. determined that butyrate (0.2 mM) and propionate (3 mM) administered in the diet as sodium salts stimulated leptin production in isolated epididymal adipocytes, whereas acetate appeared to have an inhibitory effect [107]. In contrast, acetate was more potent than butyrate at stimulating leptin production in wildtype mice. The authors did not report on the effects of propionate in the wildtype mice. The authors examined the expression of both GPR41 and GPR43 in the wildtype mice and concluded that because only GPR43 could be detected, this effect was in fact mediated by GPR43 and not GPR41 [107]. The expression of GPR43 in the adipose tissue of GPR41 knockout mice confirmed this assumption, and the authors hypothesised that the contrasting response observed between the SCFA was due to differing expression levels of GPR43 between the wildtype and knockout mice (lower expression in the knockout mice) and the greater affinity of GPR43 to acetate.

In contrast, addition of propionate, butyrate and valerate to primary cultures of mouse white adipose tissue expressing the GPR41 receptor stimulated leptin secretion whereas addition of acetate did not [106]. Propionate was the most potent SCFA with EC_{50} of 190 μM (EC_{50} of 200 and 360 μM for butyrate and valerate, respectively). Furthermore, oral administration of propionate equivalent to 25-250 μM in plasma increased plasma leptin levels by 80% in mice fed ad libitum [106]. The authors also noted that propionate administration did not affect food intake of the mice and indicated that the elevation in leptin levels may not have been adequate to affect food intake under the experimental conditions used. These results are in contrast to those of Hong et al. and Zaibi et al., who concluded that leptin secretion is due to stimulation of GPR43 [105, 107].

The contrasting outcomes of these studies seem to indicate that the mode of delivery of SCFA to the colon is important in accurately determining the relative contribution of individual SCFA to observed physiological effects and their underlying mechanisms. While the oral administration of SCFA, e.g., in the drinking water results in absorption in the upper gastrointestinal tract, production in the large bowel following dietary intake of fermentable fibre or acylated starches [37] results in localised release of SCFA specifically in the large colon leading to topical exposure to the mucosa. Although the experiments detailed here utilise SCFA concentrations in the range that is relevant to physiological levels, animal studies with appropriate modes of SCFA delivery will also help to determine their true peripheral effects and potentially support the results of in vitro experiments which imply that direct effects of SCFA on adipocytes via activation of GPR41 and/or GPR43 are possible mechanisms in the prevention of metabolic syndrome [36, 105-107].

Development of Obesity, Inflammation of Adipose Tissue and SCFA in Human Studies

Obesity is associated with a chronic inflammatory state with elevated circulating levels of pro-inflammatory cytokines such as TNF-alpha [108, 109], IL6 [110, 111] and C-reactive protein [111] and chronic low level inflammation of adipose tissue has been associated with the development of type 2 diabetes [112, 113]. Inflammation of adipose tissue is characterised by infiltration of immune cells such as macrophages, neutrophils and T cells which are the primary sources of circulating adipokines and cytokines observed in the obese state [114-118].

Human studies investigating the specific effects of SCFA on obesity, appetite regulation or satiety are scant. Recently, propionate (3 mM) was shown to increase leptin mRNA and protein expression in explanted human omental and subcutaneous adipose tissue [119]. Resistin mRNA expression but not protein expression was also reduced, and no affect was seen on adiponectin mRNA or protein expression. GPR43 and GPR41 expression levels were detected in both tissue types and the abolishment of the effects of propionate on adipokine expression by pertussis toxin indicates the involvement of signalling by these receptors, or other GPRs. In another study by the same authors, propionate (3 mM) reduced the expression of several cytokines and chemokines in omental adipose tissue derived from overweight human subjects, indicating that this SCFA has the potential to exert anti-inflammatory action on adipose tissue in overweight humans by inhibiting the migration of immune cells from the circulation into the adipose tissue [120]. The authors also showed elevated expression of genes involved with glucose and lipid metabolism (GLUT4, lipoprotein lipase and sterol regulatory-element-binding protein 1c), indicating that overweight individuals may have an enhanced ability to metabolise glucose and lipids.

These studies have only investigated the role of propionate on humans and to date, there is no data available regarding the ability of butyrate or acetate to mediate these effects. Furthermore, both studies by Al-Lahham et al. utilised propionate at concentrations in excess of physiological circulating levels in healthy humans [119, 120], indicating that SCFA derived from fermentation of dietary fibre may not be sufficient to elicit these effects on visceral tissue. Although animal studies have shown similar results with comparable levels of

SCFA [36, 107], this is in contradiction to the doses of SCFA utilised in in vitro studies which are in the micromolar range [106]. The evidence to support the role of dietary fibre in improving insulin sensitivity and prevention of diet-related obesity in humans is strong, however, the experimental data to date indicates that alternative mechanisms are likely responsible for the effects seen in visceral adipose tissue.

Future Directions

Evidence in support of dietary fibre consumption in the promotion of gastrointestinal health and its contribution to reduced risk of chronic inflammatory disease is strong and continues to grow. These positive effects have been widely attributed to production of SCFA produced by the large bowel bacterial digestion of fermentable fibre, in particular RS. Epidemiological evidence indicates a protective effect of dietary fibre in CRC prevention which has been attributed to SCFA [1]. While this has been supported by a large number of animal studies and in vitro experiments, the results of randomised human trials where participants with CRC consumed RS as a dietary supplement have shown little to no effect [121-123].

To date, determining the contribution of each SCFA to the observed effects in the colon or on peripheral organs has been hampered by the lack of specificity of delivery of SCFA to the colon. For example, supplementation of diets with fibre sources results in the generation of all three SCFA in varying amounts and observed effects cannot be attributed to any one SCFA alone. Furthermore, oral administration of SCFA, for instance in the drinking water or as the sodium salt, results in absorption in the upper gastrointestinal tract which can confound interpretation of experimental results, especially for those experiments investigating the potential effects of dietary fibre on peripheral organs. Recent studies, such as those by Fukuda et al. [71] and Furusawa et al. [70], have overcome these limitations by utilising tools that deliver specific SCFA preferentially to the large colon [37], limiting absorption in the upper gastrointestinal tract and enabling observed cellular and physiological effects to be directly attributed to an individual SCFA. Additionally, experiments in rodents involving specific delivery of butyrate to the colon using modified RS have been performed to better understand the potential of butyrate to prevent CRC [124, 125]. When coupled to systems biology approaches (e.g., next generation sequencing, gene expression arrays, proteomics, metabolomics, metagenomics), experiments such as these will be invaluable to delineate the specific role(s) of individual SCFA and the mechanisms underlying their health promoting effects.

References

[1] Food, nutrition, physical activity, and the prevention of cancer: a global perspective, 2007, World Cancer Research Fund and American Institute for Cancer Research: Washington, DC.

[2] Howarth, N. C., E. Saltzman, and S. B. Roberts, Dietary fiber and weight regulation. *Nutr. Rev.*, 2001. 59(5): p. 129-39.

[3] King, D. E., A. G. Mainous, 3rd, and C. A. Lambourne, *Trends in dietary fiber intake in the United States, 1999-2008. J. Acad. Nutr. Diet*, 2012. 112(5): p. 642-8.

[4] Tremaroli, V. and F. Backhed, Functional interactions between the gut microbiota and host metabolism. *Nature*, 2012. 489(7415): p. 242-9.

[5] Arumugam, M., et al., Enterotypes of the human gut microbiome. *Nature*, 2011. 473(7346): p. 174-80.

[6] Cotillard, A., et al., Dietary intervention impact on gut microbial gene richness. *Nature*, 2013. 500(7464): p. 585-8.

[7] Walker, A. W., et al., Dominant and diet-responsive groups of bacteria within the human colonic microbiota. *ISME J.*, 2011. 5(2): p. 220-30.

[8] Abell, G. C., et al., Phylotypes related to Ruminococcus bromii are abundant in the large bowel of humans and increase in response to a diet high in resistant starch. *FEMS Microbiol. Ecol.,* 2008. 66(3): p. 505-15.

[9] Martinez, I., et al., Resistant starches types 2 and 4 have differential effects on the composition of the fecal microbiota in human subjects. *PLoS O*ne, 2010. 5(11): p. e15046.

[10] Ze, X., et al., Ruminococcus bromii is a keystone species for the degradation of resistant starch in the human colon. *ISME J.*, 2012. 6(8): p. 1535-43.

[11] Mortensen, P. B. and M. R. Clausen, *Short-chain fatty acids in the human colon: relation to gastrointestinal health and disease. Scand. J. Gastroenterol. Suppl.*, 1996. 216: p. 132-48.

[12] Cummings, J. H., et al., Short chain fatty acids in human large intestine, portal, hepatic and venous blood. *Gut*, 1987. 28(10): p. 1221-7.

[13] Ganapathy, V., et al., Transporters and receptors for short-chain fatty acids as the molecular link between colonic bacteria and the host. *Curr. Opin. Pharmacol.*, 2013.

[14] Topping, D. L. and P. M. Clifton, Short-chain fatty acids and human colonic function: roles of resistant starch and nonstarch polysaccharides. *Physiol. Rev.*, 2001. 81(3): p. 1031-64.

[15] Sleeth, M. L., et al., Free fatty acid receptor 2 and nutrient sensing: a proposed role for fibre, fermentable carbohydrates and short-chain fatty acids in appetite regulation. *Nutr. Res. Rev.*, 2010. 23(1): p. 135-45.

[16] Weickert, M. O. and A. F. Pfeiffer, Metabolic effects of dietary fiber consumption and prevention of diabetes. *J. Nutr.*, 2008. 138(3): p. 439-42.

[17] Fung, K. Y., et al., A review of the potential mechanisms for the lowering of colorectal oncogenesis by butyrate. *Br. J. Nutr.*, 2012. 108(5): p. 820-31.

[18] Hamer, H. M., et al., Review article: the role of butyrate on colonic function. *Aliment Pharmacol. Ther.*, 2008. 27(2): p. 104-19.

[19] Havenaar, R., Intestinal health functions of colonic microbial metabolites: a review. *Benef. Microbes*, 2011. 2(2): p. 103-14.

[20] Donohoe, D. R., et al., The microbiome and butyrate regulate energy metabolism and autophagy in the mammalian colon. *Cell Metab.*, 2011. 13(5): p. 517-26.

[21] Pajak, B., B. Gajkowska, and A. Orzechowski, Sodium butyrate sensitizes human colon adenocarcinoma COLO 205 cells to both intrinsic and TNF-alpha-dependent extrinsic apoptosis. *Apoptosis*, 2009. 14(2): p. 203-17.

[22] Shao, Y., et al., Apoptotic and autophagic cell death induced by histone deacetylase inhibitors. *Proc. Natl. Acad. Sci. U. S. A.*, 2004. 101(52): p. 18030-5.

[23] Tang, Y., et al., The role of short-chain fatty acids in orchestrating two types of programmed cell death in colon cancer. *Autophagy*, 2011. 7(2): p. 235-7.

[24] Wang, L., H. S. Luo, and H. Xia, Sodium butyrate induces human colon carcinoma HT-29 cell apoptosis through a mitochondrial pathway. *J. Int. Med. Res.*, 2009. 37(3): p. 803-11.

[25] Brown, A. J., et al., The Orphan G protein-coupled receptors GPR41 and GPR43 are activated by propionate and other short chain carboxylic acids. *J. Biol. Chem.*, 2003. 278(13): p. 11312-9.

[26] Le Poul, E., et al., Functional characterization of human receptors for short chain fatty acids and their role in polymorphonuclear cell activation. *J. Biol. Chem.*, 2003. 278(28): p. 25481-9.

[27] Nilsson, N. E., et al., Identification of a free fatty acid receptor, FFA2R, expressed on leukocytes and activated by short-chain fatty acids. *Biochem. Biophys. Res. Commun.*, 2003. 303(4): p. 1047-52.

[28] Tang, Y., et al., G-protein-coupled receptor for short-chain fatty acids suppresses colon cancer. *Int. J. Cancer*, 2011. 128(4): p. 847-56.

[29] Thangaraju, M., et al., GPR109A is a G-protein-coupled receptor for the bacterial fermentation product butyrate and functions as a tumor suppressor in colon. *Cancer Res.*, 2009. 69(7): p. 2826-32.

[30] Cherbut, C., et al., Effects of short-chain fatty acids on gastrointestinal motility. *Scand. J. Gastroenterol. Suppl.*, 1997. 222: p. 58-61.

[31] Cherbut, C., et al., Short-chain fatty acids modify colonic motility through nerves and polypeptide YY release in the rat. *Am. J. Physiol.*, 1998. 275(6 Pt 1): p. G1415-22.

[32] Cuche, G., J. C. Cuber, and C. H. Malbert, Ileal short-chain fatty acids inhibit gastric motility by a humoral pathway. *Am. J. Physiol. Gastrointest. Liver Physiol.*, 2000. 279(5): p. G925-30.

[33] Karaki, S., et al., Short-chain fatty acid receptor, GPR43, is expressed by enteroendocrine cells and mucosal mast cells in rat intestine. *Cell Tissue Res.*, 2006. 324(3): p. 353-60.

[34] Lin, H. V., et al., Butyrate and propionate protect against diet-induced obesity and regulate gut hormones via free fatty acid receptor 3-independent mechanisms. *PLoS One,* 2012. 7(4): p. e35240.

[35] Samuel, B.S., et al., Effects of the gut microbiota on host adiposity are modulated by the short-chain fatty-acid binding G protein-coupled receptor, Gpr41. *Proc. Natl. Acad. Sci. U. S. A.*, 2008. 105(43): p. 16767-72.

[36] Ge, H., et al., Activation of G protein-coupled receptor 43 in adipocytes leads to inhibition of lipolysis and suppression of plasma free fatty acids. *Endocrinology*, 2008. 149(9): p. 4519-26.

[37] Annison, G., R. J. Illman, and D. L. Topping, Acetylated, propionylated or butyrylated starches raise large bowel short-chain fatty acids preferentially when fed to rats. *J. Nutr.*, 2003. 133(11): p. 3523-8.

[38] Atarashi, K., et al., Treg induction by a rationally selected mixture of Clostridia strains from the human microbiota. *Nature*, 2013. 500(7461): p. 232-6.

[39] Atarashi, K., et al., Induction of colonic regulatory T cells by indigenous Clostridium species. *Science*, 2011. 331(6015): p. 337-41.

[40] Round, J.L. and S.K. Mazmanian, Inducible Foxp3+ regulatory T-cell development by a commensal bacterium of the intestinal microbiota. *Proc. Natl. Acad. Sci. U. S. A.*, 2010. 107(27): p. 12204-9.

[41] Tanoue, T. and K. Honda, Induction of Treg cells in the mouse colonic mucosa: a central mechanism to maintain host-microbiota homeostasis. *Semin. Immunol.*, 2012. 24(1): p. 50-7.

[42] Cavaglieri, C. R., et al., Differential effects of short-chain fatty acids on proliferation and production of pro- and anti-inflammatory cytokines by cultured lymphocytes. *Life Sci.*, 2003. 73(13): p. 1683-90.

[43] Butzner, J. D., et al., Butyrate enema therapy stimulates mucosal repair in experimental colitis in the rat. *Gut*, 1996. 38(4): p. 568-73.

[44] Tarrerias, A. L., et al., Short-chain fatty acid enemas fail to decrease colonic hypersensitivity and inflammation in TNBS-induced colonic inflammation in rats. *Pain*, 2002. 100(1-2): p. 91-7.

[45] Hamer, H. M., et al., Butyrate modulates oxidative stress in the colonic mucosa of healthy humans. *Clin. Nutr.*, 2009. 28(1): p. 88-93.

[46] Hamer, H. M., et al., Effect of butyrate enemas on inflammation and antioxidant status in the colonic mucosa of patients with ulcerative colitis in remission. *Clin. Nutr.*, 2010. 29(6): p. 738-44.

[47] Kovarik, J. J., et al., Impaired anti-inflammatory efficacy of n-butyrate in patients with IBD. *Eur. J. Clin. Invest.*, 2011. 41(3): p. 291-8.

[48] Scheppach, W., Treatment of distal ulcerative colitis with short-chain fatty acid enemas. A placebo-controlled trial. German-Austrian SCFA Study Group. *Dig. Dis. Sci.*, 1996. 41(11): p. 2254-9.

[49] Haenen, D., et al., A diet high in resistant starch modulates microbiota composition, SCFA concentrations, and gene expression in pig intestine. *J. Nutr.*, 2013. 143(3): p. 274-83.

[50] Keenan, M. J., et al., High-amylose resistant starch increases hormones and improves structure and function of the gastrointestinal tract: a microarray study. *J. Nutrigenet. Nutrigenomics*, 2012. 5(1): p. 26-44.

[51] Vanhoutvin, S. A., et al., Butyrate-induced transcriptional changes in human colonic mucosa. *PLoS One*, 2009. 4(8): p. e6759.

[52] Conlon, M. A. and A. R. Bird, Interactive and individual effects of dietary non-digestible carbohydrates and oils on DNA damage, SCFA and bacteria in the large bowel of rats. *Br. J. Nutr.*, 2009. 101(8): p. 1171-7.

[53] Haenen, D., et al., Resistant starch induces catabolic but suppresses immune and cell division pathways and changes the microbiome in the proximal colon of male pigs. *J. Nutr.*, 2013. 143(12): p. 1889-98.

[54] Fung, K. Y., et al., Colorectal carcinogenesis: a cellular response to sustained risk environment. *Int. J. Mol. Sci.*, 2013. 14(7): p. 13525-41.

[55] Daly, K. and S. P. Shirazi-Beechey, Microarray analysis of butyrate regulated genes in colonic epithelial cells. *DNA Cell Biol.*, 2006. 25(1): p. 49-62.

[56] Fung, K. Y., et al., Butyrate-induced apoptosis in HCT116 colorectal cancer cells includes induction of a cell stress response. *J. Proteome Res.*, 2011. 10(4): p. 1860-9.

[57] Fung, K. Y., et al., Proteomic analysis of butyrate effects and loss of butyrate sensitivity in HT29 colorectal cancer cells. *J. Proteome Res.*, 2009. 8(3): p. 1220-7.

[58] Iacomino, G., et al., Transcriptional response of a human colon adenocarcinoma cell line to sodium butyrate. *Biochem. Biophys. Res. Commun.*, 2001. 285(5): p. 1280-9.
[59] Tan, S., et al., Proteome analysis of butyrate-treated human colon cancer cells (HT-29). *Int. J. Cancer*, 2002. 98(4): p. 523-31.
[60] Usami, M., et al., Butyrate and trichostatin A attenuate nuclear factor kappaB activation and tumor necrosis factor alpha secretion and increase prostaglandin E2 secretion in human peripheral blood mononuclear cells. *Nutr. Res.*, 2008. 28(5): p. 321-8.
[61] Vinolo, M. A., et al., Suppressive effect of short-chain fatty acids on production of proinflammatory mediators by neutrophils. *J. Nutr. Biochem.*, 2011. 22(9): p. 849-55.
[62] Kim, M. H., et al., Short-chain fatty acids activate GPR41 and GPR43 on intestinal epithelial cells to promote inflammatory responses in mice. *Gastroenterology*, 2013. 145(2): p. 396-406 e1-10.
[63] Maslowski, K. M., et al., Regulation of inflammatory responses by gut microbiota and chemoattractant receptor GPR43. *Nature*, 2009. 461(7268): p. 1282-6.
[64] Sina, C., et al., G protein-coupled receptor 43 is essential for neutrophil recruitment during intestinal inflammation. *J. Immunol.*, 2009. 183(11): p. 7514-22.
[65] Smith, P. M., et al., The microbial metabolites, short-chain fatty acids, regulate colonic Treg cell homeostasis. *Science*, 2013. 341(6145): p. 569-73.
[66] Wolever, T. M., et al., Time of day and glucose tolerance status affect serum short-chain fatty acid concentrations in humans. *Metabolism*, 1997. 46(7): p. 805-11.
[67] Pomare, E. W., W. J. Branch, and J. H. Cummings, Carbohydrate fermentation in the human colon and its relation to acetate concentrations in venous blood. *J. Clin. Invest.*, 1985. 75(5): p. 1448-54.
[68] Vinolo, M. A., et al., Short-chain fatty acids stimulate the migration of neutrophils to inflammatory sites. *Clin. Sci.* (Lond), 2009. 117(9): p. 331-8.
[69] Arpaia, N., et al., Metabolites produced by commensal bacteria promote peripheral regulatory T-cell generation. *Nature*, 2013.
[70] Furusawa, Y., et al., Commensal microbe-derived butyrate induces the differentiation of colonic regulatory T cells. *Nature*, 2013.
[71] Fukuda, S., et al., Bifidobacteria can protect from enteropathogenic infection through production of acetate. *Nature*, 2011. 469(7331): p. 543-7.
[72] Higgins, J. A., M. A. Brown, and L. H. Storlien, Consumption of resistant starch decreases postprandial lipogenesis in white adipose tissue of the rat. *Nutr. J.*, 2006. 5: p. 25.
[73] Robertson, M. D., et al., Insulin-sensitizing effects of dietary resistant starch and effects on skeletal muscle and adipose tissue metabolism. *Am. J. Clin. Nutr.*, 2005. 82(3): p. 559-67.
[74] So, P. W., et al., Impact of resistant starch on body fat patterning and central appetite regulation. *PLoS One*, 2007. 2(12): p. e1309.
[75] Vidrine, K., et al., Resistant starch from high amylose maize (HAM-RS2) and dietary butyrate reduce abdominal fat by a different apparent mechanism. *Obesity* (Silver Spring), 2013.
[76] Zheng, J., et al., Resistant starch, fermented resistant starch, and short-chain fatty acids reduce intestinal fat deposition in Caenorhabditis elegans. *J. Agric. Food Chem.*, 2010. 58(8): p. 4744-8.

[77] Zhou, J., et al., Failure to ferment dietary resistant starch in specific mouse models of obesity results in no body fat loss. *J. Agric. Food Chem.*, 2009. 57(19): p. 8844-51.

[78] Weickert, M. O., et al., Changes in dominant groups of the gut microbiota do not explain cereal-fiber induced improvement of whole-body insulin sensitivity. *Nutr. Metab.* (Lond), 2011. 8: p. 90.

[79] Bjursell, M., et al., Improved glucose control and reduced body fat mass in free fatty acid receptor 2-deficient mice fed a high-fat diet. *Am. J. Physiol. Endocrinol. Metab.*, 2011. 300(1): p. E211-20.

[80] Gao, Z., et al., Butyrate improves insulin sensitivity and increases energy expenditure in mice. *Diabetes*, 2009. 58(7): p. 1509-17.

[81] Hara, H., et al., Short-chain fatty acids suppress cholesterol synthesis in rat liver and intestine. *J. Nutr.*, 1999. 129(5): p. 942-8.

[82] Alvaro, A., et al., Gene expression analysis of a human enterocyte cell line reveals downregulation of cholesterol biosynthesis in response to short-chain fatty acids. *IUBMB Life*, 2008. 60(11): p. 757-64.

[83] Illman, R. J., et al., Hypocholesterolaemic effects of dietary propionate: studies in whole animals and perfused rat liver. *Ann. Nutr. Metab.*, 1988. 32(2): p. 95-107.

[84] Tazoe, H., et al., Expression of short-chain fatty acid receptor GPR41 in the human colon. *Biomed. Res.*, 2009. 30(3): p. 149-56.

[85] Batterham, R. L., et al., Gut hormone PYY(3-36) physiologically inhibits food intake. *Nature*, 2002. 418(6898): p. 650-4.

[86] Gutzwiller, J. P., et al., Glucagon-like peptide-1: a potent regulator of food intake in humans. *Gut*, 1999. 44(1): p. 81-6.

[87] Hussain, S. S. and S. R. Bloom, The regulation of food intake by the gut-brain axis: implications for obesity. *Int. J. Obes.* (Lond), 2013. 37(5): p. 625-33.

[88] Nauck, M. A., et al., Glucagon-like peptide 1 inhibition of gastric emptying outweighs its insulinotropic effects in healthy humans. *Am. J. Physiol.*, 1997. 273(5 Pt 1): p. E981-8.

[89] Suzuki, K., et al., The role of gut hormones and the hypothalamus in appetite regulation. *Endocr. J.*, 2010. 57(5): p. 359-72.

[90] Turton, M. D., et al., A role for glucagon-like peptide-1 in the central regulation of feeding. *Nature*, 1996. 379(6560): p. 69-72.

[91] Wettergren, A., et al., The inhibitory effect of glucagon-like peptide-1 (GLP-1) 7-36 amide on gastric acid secretion in humans depends on an intact vagal innervation. *Gut*, 1997. 40(5): p. 597-601.

[92] Batterham, R. L., et al., Inhibition of food intake in obese subjects by peptide YY3-36. *N. Engl. J. Med.*, 2003. 349(10): p. 941-8.

[93] Blundell, J. E., et al., Overconsumption and obesity: peptides and susceptibility to weight gain. *Regul. Pept.*, 2008. 149(1-3): p. 32-8.

[94] Gutzwiller, J. P., et al., Glucagon-like peptide-1 promotes satiety and reduces food intake in patients with diabetes mellitus type 2. *Am. J. Physiol.*, 1999. 276(5 Pt 2): p. R1541-4.

[95] Naslund, E., et al., Energy intake and appetite are suppressed by glucagon-like peptide-1 (GLP-1) in obese men. *Int. J. Obes. Relat. Metab. Disord.*, 1999. 23(3): p. 304-11.

[96] Naslund, E., et al., Glucagon-like peptide 1 increases the period of postprandial satiety and slows gastric emptying in obese men. *Am. J. Clin. Nutr.*, 1998. 68(3): p. 525-30.

[97] Sloth, B., et al., Effects of PYY1-36 and PYY3-36 on appetite, energy intake, energy expenditure, glucose and fat metabolism in obese and lean subjects. *Am. J. Physiol. Endocrinol. Metab.*, 2007. 292(4): p. E1062-8.

[98] Vinolo, M. A., et al., Tributyrin attenuates obesity-associated inflammation and insulin resistance in high-fat-fed mice. *Am. J. Physiol. Endocrinol. Metab.*, 2012. 303(2): p. E272-82.

[99] Egorin, M. J., et al., Plasma pharmacokinetics of butyrate after intravenous administration of sodium butyrate or oral administration of tributyrin or sodium butyrate to mice and rats. *Cancer Chemother. Pharmacol.*, 1999. 43(6): p. 445-53.

[100] Su, J., N. Zhang, and P. C. Ho, Determination of tributyrin and its metabolite butyrate in Wistar rat plasma samples by gas chromatography/mass spectrometry. *Rapid Commun. Mass Spectrom.*, 2004. 18(19): p. 2217-22.

[101] Tazoe, H., et al., Roles of short-chain fatty acids receptors, GPR41 and GPR43 on colonic functions. *J. Physiol. Pharmacol.*, 2008. 59 Suppl 2: p. 251-62.

[102] Bellahcene, M., et al., Male mice that lack the G-protein-coupled receptor GPR41 have low energy expenditure and increased body fat content. *Br. J. Nutr.*, 2013. 109(10): p. 1755-64.

[103] Dhillon, H., et al., Leptin directly activates SF1 neurons in the VMH, and this action by leptin is required for normal body-weight homeostasis. *Neuron*, 2006. 49(2): p. 191-203.

[104] Raben, A. and A. Astrup, Leptin is influenced both by predisposition to obesity and diet composition. *Int. J. Obes. Relat. Metab. Disord.*, 2000. 24(4): p. 450-9.

[105] Hong, Y. H., et al., Acetate and propionate short chain fatty acids stimulate adipogenesis via GPCR43. *Endocrinology*, 2005. 146(12): p. 5092-9.

[106] Xiong, Y., et al., Short-chain fatty acids stimulate leptin production in adipocytes through the G protein-coupled receptor GPR41. *Proc. Natl. Acad. Sci. U. S. A.*, 2004. 101(4): p. 1045-50.

[107] Zaibi, M. S., et al., Roles of GPR41 and GPR43 in leptin secretory responses of murine adipocytes to short chain fatty acids. *FEBS Lett.*, 2010. 584(11): p. 2381-6.

[108] Hotamisligil, G. S., N. S. Shargill, and B. M. Spiegelman, Adipose expression of tumor necrosis factor-alpha: direct role in obesity-linked insulin resistance. *Science*, 1993. 259(5091): p. 87-91.

[109] Kern, P. A., et al., The expression of tumor necrosis factor in human adipose tissue. Regulation by obesity, weight loss, and relationship to lipoprotein lipase. *J. Clin. Invest.*, 1995. 95(5): p. 2111-9.

[110] Bastard, J. P., et al., Adipose tissue IL-6 content correlates with resistance to insulin activation of glucose uptake both in vivo and in vitro. *J. Clin. Endocrinol. Metab.*, 2002. 87(5): p. 2084-9.

[111] Kopp, H.P., et al., Impact of weight loss on inflammatory proteins and their association with the insulin resistance syndrome in morbidly obese patients. *Arterioscler. Thromb. Vasc. Biol.*, 2003. 23(6): p. 1042-7.

[112] Weisberg, S.P., et al., Obesity is associated with macrophage accumulation in adipose tissue. *J. Clin. Invest.*, 2003. 112(12): p. 1796-808.

[113] Xu, H., et al., Chronic inflammation in fat plays a crucial role in the development of obesity-related insulin resistance. *J. Clin. Invest.*, 2003. 112(12): p. 1821-30.

[114] Cildir, G., S. C. Akincilar, and V. Tergaonkar, Chronic adipose tissue inflammation: all immune cells on the stage. *Trends Mol. Med.*, 2013. 19(8): p. 487-500.
[115] Han, J. M. and M. K. Levings, Immune regulation in obesity-associated adipose inflammation. *J. Immunol.*, 2013. 191(2): p. 527-32.
[116] Nteeba, J., et al., Diet-induced obesity alters immune cell infiltration and expression of inflammatory cytokine genes in mouse ovarian and peri-ovarian adipose depot tissues. *Mol. Reprod. Dev.*, 2013.
[117] Sun, S., et al., Mechanisms of inflammatory responses in obese adipose tissue. *Annu. Rev. Nutr.*, 2012. 32: p. 261-86.
[118] Surmi, B. K. and A. H. Hasty, Macrophage infiltration into adipose tissue: initiation, propagation and remodeling. *Future Lipidol.*, 2008. 3(5): p. 545-556.
[119] Al-Lahham, S. H., et al., Regulation of adipokine production in human adipose tissue by propionic acid. *Eur. J. Clin. Invest.*, 2010. 40(5): p. 401-7.
[120] Al-Lahham, S., et al., Propionic acid affects immune status and metabolism in adipose tissue from overweight subjects. *Eur. J. Clin. Invest.*, 2012. 42(4): p. 357-64.
[121] Dronamraju, S. S., et al., Cell kinetics and gene expression changes in colorectal cancer patients given resistant starch: a randomised controlled trial. *Gut*, 2009. 58(3): p. 413-20.
[122] Mathers, J. C., et al., Long-term effect of resistant starch on cancer risk in carriers of hereditary colorectal cancer: an analysis from the CAPP2 randomised controlled trial. *Lancet Oncol.*, 2012. 13(12): p. 1242-9.
[123] Burn, J., et al., Effect of aspirin or resistant starch on colorectal neoplasia in the Lynch syndrome. *N. Engl. J. Med.*, 2008. 359(24): p. 2567-78.
[124] Clarke, J. M., et al., Effects of high-amylose maize starch and butyrylated high-amylose maize starch on azoxymethane-induced intestinal cancer in rats. *Carcinogenesis*, 2008. 29(11): p. 2190-4.
[125] Conlon, M. A., et al., Resistant starches protect against colonic DNA damage and alter microbiota and gene expression in rats fed a Western diet. *J. Nutr.*, 2012. 142(5): p. 832-40.

In: Butyrate: Food Sources, Functions and Health Benefits ISBN: 978-1-63117-657-9
Editor: Cong-Jun Li © 2014 Nova Science Publishers, Inc.

Chapter 4

BUTYRATE ACTIONS ON CARCINOGENESIS: FOCUS ON EPIGENETIC MECHANISMS

Aline de Conti*
National Center for Toxicological Research,
FDA, Jefferson, Arkansas, US

ABSTRACT

The steady increase in the incidence and mortality of cancer signifies a crucial need for improving clinical management and prevention of this disease. Cancer is a complex disease resulting from genetic and epigenetic events that conduct to neoplastic transformation. The short chain fatty acid, butyrate, has been investigated as a potential agent for the treatment and prevention of cancer. Butyrate can contribute to the control of the main deregulated mechanisms on carcinogenesis. Studies have demonstrated the butyrate ability to impose cell cycle arrest, differentiation, and/or apoptosis in many tumor cell types. In addition, butyrate also modulates epigenetic mechanisms, as histone deacetylase inhibition. However, its short half-life considerably restricts its therapeutic application. In this regard, strategies as nanoparticles, or alternative molecules, as its pro-drug tributyrin, are currently being investigated to improve the butyrate bioavailability and allow its clinical use.

INTRODUCTION

Classically, the development of cancer has been viewed by the accumulation of genetic mutations [1]; however, a wealth of data indicates that cancer cells, in addition to a large number of genetic alterations, exhibit prominent epigenetic abnormalities [2]. The genetic path to cancer is relatively straightforward: mutation of tumor suppressors and/or oncogenes causes either loss or gain of function and abnormal expression. The epigenetic pathway to cancer is not as simple and is determined by chromatin structure, including DNA methylation,

* Email: Aline.deconti@fda.hhs.gov.

histone modifications, nucleosome remodeling, as well as, small non-coding regulatory RNAs [3]. Genetic and epigenetic mechanisms are not separate events in cancer; they intertwine and take advantage of each other during tumorigenesis. Moreover, alterations in epigenetic mechanisms can lead to genetic mutations and genetic mutations in epigenetic regulators leads to an altered epigenome. Importantly, in contrast to genetic defects, epigenetic aberrations can be reversible.

With advances in our understanding of the contribution of epigenetic modifications to the development of cancer the roles of components with epigenetic regulating properties have been recognized. In this context, butyrate has been investigated as a potential agent for the treatment and prevention of cancer. Butyrate can contribute to the control of the main deregulated mechanisms on carcinogenesis and modulates epigenetic mechanisms. In this chapter, it will be discussed how butyrate mediates its effect by altering epigenetic mechanisms and how it could be used as a strategy in the prevention and/or treatment of cancers.

Epigenetic

Epigenetics can be defined as heritable changes in gene expression that are not due to any alteration in the primary DNA sequence [3]. Epigenetic modifications include methylation of DNA, modifications of the proteins that bind to DNA, the nucleosome positioning along DNA and small non-coding RNAs [3].

DNA methylation, the best understood epigenetic modification, is the addition of a methyl group from the universal methyl donor, *S*-Adenosyl-L-methionine (SAM), to carbon 5 in the cytosine pyridine ring, resulting in the formation of 5-methylcytosine (5meC) in DNA. This reaction is catalyzed by DNA methyltransferases (DNMTs). DNA methylation is initiated and established by means of the de novo DNMT3 family (DNMT3A and DNMT3B). During DNA replication, DNA methylation is maintained by a complex, cooperative interplay of the maintenance DNMT1, de novo DNMT3A and DNMT3B, methyl-CpG-binding protein, and histone-modifying proteins [4]. Approximately 70–90% of the CpG dinucleotides in the mammalian genome are methylated; however, the CpG sites are not distributed uniformly across the genome [5] but are concentrated in short regions of DNA that contain a high G+C content and a high frequency of CpG dinucleotides called "CpG islands" and long domains that contain predominantly repetitive elements. In normal cells, CpG sites located in CpG islands are undermethylated, although most of the remaining CpG sites are methylated. Promoters and the first exons of the majority of genes (>60%) in the genome are enriched in unmethylated domains and depleted in methylated domains. Methylated domains are found predominantly in interspersed and tandem repetitive sequences and exons other than the first exons [5].

A second well-studied and more complex epigenetic mechanism that regulates chromatin structure and gene expression involves modifications of histone proteins. Histones (H2A, H2B, H3, and H4) are evolutionary conserved proteins that together with DNA constitute the nucleosomes, structural units of chromatin that are essential in packaging eukaryotic DNA. Histones have a globular C-terminal domain critical to nucleosome formation and a flexible N-terminal tail that protrudes from the nucleosome core and contacts adjacent nucleosomes in a higher-order structure. The N-terminal tails of histones are subject to different types of post-translational modifications, including acetylation, methylation, phosphorylation, ubiquitylation, sumoylation, biotinylation, and ADP ribosylation [6]. These histone modifications function by either influencing chromatin packaging or by recruiting and/or occluding other protein complexes. Chromatin functions are specified by multiple and coordinated histone modifications known by the term "histone code".

Acetylation and methylation of histone lysine residues are the best-studied post-translational histone modifications. Typically, histone acetylation, catalyzed by histone acetyltransferase (HAT) enzymes, is associated with formation of the open chromatin structure and active gene transcription. Additionally, acetylation of core histones has been correlated with other genome functions, including chromatin assembly, DNA repair and recombination. In contrast, histone lysine deacetylation, performed by several different classes of histone deacetylases (HDAC), is associated with gene silencing [7]. Deacetylated lysines are positively charged and interact strongly with the negatively charged DNA. This leads to chromatin condensation at gene promoters and transcriptional gene repression by limiting the access to transcription machinery [7]. In all of these cases, a complex spatio-temporal interplay between HATs and HDACs takes place, which is essential for the correct execution of these events [6]. Histone lysine methylation may be associated with either active or repression states depending on the modified site [8].

MicroRNAs (miRNAs) have received considerable attention in recent years. They are small single stranded RNA (ssRNA) molecules of 21-23 nucleotides in length, and it was long speculated that they are just degraded RNA fragments or non-translated small RNAs. They control gene expression by targeting mRNA in a sequence-specific manner, recognizing and triggering translation repression or RNA degradation. The biogenesis of miRNAs is a complex multi-step process. The mature miRNA strand is incorporated into a RNA-induced silencing complex (RISC), which inhibits the function of its target mRNA through degradation or, most commonly, by translational repression after binding of the RISC to the target mRNA, and in very few cases increase the expression by stabilizing the target mRNA. MiRNAs are estimated to regulate with up to 30% of all human transcripts [9].

EPIGENETIC ALTERATIONS IN CANCER

The epigenetic status is balanced in normal cells; however, a number of factors may disrupt this balance and compromise the stability of the epigenome leading to the development of a wide range of pathologies, including cancer.

A distorted epigenetic landscape is a common feature of neoplastic cells, that is characterized by global genomic hypomethylation, hypermethylation and hypomethylation of critical genes, altered histone modification patterns, and altered nucleosome positioning along DNA [3]. A mechanistic link between the loss of DNA methylation and cancer development is indicated by events that destabilize the genome, including the induction of mutations [10], chromosomal instability [11], reactivation and transposition of retrotransposable elements [12], loss of imprinting [13], and activation of normally silenced oncogenes [14]. DNA hypermethylation is the alternative state of DNA methylation and refers to the relative increase of methylation at normally undermethylated CpG islands. Hypermethylation of CpG islands containing promoters and concomitant inhibition of gene expression is the most frequently and consistently observed epigenetic abnormality in cancer cells and is regarded as a crucial event in cancer progression [15]. Similar to alterations in DNA methylation, changes in histone modifications in cancer cells occur on both the genome-wide and gene-specific scales. During the carcinogenesis, overexpression of HDAC contributes to the hallmarks of cancer by altering differentiation and apoptosis as well as contributing to proliferation, angiogenesis and metastasis [16]. It has been demonstrated that the hypermethylation of promoter CpG islands of many transcriptionally repressed genes is accompanied by deacetylation of lysines in histones H3 or H4 and/or increased methylation of histone H3 lysine 9 and histone H3 lysine 27 [17]. These histone marks are essential for organizing higher order chromatin structure, maintaining genome stability, silencing repetitive DNA elements, regulating cell-cycle progression, recognizing DNA damage sites and initiating/allowing DNA repair, and proper expression of genetic information.

MiRNAs are significant players in tumorigenesis and basically every step of carcinogenesis, including invasion, metastasis, apoptosis and drug resistance. In cancer, pathologically altered miRNA regulation can be due to mutations affecting miRNA coding loci, epigenetic alterations, or chromosomal aberrations. All of these pathologic variations of miRNA biogenesis potentially affect miRNA expression. Depending on their downstream target genes, miRNAs can act as tumor suppressors or oncogenes, and therefore miRNA expression in tumors can be either up-or downregulated [6].

Some epigenetic drugs have been approved by the US Food and Drug Administration for use in clinical oncology. Due to the crucial involvement of HDACs in cancer pathogenesis and progression, special attention has been given to HDAC inhibitors (HDACi) to restore the physiological pattern of gene expression and function in tumors. Vorinostat (suberoylanilide hydroxamic acid, SAHA, Zolinza®, Merck & Co Inc., Whitehouse Station, New Jersey) was the first commercially available HDACi for approved oncology use [18]. It has been approved for use in patients with cutaneous T-cell lymphoma who have progressive, persistent, or recurrent disease, or those following two systemic therapies [18]. The hypothesis of the mechanism for these drugs is that DNA/chromatin interactions are kept in a constrained state in the presence of HDAC/corepressor complexes, but HDACi enable histone acetyltransferase/co-activator (HAT/CoA) complexes to transfer acetyl groups to lysine 'tails' in histones, thereby loosening the interactions with DNA and facilitating transcription factor access and gene activation.

Butyrate and Cancer

Butyrate has been considered a potential molecule for cancer prevention and therapy. The anticarcinogenic potential of butyrate was observed in several *in vitro* and *in vivo* cancer models, including colon [19], prostate [20, 21], breast [22, 23], stomach [24], and liver [25]. Partial remission of acute leukemia was also observed after parenteral butyrate treatment [26, 27]. The mechanisms of action of butyrate are multiple. Studies have demonstrated the butyrate ability to impose cell cycle arrest, differentiation, and/or apoptosis in many tumor cell types. Interestingly, most of these mechanisms involve an epigenetic regulation of gene expression. There is a growing interest in butyrate because its impact on epigenetic mechanisms will lead to more specific and efficacious therapeutic strategies for the prevention and treatment of different diseases, including cancer.

Butyrate was the first compound found to cause an increase in histone acetylation [28, 29]. Butyrate acts as a weak ligand for most HDACs [30, 31], most likely because it contains a short three-carbon spacer attached to a carboxylic acid group, which likely enters into the active site of the enzyme and forms a bidentate ligand with a zinc atom [32]. Two butyrate molecules could possibly occupy the hydrophobic pocket and inhibit the enzyme [33]. Butyrate administration reduces the incidence of colorectal cancer in ICR mice, and this action is involved with the epigenetic mechanism of histone acetylation. NaBu induces the sensitization of HeLa cells towards the action of cisplatin, and it was associated with hyperacetylation of the histone core and abrogation of the cisplatin-imposed cell cycle arrest [34]. Genome-wide analyses demonstrated that butyrate-induced enterocytic differentiation is associated with H3K9 hyperacetylation at some gene promoters, indicating that this epigenetic pattern seems to be an important marker of distinct differentiation pathways [35]. Several studies have shown that butyrate, strongly activated $p21^{cip/waf}$ expression [36, 37], a tumor suppressor gene that influences multiple functional processes such as cell division, cell death, repair, and differentiation. Histone acetylation in the promoter region of this gene after butyrate treatment has been reported [38]. Studies indicate that as much as 10% of genes may be affected by butyrate either directly or indirectly. Interestingly, a similar number or even more genes are down-regulated than up-regulated by this drug. This can be explained by the specific genomic regions that can be deacetylated after butyrate exposure [39]. The promoter regions of butyrate-responsive genes contain butyrate response elements that control genes that are induced or repressed by this compound [40-43]. In this context, a bipartite butyrate-responsive element was identified in the human promoter region of *calretinin* (*CALB2*), a gene negatively regulated by butyrate and expressed in the majority of poorly differentiated colon carcinoma cells [44].

Histones are not the only substrates that can undergo post-translational modification. High-mobility group proteins, including multiple transcription factors, can be acetylated, which has a wide range of effects on their function. HDACi including butyrate reverted the resistance to chemotherapy by inducing p53 acetylation and its consequent migration towards the nucleus, thus restoring its function in neuroblastoma cells [45].

Butyrate treatment induced the differentiation of human embryonic stem cells, which was related with alterations in the miRNA profile [46]. In addition, butyrate inhibited several miRNAs induced in HCT-116 human colon cancer cells. One such miRNA is mir106b, whose target is $p21^{cip/waf}$ [47].

It is worth emphasizing that the intravenous or oral administration of butyrate and its derivatives is not associated with noticeable toxicity [26, 27, 48], however the effective butyrate blood concentrations are difficult to maintain because it is quickly metabolized [49, 50]. Bioavailability studies have demonstrated that the butyrate half-life exhibits a biphasic behavior as a consequence of its pattern of elimination from the body. During the first minutes, butyrate clearance is fast and results in a serum half-life of just 30 seconds. Butyrate then binds to serum proteins, its clearance decreases, and its half-life increases up to 14 minutes [50]. The short half-life of butyrate is, however, an important limitation to its clinical use.

The butyrate half-life may be considerably increased when it is administered as its natural prodrug, namely tributyrin (TB) [51-53]. TB, which is found in a variety of foodstuffs such as milk fat and honey [54, 55], is a triacylglycerol composed of three butyric acid molecules esterified with glycerol. Therefore, the full hydrolysis of 1 mole of TB may generate 3 moles of butyric acid. After oral administration to rodents, the TB half-life was approximately 40 minutes [56]. In addition, the oral administration of TB to rodents produced detectable serum butyrate levels five minutes later, and the levels reached their peak 15 to 60 minutes after administration [53] and could be maintained above 0.1 mM for up to 120 minutes [53, 55]. The oral administration of 2 g/Kg of TB to animals subjected to an experimental hepatocarcinogenesis model increased the BA level in the liver up to five times [57, 58]. The fact that TB may be administered per the oral route represents an advantage because, in addition to more favorable pharmacokinetic properties, it exhibits minimal toxicity [59], is better tolerated than butyrate [53, 56], and is better accepted by patients [52, 56]. Thus, TB is quite promising, and its use as a food additive has been approved in several countries including the United States, Canada, and Brazil [60, 61].

The anticarcinogenic potential of TB was shown in several *in vitro* [62-67] and *in vivo* [57, 58, 68] studies. Among its mechanisms of action in cells, the induction of apoptosis and cell differentiation are notable [69]. In addition, TB also modulates epigenetic mechanisms such as histone acetylation [69]. Moreover, the chemopreventive activity of tributyrin may be related to an increase of histone and p53 acetylation, which could lead to the induction of the p53 apoptotic pathway [70], and also, to angiogenisis inhibition [71].

Recently, nanotechnology has become an interesting technology applied to cancer treatment [72], particularly for the development of drug delivery systems that may improve the bioavailability of molecules such as butyrate. Nanoparticles obtained from cholesterol and butyrate ester i.e., cholesteryl butyrate, inhibited the proliferation of lung carcinoma cell lines [73] and induced apoptosis in melanoma cells in a dose-dependent manner [74]. It was further observed that the treatment of myeloid or lymphocytic leukemia cells with these nanoparticles more powerfully inhibited the cell proliferation and expression of the c-myc oncogene than butyrate [75].

The combination of butyrate with other agents also exhibiting anticarcinogenic potential may increase biological responses and thus be used as a promising anticancer strategy. Because of its HDAC-inhibitory effects, butyrate has been considered for combinatorial anticancer interventions with diverse agents, including dietary and synthetic DNMT inhibitors and retinoids. A combination of retinoids and HDACi was assessed in preclinical and clinical trials [76, 77]. The epigenetic reactivation of the genes involved in the metabolism of retinoids, which are silent in several types of preneoplastic and neoplastic lesions, may possibly explain the synergism between those compounds and their use in strategies for the control of cancer. It has been observed that treatment with VA and butyrate inhibited the growth of MCF-7 breast cancer cells in addition to restoring RAR-β expression [78].

CONCLUSION

Butyrate is considered a potent molecule that exhibits anticarcinogenic effects. The tumor-supressing activity of butyrate has been investigated in many model systems. Among the molecular mechanisms induced by butyrate, the induction of hyperacetylation of histones by inhibiting HDAC is notorious, and can lead to transcriptional regulation of genes that are involved in the control of cell cycle progression, differentiation, apoptosis and cancer development. Moreover, besides no toxic adverse effects observed in clinical trials its use is still limited by butyrate short half life. In this regard, alternative molecules as tributyrin or the combination of butyrate with others chemopreventive/chemotherapic compounds appears to increase butyrate efficacy and deserve to be explored in strategies for cancer control.

REFERENCES

[1] Vogelstein B, Kinzler KW. Cancer genes and the pathways they control. *Nat. Med.* 10:789-99, 2004.

[2] Feinberg PA. The epigenetic of cancer etiology. *Semin. Cancer Biol.* 14:427-432, 2004.

[3] Sharma S, Kelly TK, Jones PA. Epigenetics in cancer. *Carcinogenesis* 31:27-36, 2010.

[4] Jones PA, Liang G. Rethinking how DNA methylation *Nat. Rev. Genet.* 10:805-811, 2009.

[5] Rollins RA, Haghighi F, Edwards JR, Das R, Zhang MQ, Ju J, Bestor TH. Large-scale structure of genomic methylation patterns. *Genome Res.* 6:157-163, 2006.

[6] Lennartsson A, Ekwall K.Histone modification patterns and epigenetic codes. *Biochim. Biophys. Acta.* 1790:863-868, 2009.

[7] Ropero S, Esteller M. The role of histone deacetylase *Mol. Oncol.* 1:19-25, 2007.

[8] Moss TJ, Wallrath LL. Connections between epigenetic gene silencing and human disease. *Mutat. Res.* 618:163-74, 2007.

[9] Wiemer EA. The role of microRNAs in cancer: no small matter. *Eur. J. Cancer* 43:1529-1544, 2007.

[10] Chen RZ, Pettersson U, Beard C, Jackson-Grusby L, Jaenisch R. DNA hypomethylation leads to elevated mutation rates. *Nature* 395:89–93, 1998.

[11] Eden A, Gaudet F, Waghmare A, Jaenisch R. Chromosomal instability and tumors promoted by DNA hypomethylation. *Science* 300:455, 2003.

[12] Howard G, Eiges R, Gaudet F, Jaenisch R, Eden A. Activation and transposition of endogenous retroviral elements in hypomethylation induced tumors in mice. *Oncogene* 27:404–408, 2008.

[13] Feinberg AP. Epigenetics at the epicenter of modern medicine. *JAMA* 299:1345–1350, 2008.

[14] Sharrard RM, Royds JA, Rogers S, Shorthouse AJ. Patterns of methylation of the c-myc gene in human colorectal cancer progression. *Br. J. Cancer* 65:667–672, 1992.

[15] Jones PA, Baylin SB. The epigenomics of cancer. *Cell* 128:683–692, 2007.

[16] Dell'Aversana C, Lepore I, Altucci L. HDAC modulation and cell death in the clinic. *Exp. Cell Res.* 318:1229-1244, 2012.

[17] Kouzarides T. Chromatin modifications and their function. *Cell* 128:693–705, 2007.

[18] Mann BS, Jonhson JR, He K et al. Vorinostat for treatment of cutaneous manifestations of advancer primary cutaneous T-cell lymphoma. *Clin. Cancer Res.* 2007; 13:2318-2322.

[19] Russo GL, Della Pietra V, Mercurio C, Palumbo R, Iacomino G, Russo M, Tosto M, Zappia V. Protective effects of butyric acid in colon *Adv. Exp. Med. Biol.* 472:131-147, 1999.

[20] Kuefer R, Hofer MD, Altug V et al. Sodium butyrate and tributyrin induce in vivo growth inhibition and apoptosis in human prostate cancer. *Br. J. Cancer* 2004; 90: 535-541.

[21] Maier S, Reich E, Martin R et al. Tributyrin induces differentiation, growth arrest and apoptosis in androgen-sensitive and androgen-resistant human prostate cancer cell lines. *Int. J. Cancer* 2000; 88: 245-251.

[22] Coradini D, Biffi A, Costa A, Pellizzaro C, Pirronello E, Di Fronzo G. Effect of sodium butyrate on human breast cancer cell lines. *Cell Prolif.* 1997; 30: 149-159.

[23] Walker GE, Wilson EM, Powell D, Oh Y. Butyrate, a histone deacetylase inhibitor, activates the human IGF binding protein-3 promoter in breast cancer cells: molecular mechanism involves an Sp1/Sp3 multiprotein complex. *Endocrinology* 2001; 142: 3817-3827.

[24] Litvak DA, Hwang KO, Evers BM, Townsend CM Jr. Induction of apoptosis in human gastric cancer by sodium butyrate. *Anticancer Res.* 2000; 20:779-784.

[25] Velázquez OC, Jabbar A, Dematteo RP, Rombeau JL. Butyrate inhibits seeding and growth of colorectal metastases to the liver in mice. *Surgery* 1996; 120:440-447.

[26] Rephaeli A, Nordenberg J, Aviram A et al. Butyrate-induced differentiation in leukemic myeloid cells in vitro and in vivo studies. *Int. J. Oncol.* 1994; 4: 1387-1391.

[27] Miller AA, Kurschel, E, Osieka, R, Schmidt CG. Clinical pharmacology of sodium butyrate in patients with acute leukemia. *Eur. J. Cancer Clin. Oncol.* 1987; 23: 1283.

[28] Riggs MG, Whittaker RG, Neumann JR, Ingram VM. n-Butyrate causes histone modification in HeLa and Friend erythroleukaemia cells. *Nature* 1977; 268: 462-464.

[29] Boffa LC, Vidali G, Mann RS, Allfrey VG. Suppression of histone deacetylation in vivo and in vitro by sodium butyrate. *J. Biol. Chem.* 1978; 253:3364-3366.

[30] Davie JR. Inhibition of histone deacetylase activity by butyrate. *J. Nutr.* 2003; 133: 2485S-2493S.

[31] Sekhavat A, Sun JM, Davie JR. Competitive inhibition of histone deacetylase activity by trichostatin A and butyrate. *Biochem. Cell Biol.* 2007; 85: 751-758.

[32] Herceg Z. Epigenetics and cancer: towards an evaluation of the impact of environmental and dietary factors. *Mutagenesis* 2007; 2: 91–103.

[33] Lu R, Wang X, Sun DF et al. Folic acid and sodium butyrate prevent tumorigenesis in a mouse model of colorectal cancer. *Epigenetics* 2008; 3: 330-335.

[34] Koprinarova M, Markovska P, Iliev I, Anachkova B, Russev G. Sodium butyrate enhances the cytotoxic effect of cisplatin by abrogating the cisplatin imposed cell cycle arrest. *BMC Mol. Biol.* 2010; 11: 49.

[35] Strasak L, Bartova E, Harnicarova A, Galiova G, Krejci J, Kozubek S. H3K9 acetylation and radial chromatin positioning. *J. Cell Physiol.* 2009; 220: 91-101.

[36] Rocchi P, Tonelli R, Camerin C et al. p21 waf1/cip1 is a common target induced by short-chain fatty acid HDAC inhibitors (valproic acid, tributyrin and sodium butyrate) in neuroblastoma cells. *Oncol. Rep.* 2005; 13: 1139-1144.

[37] Ocker M, Schneider-Stock R. Histone deacetylase inhibitors: signalling towards p21cip1/waf1. *Int. J. Biochem. Cell Biol.* 2007; 39: 1367-1374.

[38] Richon VM, Sandhoff TW, Rifkind RA, Marks PA. Histone deacetylase inhibitor selectively induces p21waf1 expression and gene-associated histone acetylation. *Proc. Natl. Acad. Sci. USA* 2000; 97: 10014-10019.

[39] Rada-Iglesias A, Enroth S, Ameur A et al. Butyrate mediates decrease of histone acetylation centered on transcription start sites and down-regulation of associated genes. *Genome Res.* 2007; 17: 708-719.

[40] Yang J, Kawai Y, Hanson RW, Arinze IJ. Sodium butyrate induces transcription from the G alpha (i2) gene promoter through multiple Sp1 sites in the promoter and by activating the MEK-ERK signal transduction pathway. *J. Biol. Chem.* 2001; 276: 25742–25752.

[41] Siavoshian S, Segain JP, Kornprobst M et al. Butyrate and trichostatin A effects on the proliferation/differentiation of human intestinal epithelial cells: induction of cyclin D3 and p21 expression. *Gut* 2000; 46: 507–514.

[42] Tran CP, Familari M, Parker LM, Whitehead RH, Giraud AS. Short-chain fatty acids inhibit intestinal trefoil factor gene expression in colon cancer cells. *Am. J. Physiol.* 1998; 275: G85–G94.

[43] Lu Y, Lotan R. Transcriptional regulation by butyrate of mouse galectin-1 gene in embryonal carcinoma cells. *Biochim. Biophys. Acta* 1999; 1444: 85–91.

[44] Häner K, Henzi T, Pfefferli M, Kunzli E, Salicio V, Schwaller B. A bipartite butyrate-responsive element in the human calretinin (CALB2) promoter acts as a repressor in colon carcinoma cells but not in mesothelioma cells. *J. Cell Biochem.* 2010; 109: 519-531.

[45] Condorelli F, Gnemmi I, Vallario A, Genazzani AA, Canonico PL. Inhibitors of histone deacetylase (HDAC) restore the p53 pathway in neuroblastoma cells. *Br. J. Pharmacol.* 2008; 153: 657-668.

[46] Tzur G, Levy A, Meiri E et al. MicroRNA expression patterns and function in endodermal differentiation of human embryonic stem cells. *PloS One* 2008; 3:e3726.

[47] Hu S, Dong TS, Dalal SR et al. The microbe-derived short chain fatty acid butyrate targets miRNA-dependent p21 gene expression in human colon cancer. *PLoS One* 2011; 6:e16221.

[48] Gore SD, Carducci MA. Modifying histones to tame cancer: clinical development of sodium phenylbutyrate and other histone deacetylase inhibitors. *Expert Opin. Investig. Drugs* 2000; 9: 2923-2934.

[49] Fitch MD, Fleming SE. Metabolism of short-chain fatty acids by rat colonic mucosa in vivo. *Am. J. Physiol.* 1999; 277: G31- G40.

[50] Daniel P, Brazier M, Cerutti I et al. Pharmacokinetic study of butyric acid administered in vivo as sodium and arginine butyrate salts. *Clin. Chim. Acta* 1989; 181: 255-263.

[51] Chen ZX, Breitman TR. Tributyrin: a prodrug of butyric acid for potential clinical application in differentiation therapy. *Cancer Res.* 1994; 54: 3494-3499.

[52] Conley BA, Egorin MJ, Tait N et al. Phase I study of the orally administered butyrate prodrug, tributyrin, in patients with solid tumors. *Clin. Cancer Res.* 1998; 4: 629-634.

[53] Egorin MJ, Yuan ZM, Sentz DL, Plaisance K, Eiseman JL. Plasma pharmacokinetics of butyrate after intravenous administration of sodium butyrate or oral administration of tributyrin or sodium butyrate to mice and rats. *Cancer Chemother. Pharmacol.* 1999; 43: 445-453.

[54] Parodi PW. Cows' milk fat components as potential anticarcinogenic agents. *J. Nutr.* 1997; 127: 1055-1060.

[55] Miyoshi M, Sakaki H, Usami M et al. Oral administration of tributyrin increases concentration of butyrate in the portal vein and prevents lipopolysaccharide-induced liver injury in rats. *Clin. Nutr.* 2011; 30: 252-258.

[56] Su J, He L, Zhang N, Ho PC. Evaluation of tributyrin lipid emulsion with affinity to low-density lipoprotein: pharmacokinetics in adult male Wistar rats and cellular activity on Caco-2 and HepG2 cell lines. *J. Pharmacol. Exp. Ther.* 2006; 316: 62-70.

[57] Kuroiwa-Trzmielina J, de Conti A, Scolastici C et al. Chemoprevention of rat hepatocarcinogenesis with histone deacetylase inhibitors: efficacy of tributyrin, a butyric acid prodrug. *Int. J. Cancer* 2009; 124: 2520-2527.

[58] de Conti A, Kuroiwa-Trzmielina J, Horst MA et al. Chemopreventive effects of the dietary histone deacetylase inhibitor tributyrin alone or in combination with vitamin A during the promotion phase of rat hepatocarcinogenesis. *J. Nutr. Biochem.* 2012; 23:860-866.

[59] Edelman MJ, Bauer K, Khanwani S et al. Clinical and pharmacologic study of tributyrin: an oral butyrate prodrug. *Cancer Chemother. Pharmacol.* 2003; 51: 439-444.

[60] Clarke KO, Feinman R, Harrison LE. Tributyrin, an oral butyrate analogue, induces apoptosis through the activation of caspase-3. *Cancer Lett.* 2001; 171: 57-65.

[61] Li Y, Le Maux S, Xiao H, McClements DJ. Emulsion-based delivery systems for tributyrin, a potential colon cancer preventative agent. *J. Agric. Food Chem.* 2009; 57: 9243-9249.

[62] Watkins SM, Carter LC, Mak J, Tsau J, Yamamoto S, German JB. Butyric acid and tributyrin induce apoptosis in human hepatic tumour cells. *J. Dairy Res.* 1999; 66: 559-567.

[63] Maier S, Reich E, Martin R et al. Tributyrin induces differentiation, growth arrest and apoptosis in androgen-sensitive and androgen-resistant human prostate cancer cell lines. *Int. J. Cancer* 2000; 88: 245-251.

[64] Clarke KO, Feinman R, Harrison LE. Tributyrin, an oral butyrate analogue, induces apoptosis through the activation of caspase-3. *Cancer Lett.* 2001; 171: 57-65.

[65] Kang SN, Lee E, Lee MK, Lim SJ. Preparation and evaluation of tributyrin emulsion as a potent anti-cancer agent against melanoma. *Drug Deliv.* 2011; 18:143-149.

[66] Heerdt BG, Houston MA, Anthony GM, Augenlicht LH. Initiation of growth arrest and apoptosis of MCF-7 mammary carcinoma cells by tributyrin, a triglyceride analogue of the short-chain fatty acid butyrate, is associated with mitochondrial activity. *Cancer Res.* 1999; 59: 1584-1591.

[67] Yan J, Xu YH. Tributyrin inhibits human gastric cancer SGC-7901 cell growth by inducing apoptosis and DNA synthesis arrest. *World J. Gastroenterol.* 2003; 9: 660-664.

[68] Kuefer R, Hofer MD, Altug V et al. Sodium butyrate and tributyrin induce in vivo growth inhibition and apoptosis in human prostate cancer. *Br. J. Cancer* 2004; 90: 535-541.

[69] Heidor R, Ortega JF, de Conti A, Ong TP, Moreno FS. Anticarcinogenic *Curr. Drug Targets.* 13:1720-1729, 2012.

[70] de Conti A, Tryndyak V, Koturbash I, Heidor R, Kuroiwa-Trzmielina J, Ong TP, Beland FA, Moreno FS, Pogribny IP. The chemopreventive activity of the butyric acid prodrug tributyrin in experimental rat hepatocarcinogenesis is associated with p53

acetylation and activation of the p53 apoptotic signaling pathway. *Carcinogenesis.* 34:1900-1906, 2013.

[71] Guariento AH, Furtado KS, de Conti A, Campos A, Purgatto E, Carrilho J, Shinohara EM, Tryndyak V, Han T, Fuscoe JC, Ross SA, Beland FA, Pogribny IP, Moreno FS. Transcriptomic responses provide a new mechanistic basis for the chemopreventive effects of folic acid and tributyrin in rat liver carcinogenesis. *Int. J. Cancer.* 2013.

[72] Ferrari M. Cancer nanotechnology: opportunities and challenges. *Nat. Rev. Cancer* 2005; 5: 161-171.

[73] Pellizzaro C, Coradini D, Morel S, Ugazio E, Gasco MR, Daidone MG. Cholesteryl butyrate in solid lipid nanospheres as an alternative approach for butyric acid delivery. *Anticancer Res.* 1999; 19:3921-3925.

[74] Salomone B, Ponti R, Gasco MR et al. In vitro effects of cholesteryl butyrate solid lipid nanospheres as a butyric acid prodrug on melanoma cells: evaluation of antiproliferative activity and apoptosis induction. *Clin. Exp. Metastasis* 2000; 18: 663-673.

[75] Serpe L, Laurora S, Pizzimenti S et al. Cholesteryl butyrate solid lipid nanoparticles as a butyric acid pro-drug: effects on cell proliferation, cell-cycle distribution and c-myc expression in human leukemic cells. *Anticancer Drugs* 2004; 15: 525-536.

[76] Taimi M, Chen ZX, Breitman TR. Potentiation of retinoic acid-induced differentiation of human acute promyelocytic leukemia NB4 cells by butyric acid, tributyrin, and hexamethylene bisacetamide. *Oncol. Res.* 1998; 10: 75-84.

[77] De los Santos M, Zambrano A, Aranda A. Combined effects of retinoic acid and histone deacetylase inhibitors on human neuroblastoma SH-SY5Y cells. *Mol. Cancer Ther.* 2007; 6:1425–32.

[78] Andrade FO, Nagamine MK, Conti AD, Chaible LM, Fontelles CC, Jordão Junior AA, Vannucchi H, Dagli ML, Bassoli BK, Moreno FS, Ong TP. Efficacy of the dietary histone deacetylase *Braz. J. Med. Biol. Res.* 45:841-850, 2012.

In: Butyrate: Food Sources, Functions and Health Benefits
Editor: Cong-Jun Li
ISBN: 978-1-63117-657-9
© 2014 Nova Science Publishers, Inc.

Chapter 5

POTENTIAL BENEFICIAL EFFECTS OF BUTYRATE AGAINST FOOD ALLERGY

***Margherita Di Costanzo*[1], *Lorella Paparo*[1], *Rosita Aitoro*[1], *Linda Cosenza*[1], *Rita Nocerino*[1], *Tommaso Cozzolino*[1], *Vincenza Pezzella*[1], *Gianfranco Vallone*[2] and *Roberto Berni Canani*[1,3,*]**

[1]Food Allergy Unit, Department of Translational Medical Science, Pediatric Section, University of Naples "Federico II", Naples, Italy
[2]Department of Biomorphological and Functional Sciences, University of Naples "Federico II", Naples, Italy
[3]European Laboratory for the Investigation of Food Induced Diseases, University of Naples "Federico II", Naples, Italy

ABSTRACT

The intestinal immune system has coevolved with gut microbiota for the maintenance of body health. An imbalance in gut microbiota composition, named dysbiosis, has been associated with various gastrointestinal and extraintestinal diseases, including food allergies. Gut microbiota is a crucial factor for food oral tolerance and it regulates an appropriate balance between immune effectors and regulatory pathways. Regulatory T cells (Tregs), that express the transcription factor Foxp3, are also critical for the induction and the maintenance of food oral tolerance and for the regulation of intestinal inflammation. Short chain fatty acids (SCFAs) such as propionate, acetate and butyrate are gut microbiota derived bacterial fermentation products that selectively expand Tregs in the large intestine.

These SCFAs stimulate the expansion and immune suppressive properties of Tregs, such as the production of IL-10.

[*] Corresponding author: Roberto Berni Canani. Food Allergy Unit, Department of Translational Medical Science, Pediatric Section, University of Naples "Federico II". European Laboratory for the Investigation of Food Induced Diseases (ELFID), University of Naples "Federico II", Via S. Pansini, 5 - 80131, Naples, Italy. E-Mail: berni@unina.it.

Among the SCFAs, butyrate has received particular attention for its multiple beneficial effects from the intestinal tracts to the peripheral tissues.

The mechanisms of action of butyrate are multiple and involve also an epigenetic regulation of gene expression through the inhibition of histone deacetylase. In particular, the inhibition of histone deacetylase 9 and 6 increases Foxp3 gene expression, as well as the production and suppressive function of Tregs.

The identification of bacterial metabolites, that affect host immunity, may be an interesting strategy to prevent and/or to treat food allergy and promote human health.

THE CHANGING PATTERN OF FOOD ALLERGY

Food allergy (FA) is a major health issue in Western countries with a substantial effect on quality of life of both patients and their relatives. Some evidence has suggested that the prevalence of the disorder in childhood has increased in recent years, affecting between 5 and 10% of young children in Western countries [1]. During the last decade in the United States pediatric FA diagnosis rates increased by 18%. However, it cannot be determined how much of the increases in estimates are truly attributable to increases in clinical disease and how much are attributable to increased awareness by physicians, other health care providers, and parents. However, the consistent increases across surveys and among children in all age, gender, and race/ethnicity groups provide evidence that the increases are not limited to a certain setting, reporting mechanism, or demographic group [2]. Although any food can provoke a reaction, relatively few foods are responsible for the vast majority of significant food induced allergic reactions in children: cow's milk, hen's eggs, soy, wheat, fish, peanuts, and shellfish [3]. Features common to major food allergens are that they are water soluble glycoproteins ranging from 10 to 70 kDa in size and are relatively stable to heat, acid and proteases [4]. Cow's milk allergy (CMA) is the most common FA in early childhood, with an estimated incidence ranging between 2% and 3% in infants and marginally lower in older children [5]. The majority of children will regain tolerance to cow's milk proteins (CMP) within the first 5 years of life [6]. However during the last decade, we observed a changing pattern in CMA with an increased prevalence, severity of clinical manifestations and risk of persistence until later ages in Western countries [7]. Over the last twenty years rates of potentially life threatening reactions to food (anaphylaxis) have steadily risen in the developed world [8]. For all these reasons, there is a strong need to develop effective strategies to stimulate oral tolerance acquisition and maintenance.

FOOD ORAL TOLERANCE AND FOOD ALLERGY

Food antigens and intestinal microflora constitute the majority of the antigen load in the intestine, and the "default" reaction of the immune system confronted with them leads to systemic unresponsiveness. This phenomenon is known as oral tolerance and is a key feature of intestinal immunity [9]. The systemic unresponsiveness to dietary antigens is induced in mesenteric lymph nodes as a result of inactivation of antigen specific T cells when antigen loaded dendritic cells (DCs) seed antigens from the intestinal mucosa [10]. A subset of DCs mediates the selective induction of Treg cells in response to an antigen encountered in the gastrointestinal mucosa.

CD103+ DCs are migratory and traffic to the mesenteric lymph nodes where gut intraluminal antigens are presented by CD103+ DCs [11]. These DCs also induce the development of Treg cells through mechanisms dependent on factors such as anti-inflammatory cytokine transforming growth factor–β (TGF-β), which is necessary for the development of food oral tolerance [12]. In a broader view, the complex interaction between intestinal contents and immune and non-immune cells result in an environment that favors the tolerance by the induction of IgA antibodies and CD4+ T regulatory cells (producing IL-10 and IFN-γ) [13]. This ensures that a homeostatic balance is maintained between the intestinal immune system and its antigen load, so that it retains the ability to recognize dangerous and harmless antigens as foreign and preserves the integrity of the intestinal mucosa. The inappropriate immune responses to food and intestinal microflora that are responsible for FA are a result of a deregulation of these crucial processes [14]. An allergic reaction mainly corresponds to the activation of Th2 cells against food allergens and occurs in two phases: the first phase corresponds to transport of the allergen through the intestinal barrier, its capture by antigen presenting cells (DCs or enterocyte), and its presentation to naive Th0 cells, which differentiate in the presence of IL-4 into Th2 cells. Activated Th2 cells then produce an IL-4 cytokine that enables the production of allergen-specific IgE by B cells [15]. These secreted IgEs then bind to mast cells via the IgE receptor FcεRI. The activation phase corresponds to the degranulation of mast cells after further exposure to the same allergen that links directly with specific IgE on the surface of these cells. This phenomenon triggers a release of the allergic mediators involved in clinical manifestations of allergy. In addition to acute allergic reactions triggered by IgE-mediated immune responses to food proteins, there are cell-mediated manifestations. Non-IgE mediated reactions or cell mediated responses include those reactions in which specific cells, different from mastocytes (and basophils), are responsible for the allergic reaction, and they mostly involve the gastrointestinal tract; mixed IgE mediated and cell mediated responses are those reactions in which both IgEs and immune cells are involved. The symptoms of food allergies may vary according to age: in early childhood, gut and skin involvement is common, whereas respiratory and the oral allergy syndrome are more frequent in older children and adults [16].

RECENT EVIDENCES IN THE PATHOGENESIS OF FOOD ALLERGY

Microbial gut colonization begins after birth and this process is affected by the newborn infant's gestational age, mode of delivery and first feeding strategies. The colonizing bacteria originate mainly from the mother's gut and vaginal tract [17]. After delivery, breast feeding continues to enhance the original inoculum by the introduction of specific lactic acid bacteria, Bifidobacteria and other bacteria from the mother's skin. These bacteria set the basis for intestinal microflora development and modulation. An imbalance in the compositional configuration of the gut microbiota, dysbiosis, alters the host-microbiota homeostasis, which is a requisite for the development and function of immune cells in the gut associated lymphoid tissue. The importance of this reciprocal regulation of the microbiota and immune system culminates in early infancy, when the balance between homeostasis and inflammation programs later disease risk. In particular, early exposure to commensal bacteria plays a crucial role in Th1/Th2 polarization and proper immune regulatory mechanisms.

Germ free animals do not develop oral tolerance and maintained a T helper 2 type immune response to orally administered ovalbumin. This could be corrected by the reconstitution of the microbiota at the neonatal stages, but not any reconstitution implemented at a later ages [18]. These findings documented a decisive role of the gut microbiota for the acquisition of food oral tolerance in early life.

Exposure to a normal intestinal microflora in early life allows for a change in the lymphocyte T-helper 1/lymphocyte T-helper 2 balance, favoring a T-helper 1 cell response [19]; while an imbalance in the compositional configuration of the gut microbiota, dysbiosis, alters the host-microbiota homeostasis, producing a shift of the T-helper 1/T-helper 2 cytokine balance toward a T-helper 2 response and a consequent activation of T-helper 2 cytokines with an increased production of immunoglobulin E [20]. Imbalance in intestinal microbiota composition have been documented in patients with food allergy. Recently, Nakayama J et al. [21] profiled the fecal bacteria compositions in allergic and non-allergic infants by using the 16S rRNA gene short-tag pyrosequencing approach and correlated some anomalies in the microbiota with allergy development in later years. The comparative analysis of genus-level composition data identified population differences in some genera between the allergic and non-allergic groups. Interestingly, allergic infants who showed high colonization of Bacteroides and/or Klebsiella showed less colonization of Clostridium perfringens/butyricum, suggesting antagonism between these bacterial groups in the gastro-intestinal tract. This finding is different from that of previous studies in which Clostridium was more abundant in allergic infants [22-24]. This discrepancy may be attributable to species differences, because Clostridium contains a highly diverse group of bacteria.

Recently, a new link between dysbiosis and food allergy development has been provided. Maternal use of antibiotics before and during pregnancy was associated with an increased risk of cow's milk allergy in the offspring and the risk of cow's milk allergy increased with increasing number of child's antibiotics used from birth to diagnosis [25]. Antibiotics alters intestinal eubiosis and several intestinal microbiota-associated characteristics, such as short-chain fatty acid (SCFA) pattern. In fact, patients with antibiotic-associated diarrhoea showed an imbalance in gut microbiota and the amounts of faecal SCFAs were reduced [26].

In addition to antibiotic exposure, there are a range of factors in the modern environment that may be associated with changes to both the microbiome and risk of FA, such as mode of delivery, infant feeding practices, farming environment and country of origin. The role of the prenatal maternal environment in early immune programming is also important. In particular, the effects of maternal microbial exposure on offspring are multifaceted, including direct effects on maternal immune system and the more obvious effects on postnatal colonization of the infant.

The Role of Clostridia Species in the Protection against Food Allergy

CD4+ T regulatory cells (Tregs), which express the Foxp3 transcription factor, play a critical role in the maintenance of immune homeostasis and oral tolerance. Atarashi K. et al.

[27] showed that in mice the spore-forming component of indigenous intestinal microbiota, particularly clusters IV and XIVa of the genus Clostridium, promotes Treg cell accumulation in the colonic mucosa. Colonization of mice by a defined mix of Clostridium strains provided an environment rich in TGF-β and affected Foxp3+ Treg number and function in the colon. In a subsequent study, Atarashi K. et al. [28] isolated 17 strains within Clostridia clusters XIVa, IV and XVIII from a human faecal sample and demonstrated that these strains affect Treg cell differentiation, accumulation and function in the mouse colon (Table 1). Oral inoculation of Clostridium during the early life of conventionally reared mice resulted in resistance to colitis and downregulation of systemic immunoglobulin E responses in adult mice, suggesting a new therapeutic approach to autoimmunity and allergy.

BUTYRATE AS A PROTECTIVE FACTOR AGAINST FOOD ALLERGY

Clostridia species belonging to cluster IV and XIVa are the prominent source of acetate, butyrate, and to a lesser extent propionate in the colon [28]. Smith et al. [29] observed that feeding germ free mice three short-chain fatty acids (propionate, acetate, butyrate), individually or in combination, increased the number of Foxp3 Treg cells in the large intestine to an amount similar to that observed in conventionally reared animals (Figure 1). The majority of the expanded Treg cell population expressed the transcription factor Helios, which suggests that they acquired Foxp3 expression in the thymus. This is of particular interest because bacterial-driven Treg cell generation in the intestine is thought to occur locally and result in Treg cells that do not express Helios. This suggests that there are distinct pathways through which intestinal bacteria can influence intestinal Treg cells.

Table 1. Isolated Treg-cell inducing strains

Closest species/strain	Corresponding strain number
Clostridium asparagiforme	Strain 15
Anaerotruncus colihominis	Strain 13
Clostridiaceae JC13	Strain 8
Clostridium bolteae	Strain 7
Clostridiales 1_7_47FAA	Strain 28
Lachnospiraceae 7 1 58FAA	Strain 3
Clostridium scindens	Strain 26
Clostridium 7 3 54FAA	Strain 16
Ruminococcus sp. ID8	Strain 14
Clostridium indolis	Strain 9
Eubacterium fissicatena	Strain 21
Clostridium ramosum	Strain 18
Lachnospiraceae 3_1_57FAA	Strain 29
Clostridium sp. 14774	Strain 1
Lachnospiraceae 3_1_57FAA	Strain 27
Blautia product	Strain 6
Clostridium hathewayi	Strain 4

Note: The composition of the gut microbiota was analysed by 16S ribosomal RNA (rRNA) gene amplicon sequencing using a 454 sequencer (see reference [16]).

A combination of clostridia species (cluster IV and XIVa) stimulates local differentiation of Treg cells, whereas administration of short-chain fatty acids leads to accumulation of thymus-derived Treg cell populations [30].

The mechanisms of action of butyrate are multiple, but many of these involve an epigenetic regulation of gene expression through the inhibition of histone deacetylase. The inhibition of histone deacetylase 9 and 6 increases Foxp3 gene expression, as well as the production and suppressive function of Tregs [31].

The identification of bacterial metabolites, that affect host immunity, may be an interesting strategy to prevent and/or to treat food allergy and promote human health.

Clinical Findings

Recently, we demonstrated that treatment of CMA infants with an extensively hydrolyzed casein formula (eHCF) supplemented with the probiotic *Lactobacillus rhamnosus* GG (LGG) accelerates oral tolerance acquisition to cow's milk [32, 33]. Subsequently, we tested the hypothesis that eHCF plus LGG induced effect on oral tolerance thanks to an influence of this dietary intervention on the composition of the gut microbiota [34, submitted].

High throughput sequencing technology (16S rRNA-based sequence analysis) was used to compare fecal samples from newly diagnosed CMA infants, collected before and after treatment with eHCF plus LGG, to those obtained from controls. Moreover, production of the SCFA butyrate was assessed in the same stool samples by gas chromatography. Treatment with eHCF plus LGG expanded gut microbiota populations associated with immunoregulatory effects and significantly increased butyrate production at intestinal level ($p<.05$). Statistically significant positive correlations were found between fecal butyrate concentration and the abundance of four clostridial genera: Faecalibacterium, Blautia, Roseburia, and

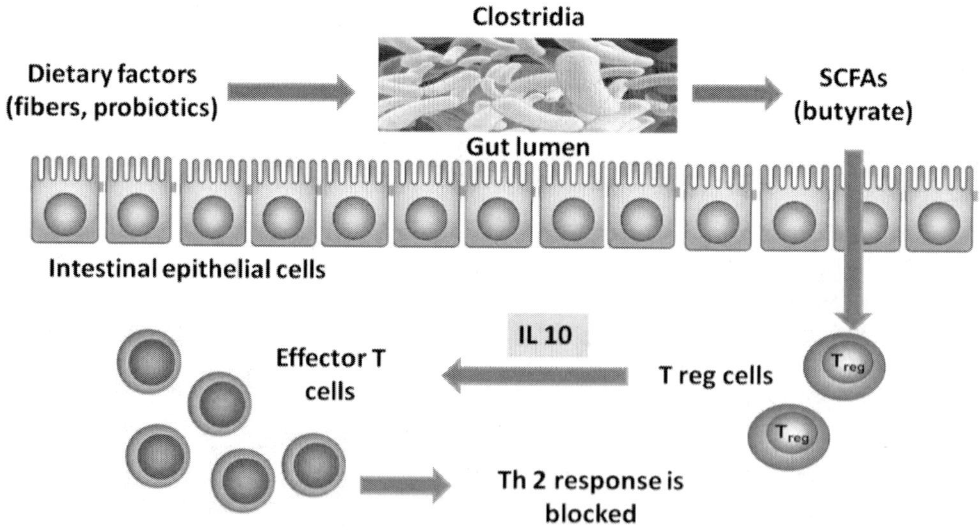

Figure 1. Intestinal microbiota that metabolizes dietary fibers can generate short chain fatty acids (SCFAs), such as butyrate, that enforce regulatory T cells in the gut.

Coprococcus ($p<.05$). All four genera increased in CMA infants after treatment with eHCF plus LGG. The protective effects of butyrate were also explored in a mouse model of CMA (5 week old female C3H/HeOuJ mice). Oral butyrate treatment (20 mg/kg/day) alleviates the allergic response in β-lactoglobulin sensitized mice, as demonstrated by a significant inhibition of acute allergic skin reaction, anaphylactic symptom score, body temperature decrease, intestinal permeability increase, and specific-IgE production ($p<.05$). Our data suggests that eHCF containing LGG promotes oral tolerance, in part, through its influence on the gut microbiome (Figure 2). These findings suggest a potential innovative therapeutic approach for infants affected by CMA, based on the effect of bacterial metabolites on host immunity and human health.

CONCLUSION

Food allergy rates in children have rapidly increased with significant direct medical costs for the health care system and even larger costs for families with a food-allergic child. The possible causes of food allergy become the target of intense scrutiny in recent years [35]. Increasing evidence underline the importance of gut microbiome in the development of allergic diseases. It has been demonstrated that in early life the gut microbiome influence immune development, balance of Treg cells and bacterial metabolites which may increase the risk of food allergy.

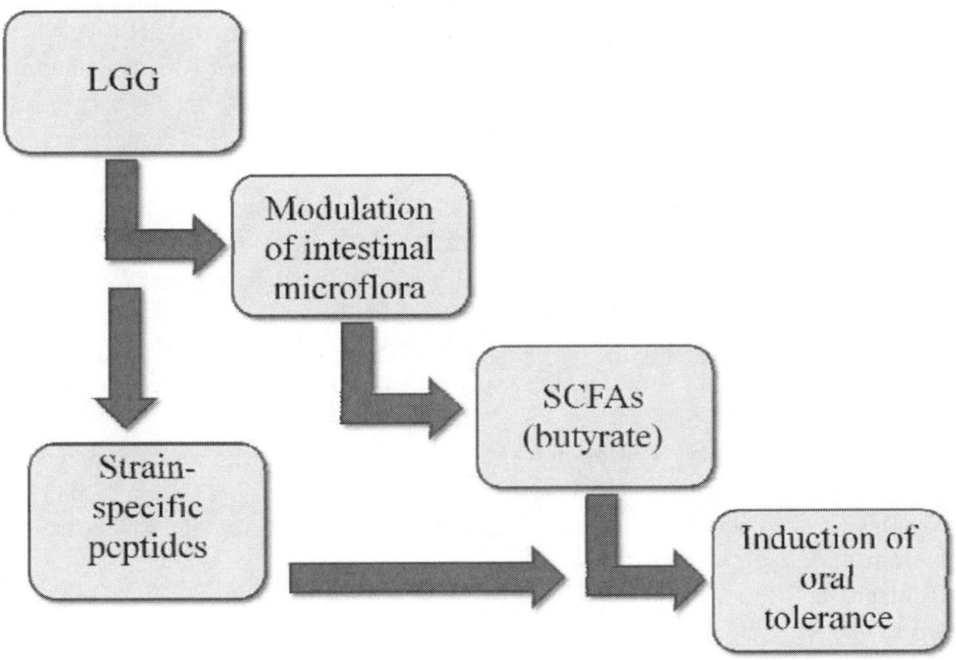

Figure 2. A schematic representation of probiotic mechanisms of actions, which explain the potential benefits of probiotics in allergy prevention and treatment.

There are a range of factors in the modern environment that may be associated with changes to both the gut microbiome and risk of FA, such as mode of delivery, antibiotic exposure, infant feeding practices, farming environment and country of origin.

Knowledge of the relationship between early life gut microbiome and allergic diseases may facilitate development of novel preventive and treatment strategies.

REFERENCES

[1] Kuehn, B. M. Food allergies becoming more common. *JAMA*. 2008;300:2358.

[2] Branum, A. M., Lukacs, S. L. Food allergy among children in the United States. *Pediatrics* 2009;124:1-7.

[3] Allen, K. J., Koplin, J. J. The epidemiology of IgE-mediated food allergy and anaphylaxis Immun. *Allergy Clin. North Am*. 2012;32:35-50.

[4] Ferreira, C. T., Seidman, E. Food allergy: a practical update from the gastroenterological viewpoint. *J. Pediatr*. (Rio J.). 2007;83:7-20.

[5] Apps, J. R., Beattie, R. M. Cow's milk allergy in children. *Cont. Med. Educ*. 2009;339: b2275.

[6] Høst, A., Halken, S., Jacobsen, H. P., Christensen, A. E., Herskind, A. M., Plesner, K. Clinical course of cow's milk protein allergy/intolerance and atopic diseases in childhood. Pediatr. *Allergy Immun*. 2002;13:23-28.

[7] Skripak, J. M., Matsui, E. C., Mudd, K., Wood, R. A. The natural history of IgE-mediated cow's milk allergy. *J. Allergy Clin. Immun*. 2007; 120:1172-1177.

[8] Berni Canani, R., Nocerino, R., Terrin, G., Leone, L., Troncone, R. Hospital admissions for food-induced anaphylaxis in Italian children. *Clin. Exp. Allergy* 2012;42:1813-1814.

[9] Mowat, A. M. Anatomical basis of tolerance and immunity to intestinal antigens. *Nat. Rev. Immun*. 2003;3:331-341.

[10] Chen, W. Dendritic cells and (CD4+) CD25+ T regulatory cells: crosstalk between two professionals in immunity versus tolerance. *Front Biosci*. 2006;11:1360-70.

[11] Schulz, O., Jaensson, E., Persson, E. K., Liu, X., Worbs, T., Agace, W. W., Pabst, O. Intestinal CD103 *J. Exp. Med*. 2009;206:3101-14.

[12] Coombes, J. L., Siddiqui, K. R., Arancibia-Cárcamo, C. V., Hall, J., Sun, C. M., Belkaid, Y., Powrie, F. A functionally specialized population of mucosal CD103 *J. Exp. Med*. 2007;204:1757-64.

[13] Gourbeyre, P., Denery, S., Bodinier, M. Probiotics, prebiotics, and synbiotics: Impact on the gut immune system and allergic reactions. *J. Leukoc. Biol*. 2011; 89:685-695.

[14] Vighi, G., Marcucci, F., Sensi, L., Di Cara, G., Frati, F. Allergy and the gastrointestinal system. *Clin. Exp. Immun*. 2008; 153:3-6.

[15] Romagnani, S. Regulation of the development of type 2 T-helper cells in allergy. *Curr. Opin. Immun*. 1994; 6:838-846.

[16] Berni Canani, R., Nocerino, R., Pezzella, V., Leone, L., Cozzolino, T., Aitoro, R., Paparo, L., Di Costanzo, M., Cosenza, L., Troncone, R. Diagnosing and treating food allergy. *Curr. Pediatr. Rep*. 2013; 1:189-197.

[17] Björkstén, B., Sepp, E., Julge, K., Voor, T., Mikelsaar, M. Allergy development and the intestinal microflora during the first year of life. *J. Allergy Clin. Immunol.* 2001; 108: 516-520.

[18] Sudo, N., Sawamura, S., Tanaka, K., Aiba, Y., Kubo, C., Koga, Y. The requirement of intestinal bacterial flora for the development of an IgE *J. Immunol.* 1997;159(4):1739-45.

[19] Kirjavainen, P. V., Arvola, T., Salminen, S. J., Isolauri, E. Aberrant composition of gut microbiota of allergic infants: a target of bifidobacterial therapy at weaning? *Gut.* 2002; 51(1):51–55.

[20] Winkler, P., Ghadimi, D., Schrezenmeir, J., Kraehenbuhl, J. P. Molecular and cellular basis of microflora-host interactions. *J. Nutr.* 2007;137:756S–772S.

[21] Nakayama, J., Kobayashi, T., Tanaka, S., Korenori, Y., Tateyama, A., Sakamoto, N., Kiyohara, C., Shirakawa, T., Sonomoto, K. Aberrant structures of fecal bacterial community in allergic infants profiled by 16S rRNA gene pyrosequencing. *FEMS Immunol. Med. Microbiol.* 2011;63(3):397-406.

[22] Bjorksten, B., Sepp, E., Julge, K., Voor, T., and Mikelsaar, M. Allergy development and the intestinal microflora during the first year of life. *J. Allergy Clin. Immunol.* 2001;108:516-520.

[23] Kalliomaki, M., Kirjavainen, P., Eerola, E., Kero, P., Salminen, S., and Isolauri, E. Distinct patterns of neonatal gut microflora in infants in whom atopy was and was not developing. *J. Allergy Clin. Immunol.* 2001;107:129-134.

[24] Smehilova, M., Vlkova, E., Nevoral, J., Flajsmanova, K., Killer, J., and Rada, V. Comparison of intestinal microflora in healthy infants and infants with allergic colitis. *Folia Microbiol.* (Praha) 2008;53:255-258.

[25] Metsälä, J., Lundqvist, A., Virta, L. J., Kaila, M., Gissler, M., Virtanen, S. M. Mother's and offspring's use of antibiotics and infant allergy to cow's milk. *Epidemiology.* 2013; 24:303-309.

[26] Gustafsson, A., Lund-Tønnesen, S., Berstad, A., Midtvedt, T., Norin, E. Faecal short-chain fatty acids in patients with antibiotic-associated diarrhoea, before and after faecal enema treatment. *Scand. J. Gastroenterol.* 1998;33:721-727.

[27] Atarashi, K., Tanoue, T., Shima, T., Imaoka, A., Kuwahara, T., Momose, Y., Cheng, G., Yamasaki, S., Saito, T., Ohba, Y., Taniguchi, T., Takeda, K., Hori, S., Ivanov, I. I., Umesaki, Y., Itoh, K., Honda, K. Induction of colonic regulatory T cells by indigenous Clostridium species. *Science.* 2011;331(6015):337-41.

[28] Atarashi, K., Tanoue, T., Oshima, K., Suda, W., Nagano, Y., Nishikawa, H., Fukuda, S., Saito, T., Narushima, S., Hase, K., Kim, S., Fritz, J. V., Wilmes, P., Ueha, S., Matsushima, K., Ohno, H., Olle, B., Sakaguchi, S., Taniguchi, T., Morita, H., Hattori, M., Honda, K. Treg induction by a rationally selected mixture of Clostridia strains from the human microbiota *Nature* 2013;500(7461):232-6.

[29] Smith, P. M., Howitt, M. R., Panikov, N., Michaud, M., Gallini, C. A., Bohlooly-Y. M., Glickman, J. N., Garrett, W. S. The microbial metabolites, short-chain fatty acids, regulate colonic Treg cell homeostasis. *Science.* 2013;341(6145):569-73.

[30] Bollrath, J., Powrie, F. Immunology. Feed your Tregs more fiber. *Science.* 2013;341 (6145):463-4.

[31] Tao, R., de Zoeten, E. F., Ozkaynak, E., Chen, C., Wang, L., Porrett, P. M., Li, B., Turka, L. A., Olson, E. N., Greene, M. I., Wells, A. D., Hancock, W. W. Deacetylase

inhibition promotes the generation and function of regulatory T cells. *Nat. Med.* 2007; 13(11):1299-307.

[32] Berni Canani, R., Nocerino, R., Terrin, G., Coruzzo, A., Cosenza, L., Leone, L., Troncone, R. Effect of Lactobacillus GG on tolerance acquisition in infants with cow's milk allergy: a randomized trial. *J. Allergy Clin. Immunol.* 2012;129:580-2, 582.e1-5.

[33] Berni Canani, R., Nocerino, R., Terrin, G., Frediani, T., Lucarelli, S., Cosenza, L., Passariello, A., Leone, L., Granata, V., Di Costanzo, M., Pezzella, V., Troncone, R. Formula selection for management of children with cow's milk allergy influences the rate of acquisition of tolerance: a prospective multicenter study. *J. Pediatr.* 2013; 163: 771-7.e1.

[34] Berni Canani, R., Stefka, A. T., Patton, T. J., Nocerino, R., Aitoro, R., Paparo, L., Calignano, A., Meli, R., Mattace Raso, G., Simeoli, R., Di Costanzo, M., Guandalini, S., Antonopoulos, D., Nagler, C. R. Lactobacillus rhamnosus GG intervention expands immunoregulatory bacterial populations in the intestines of infants with cow's milk allergy. Abstract book: 47th Annual Meeting of The European Society for Paediatric Gastroenterology, Hepatology and Nutrition 9 - 12 June 2014 Jerusalem, Israel.

[35] Gupta, R., Holdford, D., Bilaver, L., Dyer, A., Holl, J.L., Meltzer, D. The economic impact of childhood food allergy in the United States. *JAMA Pediatr.* 2013; 167: 1026-31.

In: Butyrate: Food Sources, Functions and Health Benefits
Editor: Cong-Jun Li
ISBN: 978-1-63117-657-9
© 2014 Nova Science Publishers, Inc.

Chapter 6

Short Chain Fatty Acids in Regulation of the Immune System and Tissue Inflammation in the Intestine

Myung H. Kim and Chang H. Kim*

Laboratory of Immunology and Hematopoiesis, Department of Comparative Pathobiology, Weldon School of Biomedical Engineering, Center for Cancer Research, Purdue University, West Lafayette, IN, US

Abstract

Intestinal epithelial cells (ECs) and immune cells are regulated by host and microbial factors. Among the microbial metabolites, short chain fatty acids (SCFAs) are the most abundant metabolites, produced in the intestine. SCFAs regulate ECs in G-protein-coupled receptor-dependent and independent manners. SCFAs prepare ECs to efficiently mount immune responses to pathogens to prevent chronic infection and subsequent inflammation in the intestine. At the same time, SCFAs suppress inflammatory responses by regulating a number of immune and non-immune cell types including ECs in the intestine. Moreover, SCFAs regulate the differentiation and activation of immune cells in the intestine for promotion of both immunity and immune tolerance. We discuss the recent progress in our understanding of the functions of SCFAs and their receptors in regulation of intestinal immunity and inflammation.

Keywords: Short chain fatty acids, epithelial cells, GPR41, GPR43, histone deacetylase inhibitors, cytokines, chemokines, inflammation, immunity, dietary fibers, intestine

---

* Corresponding author: C. H. Kim, Laboratory of Immunology and Hematopoiesis, Purdue University. 725 Harrison St., West Lafayette, IN 47906. E-mail: chkim@purdue.edu.

1. Introduction

Short chain fatty acids (SCFAs) are produced mainly from carbohydrates in the colon. SCFAs are mainly produced from resistant starch and dietary fibers including fructans, cellulose, galactomannans, xylans and pectins, which survive the digestion in the stomach and small intestine, and reach the microbes in the colon. Formate (C1), acetate (C2), propionate (C3), and butyrate (C4) are the most abundant SCFAs. Other SCFAs include valerate (C5) and branched SCFAs such as isobutyric acid and isovaleric acid. SCFAs are generated by fermentation of carbohydrates by bacteria through the glycolytic pathway and the pentose phosphate pathway [1, 2]. C2, C3, and C4 are found in the intestine of humans and rodents at low concentrations (~10 mM) in the terminal ileum but at high concentrations (~100 mM) in the caecum and the descending colon [3]. Of course, the concentrations of gut SCFAs can change depending on the composition of diets. These metabolites are a major energy source for enterocytes. SCFAs are important for absorption of water and ions and for maintaining pH in the gut lumen. SCFAs are also important for epithelial homeostasis, gut barrier function, and innate immunity. A mounting body of evidence now suggests that SCFAs control even the cells of adaptive immunity. The gut immune system needs to effectively mount immune responses to pathogens but should maintain immune tolerance to commensal bacteria and food antigens in the absence of infection [4]. Mechanisms for the SCFA functions are likely to be dependent on cell types, but a bulk of these functions are mediated through histone deacetylase (HDAC) inhibition and activation of GPR41 and GPR43 by SCFAs. The balance between immunity and immune tolerance is critical for maintaining a functional immune system free of chronic infection and inflammation. SCFAs apparently regulate both immunity and immune tolerance in the intestine by regulating a number of cell types in the intestine. In this review, we will discuss the functions of SCFAs in regulation of epithelial cells (ECs), the gut immune system, and tissue inflammation.

2. Transporters and Receptors of SCFAs

SCFAs, produced in the colon, are readily absorbed into ECs. Absorption of SCFAs into cells allows SCFAs to be further metabolized and integrated into cellular metabolism. At the same time, SCFAs regulate key signaling molecules to regulate various aspects of cell biology. Most of the absorbed C4 is utilized by colonocytes. C4 accounts for 5-10% of the human basal energy requirement [1, 5]. C2 and C3 are absorbed into ECs and further transported into the liver, skeletal muscle, pancreas, and other organs. SCFAs are absorbed into intestinal ECs through several different passive and active transportation processes [6-8].

SCFAs are transported into colonocytes by simple diffusion as anionic forms and facilitated transport through solute carriers (Figure 1). MCT1 and SMCT1 are the major membrane transporters of SCFAs. Monocarboxylate transporter isoform 1 (MCT1; also called SLC16A1) is involved in the SCFA-HCO_3 exchange [9-11]. Sodium-coupled monocarboxylate transporter 1 (SMCT1, also called SLC5A8) is a Na(+)-coupled transporter for SCFAs, co-transporting NA+ ion and SCFAs from the lumen into colonocytes [12, 13]. Because of their function in transporting SCFAs into cells, SMCT1 is required for the HDAC inhibitor activity of C4 in colonocytes and other cells such as dendritic cells [14, 15].

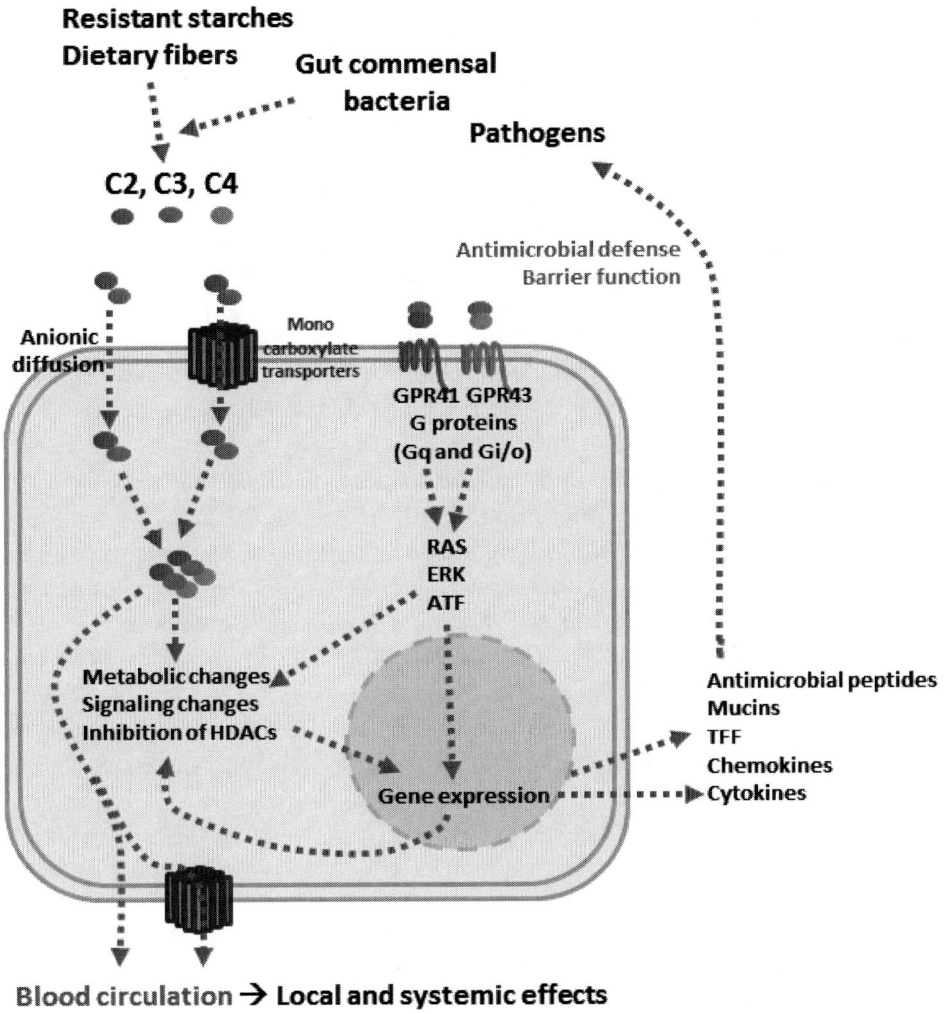

Figure 1. Interaction points of SCFAs and epithelial cells in antimicrobial defense. Resistant starch and dietary fibers reach the colon where commensal bacteria are concentrated. From these dietary materials, SCFAs such as C2, C3, and C4 are produced. SCFAs are absorbed as anionic forms or actively transported via monocarboxyl transporters (MCT1 and SMCT1). The luminal SCFAs activate membrane GPRs such as GPR41 and GPR43 expressed on colonocytes. Intracellular SCFAs are metabolized through the TCA cycle or further transported out of colonocytes into interstitial tissues and the blood circulation. Intracellular SCFAs also regulate HDACs for changes in gene expression and signal transduction. HDAC inhibition mediates the regulatory activities of SCFAs in regulating diverse cellular processes. Activation of GPR41 and GPR43 by SCFAs induces a cascade of signaling events for activation of ERKs/MAPKs and ATF. These events also regulate gene expression and other cellular processes such as induction of antimicrobial peptides, mucins, trefoil factors (TFF), chemokines, and cytokines, which together promote gut immunity and mediate intestinal inflammation.

SMCT1 preferentially transports lactate, pyruvate, propionate, butyrate, and acetate in a decreasing order [14, 16, 17]. Once absorbed into colon, SCFAs are utilized within colonocytes (metabolized through the TCA cycle) or further transported to interstitial tissues in the intestine or the systemic blood circulation.

SCFAs also function without having to enter cells (Figure 1). This is mediated through binding and activating cell surface G-protein-coupled seven transmembrane receptors (GPR). C2, C3 and C4 are major activators of GPR41 and GPR43 [18].

GPR43 (also called free fatty acid receptor 2 or FFA2) is expressed by intestinal ECs [19]. GPR43 is expressed also by neutrophils [20, 21], peptide YY-expressing endocrine cells [19], mast cells [19], and adipose tissue [22]. SCFAs bind GPR43 in the following order of affinity: C3 ≥ C2 ≥ C4 > C5 > C1. GPR41 is best activated by C3 and C4 and to a lesser degree by C2 [18, 20, 21]. GPR41 is broadly expressed in various tissues, including the intestine, pancreas, spleen, and adipose tissues [18, 23]. Enteroendocrine cells in the intestine highly express GPR41 [19, 24]. GPR41 uses the Gi/o family of proteins for signaling, whereas GPR43 signals through Gq and Gi/o families [18, 20, 21]. Gi/o and Gq regulate the adenylate cyclase pathway and the phospholipase C (PLC) pathway, respectively [25, 26]. Another receptor for SCFAs is GPR109A (also called hydroxycarboxylic acid receptor 2 or HCA2), which is a receptor for nicotinic acid and induced by IFN-γ in macrophages [27, 28]. C4 is a physiological agonist for GPR109A [29, 30]. However, C2 and C3 do not appear to activate this receptor [30]. GPR109A is expressed by adipocytes, macrophages, and colonic ECs [30-32]. In addition to GPR41, GPR43, and GPR109A, Olfr78 can serve as a receptor for C2 and C3 [33]. Olfr78 is expressed by vascular smooth muscle cells of various organs including kidney and heart.

Binding of GPR41 or GPR43 by SCFAs triggers activation of mitogen-activated protein kinases (MAPKs) (p38 and ERK), protein kinase C, Rac1/2 GTPases, phosphorylation of ribosomal protein S6, and transcriptional factors such as activating transcriptional factor-2 (ATF-2) [4, 34, 35]. Activation of these pathways promotes key cellular processes such as cell proliferation, regulation of gene expression (e.g., expression of cytokines and chemokines), and cell motility.

3. Regulation of ECs and the Intestinal Barrier Function by SCFAs

C4 fuels colonic EC growth and maintenance. It is believed that abnormally low C4 causes nutritional deficiency and mucosal atrophy in the colon [36]. C4 also regulates EC survival [37].

For transformed colonic ECs, however, C4 induces differentiation, cell cycle arrest, and apoptosis. C4 modulates expression of the cell cycle inhibitor p21Waf1/Cip1 and the proapoptotic protein BAK [38-40]. The mechanisms regulating these functions are currently unclear but likely to be diverse. A key biological feature of SCFAs is their ability to influence gene expression, which is often attributed to their HDAC inhibitor activity [41, 42]. SCFAs promote hyperacetylation of histones, resulting in enhanced accessibility of the transcriptional machinery to certain genes that regulate cell proliferation, survival and differentiation [43]. In addition to histone proteins, non-histone proteins including NFκB [44], MyoD [45], p53 [45] and N-FAT are targets of HDACs and regulated by SCFAs [46]. C4 also can regulate DNA methylation and histone phosphorylation [42]. SCFAs regulate a number of signaling pathways such as AP-1 [47-49], PKC [50], NF-κB [51], c-Fos, and ERK1/2 in ECs [49]. C4 also induces the expression of certain heat shock proteins such as HSP70 and HSP25 in ECs

[52-54]. This activity is relevant to the protective effect of SCFAs on intestinal epithelial cells from oxidative or other types of stresses [54].

Intestinal ECs provide a physical barrier between luminal content and tissues. This is important to keep not only pathogens but also commensal bacteria out of tissues and away from the immune system. Defective gut barrier functions lead to invasion by gut commensal microbes into tissues and induction of inflammatory responses. A temporary increase in gut permeability, however, occurs during normal immune responses to pathogens. However, chronically high gut permeability due to defective gut barrier functions leads to unresolving inflammatory conditions typically seen in inflammatory bowel diseases. A healthy gut barrier requires both physical and chemical barriers. Physical barrier factors include epithelial-cell tight junctions, actin-rich microvilli, a protective mucous layer, and production of antimicrobial peptides. Inter-cellular tight junctions between ECs prevent paracellular entry of the gut luminal content. Epithelial tight junctions are connected to actin-rich microvillus extensions (i.e., brush borders) that impede microbial attachment to epithelial cells [55]. Goblet cells produce mucins to form the mucous layer [56, 57]. Paneth cells secrete a number of antimicrobial peptides such as defensins, calprotectins and cathelicidins. Antimicrobial peptides are rich in hydrophobic and basic amino acid residues and, therefore, can make leaky pores on a wide range of bacterial species [58, 59].

A mounting body of evidence indicates that SCFAs strengthen the gut barrier function (Figure 1). Intestinal ECs are bathed in high concentrations of SCFAs, produced by commensal bacteria. C4 upregulates the expression of anti-microbial factors such as cathelicidin (LL-37) in intestinal ECs [60]. This effect is mediated through activation of AP-1 pathway and HDAC inhibition [48]. C4 can either decrease or increase tight junction protein expression and gut permeability depending on C4 levels. At low concentrations (up to 2 mmol/L), C4 increased tight junction proteins and decreased permeability of cultured Caco-2 and HT-29 cell lines [61-63]. In contrast, C4 increased permeability of cultured Caco-2 cells at high concentrations (8 mmol/L). This was confirmed with rat distal colon tissues mounted on an Ussing chamber [64]. C4 at 10 mmol/L, but not at lower concentrations (1-5 mmol/L), increased para-cellular permeability of rat colon tissues.

The intestinal mucous layer is formed by the products of several mucin genes [65], and SCFAs promote mucin gene expression. C4 increases MUC2 gene expression in ECs [66-69]. This effect appears to be mediated through up-regulation of MUC2-inducing prostaglandins E2 (PGE2) by SCFAs in intestinal fibroblasts [69]. C4 can stimulate mucin production in human colonic biopsy specimens [70]. Luminal C4 administration at 5 mmol/L increased mucus secretion in rat colon tissues [71]. Interestingly, C4 at a higher concentration (100 mmol/L) suppressed MUC2 gene expression through HDAC inhibition, changing the cell phenotype from a secretory to an absorptive EC phenotype [72].

Thus, SCFAs appear to regulate EC function and differentiation depending on concentrations. Trefoil factors (TFFs), secreted by intestinal goblet cells [73], increase the viscoelastic properties of mucous and help maintain the intestinal mucosa [74]. Interestingly, C4 increases trefoil factor 3 (TFF3) expression [75].

Rats, fed with fructo-oligosaccharides (FOS) for enhanced SCFA production in the intestine, had increased gut permeability and translocation of Salmonella [76]. Our group reported that mice fed with C2 did not have any changes in basal gut permeability and tight junction protein expression. However, C2 feeding accelerated the gut permeability increase induced during infection with *C. rodentium*. We determined that it is primarily the immune response not SCFAs that increased gut permeability. In other words, the gut permeability increase is a part of the normal immune response to pathogens and facilitates clearance of pathogens. Interestingly, mice deficient in GPR41 or GPR43 expression were delayed in the increase of gut permeability upon infection with *C. rodentium*. Thus, the SCFA signals mediated by the surface receptors play critical roles in conditioning ECs to change gut permeability and mount prompt immune responses.

4. Regulation of Intestinal EC Cytokines and Chemokines by SCFAs

Intestinal ECs respond to commensal bacteria and pathogens, and produce factors that activate and maintain the gut immune system. An example is production of cytokines and chemokines by ECs in addition to anti-microbial factors. IL-6 is an acute phase proinflammatory cytokine. We found that C2 and C3 enhance IL-6 production by primary ECs upon LPS stimulation in vitro [4]. For this, SCFA receptors (GPR41 and GPR43) and ERK signaling are required. C2 feeding increased IL-6 production at the initial phase of the immune response to *C. rodentium* infection. SCFAs also promote the production other proinflammatory cytokines such as IL-1β and TNF-α during infection. In line with this, SCFA-supplementation increased intestinal production of IL-6, IL-1β, and TNF-α [77]. Thus, SCFAs promote immune responses to pathogens by boosting acute cytokine production.

SCFAs regulate leukocyte trafficking during tissue inflammation (Figure 2). This is mediated by two different mechanisms. Leukocyte recruitment can be mediated through induction of chemokines that attract T cells and neutrophils. This is dependent on GPR43 expression on neutrophils [20, 35, 78, 79]. On the other hand, C4 can suppress the expression of chemokines (e.g., CXCL1, CXCL8, and MCP-1) by ECs in response to cytokines and microbe-associated molecular patterns (MAMPs) such as peptidoglycan [80-83]. C4, but not C2 and C3, blocked the expression of CXCL10 by colonic subepithelial myofibroblasts [84]. CXCL10 is a chemoattractant for T lymphocytes and monocytes.

Another mechanism is direct chemotactic attraction of leukocytes by SCFAs. SCFAs, themseleves, induce chemotaxis of neutrophils in a gradient-dependent manner through their G-protein-coupled chemoattractant receptor GPR43 [78]. This effect will be discussed in more details in the next section.

5. Regulation of Intestinal Immune Cells by SCFAs

The intestinal immune system is mainly composed of ECs, other tissue cells, and immune cells. Among immune cells, SCFAs regulate neutrophils, T cells, and macrophages. This list can grow as more cell types would be identified as targets of SCFAs in the future. SCFAs can control immune cells through cell surface receptors but they can also regulate these cells without involving the cell surface receptors. SCFAs activate neutrophils through GPR43. As a consequence, mitogen-activated protein kinases (MAPKs) (p38 and ERK), protein kinase C, ribosomal protein S6, and activating transcriptional factor-2 (ATF-2) are activated [34, 35].

Transient activation of Rac1/2 GTPase is an integral part of cell migration to chemoattractants such as SCFAs.

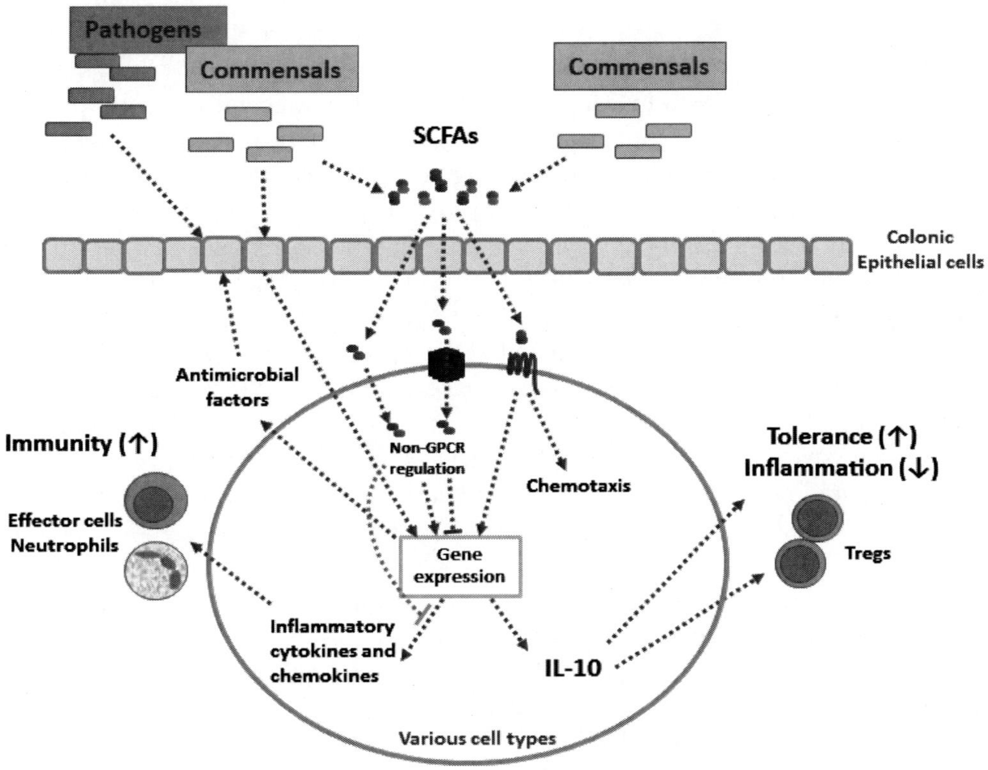

Figure 2. Functions of SCFAs in regulation of the immunity, tolerance, and inflammation in the intestine. SCFAs profoundly regulate the gut immune system in both positive and negative ways. Immune cells and epithelial cells receive signals from SCFA-GPCR signals, non-GPCR intracellular SCFA signals and MAMPs/other signals. These signals are combined to regulate the overall gene expression process for the expression of cytokines, chemokines and other factors. The combined signals are further modified by SCFA-induced HDAC inhibition. As the consequence, IL-10 and effector cytokines are produced in response to SCFAs for homeostatic promotion of immunity and immune tolerance in the intestine. In infection, the combined SCFA and MAMP signals are modified to shift the balance toward inflammatory responses. Therefore, prolonged exposure of the gut immune system to invading microbes due to defects in immunity or barrier functions can lead to uncontrolled production of inflammatory mediators. It is also important to emphasize that the regulation of the gut immune system by SCFAs is often defective in chronic inflammation due to decreased production and absorption of SCFAs.

SCFAs, while they promote immune responses to pathogens, can dampen inflammatory responses perhaps to prevent excessive tissue inflammation. SCFAs (C2, C3, and C4) inhibit TNF-α production by neutrophils in response to LPS [85, 86]. C3 and C4 attenuated NF-κB activation and inhibited the expression of TNF-α, CXCL3, and nitric oxide in neutrophils [85].

Interestingly, SCFAs can negatively regulate leukocyte migration. SCFAs reduced leukocyte adherence to endothelial cells [87, 88]. C4 decreased the neutrophil interaction with endothelial cells, induced by IL-1β and fMLP [89]. A potential mechanism for this effect is attenuation of NFκB and PPARγ activities by SCFAs, leading to decreased expression of

ICAM-1 and VCAM-1 in endothelial cells. In addition, C3 and C4 reduced the expression of L-selectin by neutrophils [79]. Thus, SCFAs can prevent unnecessary recruitment of neutrophils and inflammatory leukocytes to the intestine in the absence of any infection.

SCFAs also affect macrophages. SCFAs suppressed the production of inflammatory cytokines (IL-6, TNF-α, and IL-1β), chemokines, and nitric oxide by macrophages after activetion with LPS or IFN-γ. In contrast, C4 increased production of IL-10, a key anti-inflammatory cytokine [90, 91]. Induction of LFA-3 and ICAM-1 by IFN-γ in monocytes was decreased by C4 [92]. IL-10 production by monocytes is also decreased by SCFAs [93]. SCFAs increased production of the inflammatory mediator PGE2 and PGF1α by monocytes and Kupffer cells [90, 93-95]. PGE2, through activation of the receptor EP4, positively and negatively regulates immune responses [96].

Phagocytes such as neutrophils and macrophages ingest pathogens and produce reactive oxygen species (ROS) to kill ingested microbes. SCFAs regulate both ROS production and phagocytic acitivty [34, 97]. C4 inhibits macrophage differentiation to active phagocytes [98]. For neutrophils, some reported inhibitory effects of SCFAs [85, 99-101], while others reported suppressive effects on phagocytosis and ROS production [34, 102, 103]. More studies are required to sort out this discrepancy, but these results indicate that SCFAs appear to regulate neutrophil activation in both ways depending on immunological conditions of tissues.

SCFAs can affect cells of adaptive immunity such as T cells. C4 inhibits lymphocyte proliferation [104]. C4 reduces the production of IL-2 and IFN-γ by activated lymphocytes [105, 106]. C4 can enhance IL-10 production by activated lymphocytes [104]. C2 and C3 increased IFN-γ production in cultured lymphocytes [104]. C3 can expand the colonic FoxP3$^+$ pool and protect mice from T-cell-induced colitis [107]. C4 can induce FoxP3$^+$ T cells [108, 109]. The mechanism is unclear but HDAC inhibitory activity of SCFAs is likely to be involved [105]. Overall, these reports indicate that SCFAs regulate lymphocyte activation in both positive and negative ways.

6. Regulation of Intestinal Inflammation by SCFAs

SCFAs regulate inflammatory responses and, therefore, can greatly affect tissue inflammation in the intestine. A strong body of evidence suggests that SCFAs have beneficial effects on intestinal inflammation. SCFA levels are decreased in patients of inflammatory bowel disease such as ulcerative colitis and Crohn's disease [110, 111]. Not only the levels of SCFAs but their metabolism is generally decreased in IBD patients [112, 113]. Administration of C4 via enemas into IBD patients attenuated inflammation [114-118].

Others observed no significant effect of C3 enema on colitis patients or TNBS-induced colitis [119, 120]. C3 or C4 administration had suppressive effects on T-cell induced colitis in animal models through induction of Tregs [107, 109].

C2 administration into mice ameliorated *C. rodentium*-induced inflammation in the intestine [4]. This effect is mediated, in part, by the effect of C2 in activating intestinal ECs, which enhances the clearance of pathogens and maintenance of the barrier function, resulting in decreased tissue infiltration by commensal bacteria and tissue inflammation. Mice deficient in GPR43 were more susceptible to DSS-induced colitis [34, 121], suggesting a positive role of GPR43 in regulation of inflammation. It is also reported that GPR43-deficient animals are less susceptible to DSS-induced colitis [79]. A difference between these studies is the employment of acute versus chronic methods of inducing intestinal inflammation. The former study employed a chronic whereas the latter utilized an acute DSS model. This indicates that SCFAs and their receptors may facilitate acute immune responses but ameliorate chronic inflammatory conditions.

Similar to the beneficial effects of SCFA administration, dietary supplementation with resistant starches can decrease intestinal inflammation. Dietary fibers had significant positive effects in ameliorating intestinal inflammation in animals and humans [122-125]. For example, cellobiose is a digestion resistant disaccharide derived from cellulose and consisted of two glucose molecules linked by a $\beta(1\rightarrow4)$ bond. Feeding animals with cellobiose suppressed the development of DSS-induced colitis. [126, 127]. Many GI cancers are linked to intestinal inflammation. SCFAs and resistant starches have protective effects in development of GI cancer in humans and animals. [128-131]. We don't discuss this topic in details in this chapter as it has been covered elsewhere.

Conclusion and Future Perspectives

In this chapter, we discussed key functions of SCFAs in regulation of intestinal ECs and immune cells. SCFAs can promote both immunity and immune tolerance through various cell types in the intestine (Figure 2). SCFAs prepare tissue and immune cells in the intestine for prevention of infection. Upon infection, SCFAs promote efficient clearance of pathogens.

These functions are mediated, in part, by regulating gut-barrier functions, phagocytes, and cells of adaptive immunity. At the same time, SCFAs promote immune tolerance through induction of the immunosuppressive cytokine IL-10 and suppression of inflammatory cytokines and chemokines. More work is required to fully understand how SCFAs regulate both immunity and immune tolerance in a highly coordinated manner. Possible mechanisms may involve cell- and condition-specific actions of SCFAs. Cross-talks between SCFAs and MAMPs would occur for controlled regulation of various inflammatory and tolerogenic factors. It is important to delineate GPR41 and GPR43-dependent and independent signaling processes in individual immune and non-immune cell types. Also, important are the studies to determine HDAC-dependent and independent biological processes of SCFAs in each cell type.

Acknowledgments

This study was supported, in part, by grants from NIH (R01AI074745, R01DK076616, 1R01AI080769, and 1S10RR028293), The Crohn's and Colitis Foundation of America, and The National Multiple Sclerosis Society to CHK.

REFERENCES

[1] Vinolo, M. A., Rodrigues, H. G., Nachbar, R. T., Curi, R. Regulation of inflammation by short chain fatty acids. *Nutrients*. 2011;3(10):858-76.

[2] Macfarlane, S., Macfarlane, G. T. Regulation of short-chain fatty acid production. *Proceedings of the Nutrition Society*. 2003;62(01):67-72.

[3] Cummings, J. H., Pomare, E. W., Branch, W. J., Naylor, C. P., Macfarlane, G. T. Short chain fatty acids in human large intestine, portal, hepatic and venous blood. *Gut*. 1987; 28(10):1221-7.

[4] Kim, M. H., Kang, S. G., Park, J. H., Yanagisawa, M., Kim, C. H. Short-chain fatty acids activate GPR41 and GPR43 on intestinal epithelial cells to promote inflammatory responses in mice. *Gastroenterology*. 2013;145(2):396-406 e1-10.

[5] McNeil, N. I. The contribution of the large intestine to energy supplies in man. *Am. J. Clin. Nutr*. 1984;39(2):338-42.

[6] Schmitt, M. G., Jr., Soergel, K. H., Wood, C. M. Absorption of short chain fatty acids from the human jejunum. *Gastroenterology*. 1976;70(2):211-5.

[7] Sellin, J. H., DeSoignie, R. Short-chain fatty acid absorption in rabbit colon in vitro. *Gastroenterology*. 1990;99(3):676-83.

[8] Binder, H. J. Role of colonic short-chain fatty acid transport in diarrhea. *Annual review of physiology*. 2010;72:297-313.

[9] Hadjiagapiou, C., Schmidt, L., Dudeja, P. K., Layden, T. J., Ramaswamy, K. Mechanism(s) of butyrate transport in Caco-2 cells: role of monocarboxylate transporter 1. *Am. J. Physiol. Gastrointest. Liver Physiol*. 2000;279(4):G775-80.

[10] Alrefai, W. A., Tyagi, S., Gill, R., Saksena, S., Hadjiagapiou, C., Mansour, F., et al. Regulation of butyrate uptake in Caco-2 cells by phorbol 12-myristate 13-acetate. *Am. J. Physiol. Gastrointest. Liver Physiol*. 2004;286(2):G197-203.

[11] Ritzhaupt, A., Ellis, A., Hosie, K. B., Shirazi-Beechey, S. P. The characterization of butyrate transport across pig and human colonic luminal membrane. *The Journal of physiology*. 1998;507(3):819-30.

[12] Gopal, E., Miyauchi, S., Martin, P. M., Ananth, S., Roon, P., Smith, S. B., et al. Transport of nicotinate and structurally related compounds by human SMCT1 (SLC 5A8) and its relevance to drug transport in the mammalian intestinal tract. *Pharm. Res*. 2007;24(3):575-84.

[13] Coady, M. J., Chang, M.-H., Charron, F. M., Plata, C., Wallendorff, B., Sah, J. F., et al. The human tumour suppressor gene SLC5A8 expresses a Na+—monocarboxylate cotransporter. *The Journal of physiology*. 2004;557(3):719-31.

[14] Miyauchi, S., Gopal, E., Fei, Y. J., Ganapathy, V. Functional identification of SLC5A8, a tumor suppressor down-regulated in colon cancer, as a Na(+)-coupled transporter for short-chain fatty acids. *J. Biol. Chem*. 2004;279(14):13293-6.

[15] Singh, N., Thangaraju, M., Prasad, P. D., Martin, P. M., Lambert, N. A., Boettger, T., et al. Blockade of dendritic cell development by bacterial fermentation products butyrate and propionate through a transporter (Slc5a8)-dependent inhibition of histone deacetylases. *Journal of Biological Chemistry*. 2010;285(36):27601-8.

[16] Gopal, E., Fei, Y. J., Sugawara, M., Miyauchi, S., Zhuang, L., Martin, P., et al. Expression of slc5a8 in kidney and its role in Na(+)-coupled transport of lactate. *J. Biol. Chem.* 2004;279(43):44522-32.

[17] Thangaraju, M., Cresci, G., Itagaki, S., Mellinger, J., Browning, D. D., Berger, F. G., et al. Sodium-coupled transport of the short chain fatty acid butyrate by SLC5A8 and its relevance to colon cancer. *J. Gastrointest. Surg.* 2008;12(10):1773-81; discussion 81-2.

[18] Brown, A. J., Goldsworthy, S. M., Barnes, A. A., Eilert, M. M., Tcheang, L., Daniels, D., et al. The Orphan G protein-coupled receptors GPR41 and GPR43 are activated by propionate and other short chain carboxylic acids. *J. Biol. Chem.* 2003;278(13):11312-9.

[19] Karaki, S., Mitsui, R., Hayashi, H., Kato, I., Sugiya, H., Iwanaga, T., et al. Short-chain fatty acid receptor, GPR43, is expressed by enteroendocrine cells and mucosal mast cells in rat intestine. *Cell Tissue Res.* 2006;324(3):353-60.

[20] Le Poul, E., Loison, C., Struyf, S., Springael, J. Y., Lannoy, V., Decobecq, M. E., et al. Functional characterization of human receptors for short chain fatty acids and their role in polymorphonuclear cell activation. *J. Biol. Chem.* 2003;278(28):25481-9.

[21] Nilsson, N. E., Kotarsky, K., Owman, C., Olde, B. Identification of a free fatty acid receptor, FFA2R, expressed on leukocytes and activated by short-chain fatty acids. *Biochem. Biophys. Res. Commun.* 2003;303(4):1047-52.

[22] Hong, Y. H., Nishimura, Y., Hishikawa, D., Tsuzuki, H., Miyahara, H., Gotoh, C., et al. Acetate and propionate short chain fatty acids stimulate adipogenesis via GPCR43. *Endocrinology.* 2005;146(12):5092-9.

[23] Xiong, Y., Miyamoto, N., Shibata, K., Valasek, M. A., Motoike, T., Kedzierski, R. M., et al. Short-chain fatty acids stimulate leptin production in adipocytes through the G protein-coupled receptor GPR41. *Proc. Natl. Acad. Sci. US.* 2004;101(4):1045-50.

[24] Tazoe, H., Otomo, Y., Karaki, S.-I., Kato, I., Fukami, Y., Terasaki, M., et al. Expression of short-chain fatty acid receptor GPR41 in the human colon. *Biomedical Research.* 2009;30(3):149-56.

[25] Lee, T., Schwandner, R., Swaminath, G., Weiszmann, J., Cardozo, M., Greenberg, J., et al. Identification and functional characterization of allosteric agonists for the G protein-coupled receptor FFA2. *Molecular pharmacology.* 2008;74(6):1599-609.

[26] Wettschureck, N., Offermanns, S. Mammalian G proteins and their cell type specific functions. *Physiological reviews.* 2005;85(4):1159-204.

[27] Schaub, A., Futterer, A., Pfeffer, K. PUMA-G, an IFN-gamma-inducible gene in macrophages is a novel member of the seven transmembrane spanning receptor superfamily. *Eur. J. Immunol.* 2001;31(12):3714-25.

[28] Offermanns, S. The nicotinic acid receptor GPR109A (HM74A or PUMA-G) as a new therapeutic target. *Trends Pharmacol. Sci.* 2006;27(7):384-90.

[29] Wise, A., Foord, S. M., Fraser, N. J., Barnes, A. A., Elshourbagy, N., Eilert, M., et al. Molecular identification of high and low affinity receptors for nicotinic acid. *J. Biol. Chem.* 2003;278(11):9869-74.

[30] Taggart, A. K., Kero, J., Gan, X., Cai, T. Q., Cheng, K., Ippolito, M., et al. (D)-beta-Hydroxybutyrate inhibits adipocyte lipolysis via the nicotinic acid receptor PUMA-G. *J. Biol. Chem.* 2005;280(29):26649-52.

[31] Tunaru, S., Kero, J., Schaub, A., Wufka, C., Blaukat, A., Pfeffer, K., et al. PUMA-G and HM74 are receptors for nicotinic acid and mediate its anti-lipolytic effect. *Nat. Med.* 2003;9(3):352-5.

[32] Cresci, G. A., Thangaraju, M., Mellinger, J. D., Liu, K., Ganapathy, V. Colonic gene expression in conventional and germ-free mice with a focus on the butyrate receptor GPR109A and the butyrate transporter SLC5A8. *J. Gastrointest. Surg.* 2010;14(3):449-61.

[33] Pluznick, J. L., Protzko, R. J., Gevorgyan, H., Peterlin, Z., Sipos, A., Han, J., et al. Olfactory receptor responding to gut microbiota-derived signals plays a role in renin secretion and blood pressure regulation. *Proc. Natl. Acad. Sci. US.* 2013;110(11):4410-5.

[34] Maslowski, K. M., Vieira, A. T., Ng, A., Kranich, J., Sierro, F., Yu, D., et al. Regulation of inflammatory responses by gut microbiota and chemoattractant receptor GPR43. *Nature*. 2009;461(7268):1282-6.

[35] Vinolo, M. A., Ferguson, G. J., Kulkarni, S., Damoulakis, G., Anderson, K., Bohlooly, Y. M., et al. SCFAs induce mouse neutrophil chemotaxis through the GPR43 receptor. *PloS one.* 2011;6(6):e21205.

[36] Mortensen, F. V., Langkilde, N. C., Joergensen, J. C., Hessov, I. Short-chain fatty acids stimulate mucosal cell proliferation in the closed human rectum after Hartmann's procedure. *Int. J. Colorectal Dis.* 1999;14(3):150-4.

[37] Hague, A., Singh, B., Paraskeva, C. Butyrate acts as a survival factor for colonic epithelial cells: further fuel for the in vivo versus in vitro debate. *Gastroenterology.* 1997;112(3):1036-40.

[38] Chirakkal, H., Leech, S. H., Brookes, K. E., Prais, A. L., Waby, J. S., Corfe, B. M. Upregulation of BAK by butyrate in the colon is associated with increased Sp3 binding. *Oncogene*. 2006;25(54):7192-200.

[39] Hinnebusch, B. F., Meng, S., Wu, J. T., Archer, S. Y., Hodin, R. A. The effects of short-chain fatty acids on human colon cancer cell phenotype are associated with histone hyperacetylation. *J. Nutr.* 2002;132(5):1012-7.

[40] Davie, J. R. Inhibition of histone deacetylase activity by butyrate. *J. Nutr.* 2003;133(7 Suppl.):2485S-93S.

[41] Gibson, P. R., Rosella, O., Wilson, A. J., Mariadason, J. M., Rickard, K., Byron, K., et al. Colonic epithelial cell activation and the paradoxical effects of butyrate. *Carcinogenesis*. 1999;20(4):539-44.

[42] Daly, K., Shirazi-Beechey, S. P. Microarray analysis of butyrate regulated genes in colonic epithelial cells. *DNA Cell Biol.* 2006;25(1):49-62.

[43] Gibson, P. R. The intracellular target of butyrate's actions: HDAC or HDON'T? *Gut.* 2000;46(4):447-8.

[44] Chen, L., Fischle, W., Verdin, E., Greene, W. C. Duration of nuclear NF-kappaB action regulated by reversible acetylation. *Science*. 2001;293(5535):1653-7.

[45] Polesskaya, A., Duquet, A., Naguibneva, I., Weise, C., Vervisch, A., Bengal, E., et al. CREB-binding protein/p300 activates MyoD by acetylation. *J. Biol. Chem.* 2000;275 (44):34359-64.

[46] Glozak, M. A., Sengupta, N., Zhang, X., Seto, E. Acetylation and deacetylation of non-histone proteins. *Gene*. 2005;363:15-23.

[47] Mandal, M., Olson, D. J., Sharma, T., Vadlamudi, R. K., Kumar, R. Butyric acid induces apoptosis by up-regulating Bax expression via stimulation of the c-Jun N-terminal kinase/activation protein-1 pathway in human colon cancer cells. *Gastroenterology*. 2001;120(1):71-8.

[48] Kida, Y., Shimizu, T., Kuwano, K. Sodium butyrate up-regulates cathelicidin gene expression via activator protein-1 and histone acetylation at the promoter region in a human lung epithelial cell line, EBC-1. *Molecular immunology*. 2006;43(12):1972-81.

[49] Nepelska, M., Cultrone, A., Béguet-Crespel, F., Le Roux, K., Doré, J., Arulampalam, V., et al. Butyrate produced by commensal bacteria potentiates phorbol esters induced AP-1 response in human intestinal epithelial cells. *PloS one*. 2012;7(12):e52869.

[50] Rivero, J. A., Adunyah, S. E. Sodium butyrate stimulates PKC activation and induces differential expression of certain PKC isoforms during erythroid differentiation. *Biochemical and biophysical research communications*. 1998;248(3):664-8.

[51] Inan, M. S., Rasoulpour, R. J., Yin, L., Hubbard, A. K., Rosenberg, D. W., Giardina, C. The luminal short-chain fatty acid butyrate modulates NF-κB activity in a human colonic epithelial cell line. *Gastroenterology*. 2000;118(4):724-34.

[52] Arvans, D. L., Vavricka, S. R., Ren, H., Musch, M. W., Kang, L., Rocha, F. G., et al. Luminal bacterial flora determines physiological expression of intestinal epithelial cytoprotective heat shock proteins 25 and 72. *Am. J. Physiol. Gastrointest. Liver Physiol*. 2005;288(4):G696-704.

[53] Malago, J. J., Koninkx, J. F., Tooten, P. C., van Liere, E. A., van Dijk, J. E. Anti-inflammatory properties of heat shock protein 70 and butyrate on Salmonella-induced interleukin-8 secretion in enterocyte-like Caco-2 cells. *Clin. Exp. Immunol*. 2005;141 (1):62-71.

[54] Ren, H., Musch, M. W., Kojima, K., Boone, D., Ma, A., Chang, E. B. Short-chain fatty acids induce intestinal epithelial heat shock protein 25 expression in rats and IEC 18 cells. *Gastroenterology*. 2001;121(3):631-9.

[55] Shen, L., Turner, J. R. Role of epithelial cells in initiation and propagation of intestinal inflammation. Eliminating the static: tight junction dynamics exposed. *Am. J. Physiol. Gastrointest. Liver Physiol*. 2006;290(4):G577-82.

[56] Frey, A., Giannasca, K. T., Weltzin, R., Giannasca, P. J., Reggio, H., Lencer, W. I., et al. Role of the glycocalyx in regulating access of microparticles to apical plasma membranes of intestinal epithelial cells: implications for microbial attachment and oral vaccine targeting. *J. Exp. Med*. 1996;184(3):1045-59.

[57] McAuley, J. L., Linden, S. K., Png, C. W., King, R. M., Pennington, H. L., Gendler, S. J., et al. MUC1 cell surface mucin is a critical element of the mucosal barrier to infection. *J. Clin. Invest*. 2007;117(8):2313-24.

[58] Salzman, N. H., Ghosh, D., Huttner, K. M., Paterson, Y., Bevins, C. L. Protection against enteric salmonellosis in transgenic mice expressing a human intestinal defensin. *Nature*. 2003;422(6931):522-6.

[59] Ganz, T. Defensins: antimicrobial peptides of innate immunity. *Nat. Rev. Immunol*. 2003;3(9):710-20.

[60] Schauber, J., Svanholm, C., Termen, S., Iffland, K., Menzel, T., Scheppach, W., et al. Expression of the cathelicidin LL-37 is modulated by short chain fatty acids in colonocytes: relevance of signalling pathways. *Gut*. 2003;52(5):735-41.

[61] Peng, L., He, Z., Chen, W., Holzman, I. R., Lin, J. Effects of butyrate on intestinal barrier function in a Caco-2 cell monolayer model of intestinal barrier. *Pediatr. Res.* 2007;61(1):37-41.

[62] Ohata, A., Usami, M., Miyoshi, M. Short-chain fatty acids alter tight junction permeability in intestinal monolayer cells via lipoxygenase activation. *Nutrition.* 2005; 21(7–8):838-47.

[63] Wang, H. B., Wang, P. Y., Wang, X., Wan, Y. L., Liu, Y. C. Butyrate enhances intestinal epithelial barrier function via up-regulation of tight junction protein Claudin-1 transcription. *Dig. Dis. Sci.* 2012;57(12):3126-35.

[64] Mariadason, J. M., Kilias, D., Catto-Smith, A., Gibson, P. R. Effect of butyrate on paracellular permeability in rat distal colonic mucosa ex vivo. *J. Gastroenterol. Hepatol.* 1999;14(9):873-9.

[65] Einerhand, A. W. C., Renes, I. B., Makkink, M. K., van der Sluis, M., Büller, H. A., Dekker, J. Role of mucins in inflammatory bowel disease: important lessons from experimental models. *European Journal of Gastroenterology and Hepatology.* 2002;14 (7):757-65.

[66] Gaudier, E., Jarry, A., Blottiere, H. M., de Coppet, P., Buisine, M. P., Aubert, J. P., et al. Butyrate specifically modulates MUC gene expression in intestinal epithelial goblet cells deprived of glucose. *Am. J. Physiol. Gastrointest. Liver Physiol.* 2004;287(6): G1168-74.

[67] Augenlicht, L., Shi, L., Mariadason, J., Laboisse, C., Velcich, A. Repression of MUC2 gene expression by butyrate, a physiological regulator of intestinal cell maturation. *Oncogene.* 2003;22(32):4983-92.

[68] Hatayama, H., Iwashita, J., Kuwajima, A., Abe, T. The short chain fatty acid, butyrate, stimulates MUC2 mucin production in the human colon cancer cell line, LS174T. *Biochem. Biophys. Res. Commun.* 2007;356(3):599-603.

[69] Willemsen, L., Koetsier, M., Van Deventer, S., Van Tol, E. Short chain fatty acids stimulate epithelial mucin 2 expression through differential effects on prostaglandin E1 and E2 production by intestinal myofibroblasts. *Gut.* 2003;52(10):1442-7.

[70] Finnie, I. A., Dwarakanath, A. D., Taylor, B. A., Rhodes, J. M. Colonic mucin synthesis is increased by sodium butyrate. *Gut.* 1995;36(1):93-9.

[71] Barcelo, A., Claustre, J., Moro, F., Chayvialle, J., Cuber, J., Plaisancie, P. Mucin secretion is modulated by luminal factors in the isolated vascularly perfused rat colon. *Gut.* 2000;46(2):218-24.

[72] Augenlicht, L., Shi, L., Mariadason, J., Laboisse, C., Velcich, A. Repression of MUC2 gene expression by butyrate, a physiological regulator of intestinal cell maturation. *Oncogene.* 2003;22(32):4983-92.

[73] Thim, L. Trefoil peptides: from structure to function. *Cellular and Molecular Life Sciences CMLS.* 1997;53(11-12):888-903.

[74] Zhu, Y.-Q., Tan, X.-D. TFF3 modulates NF-κB and a novel negative regulatory molecule of NF-κB in intestinal epithelial cells via a mechanism distinct from TNF-α. *American Journal of Physiology-Cell Physiology.* 2005;289(5):C1085-C93.

[75] Song, M., Xia, B., Li, J. Effects of topical treatment of sodium butyrate and 5-aminosalicylic acid on expression of trefoil factor 3, interleukin 1β, and nuclear factor κB in trinitrobenzene sulphonic acid induced colitis in rats. *Postgraduate medical journal.* 2006;82(964):130-5.

[76] Ten Bruggencate, S. J., Bovee-Oudenhoven, I. M., Lettink-Wissink, M. L., Van der Meer, R. Dietary fructooligosaccharides increase intestinal permeability in rats. *The Journal of nutrition*. 2005;135(4):837-42.

[77] Tappenden, K. A., Thomson, A., Wild, G. E., McBurney, M. I. Short-chain fatty acid-supplemented total parenteral nutrition enhances functional adaptation to intestinal resection in rats. *Gastroenterology*. 1997;112(3):792-802.

[78] Vinolo, M., Rodrigues, H., Hatanaka, E., Hebeda, C., Farsky, S., Curi, R. Short-chain fatty acids stimulate the migration of neutrophils to inflammatory sites. *Clinical Science*. 2009;117:331-8.

[79] Sina, C., Gavrilova, O., Förster, M., Till, A., Derer, S., Hildebrand, F., et al. G protein-coupled receptor 43 is essential for neutrophil recruitment during intestinal inflammation. *The Journal of Immunology*. 2009;183(11):7514-22.

[80] Blais, M., Seidman, E. G., Asselin, C. Dual Effect of Butyrate on IL-1 β-Mediated Intestinal Epithelial Cell Inflammatory Response. *DNA and cell biology*. 2007;26(3): 133-47.

[81] Leung, C. H., Lam, W., Ma, D. L., Gullen, E. A., Cheng, Y. C. Butyrate mediates nucleotide-binding and oligomerisation domain (NOD) 2-dependent mucosal immune responses against peptidoglycan. *European journal of immunology*. 2009;39(12):3529-37.

[82] Böcker, U., Nebe, T., Herweck, F., Holt, L., Panja, A., Jobin, C., et al. Butyrate modulates intestinal epithelial cell-mediated neutrophil migration. *Clinical and Experimental Immunology*. 2003;131(1):53-60.

[83] Fusunyan, R. D., Quinn, J. J., Fujimoto, M., MacDermott, R. P., Sanderson, I. R. Butyrate switches the pattern of chemokine secretion by intestinal epithelial cells through histone acetylation. *Molecular medicine*. 1999;5(9):631.

[84] Inatomi, O., Andoh, A., Kitamura, K.-I., Yasui, H., Zhang, Z., Fujiyama, Y. Butyrate blocks interferon-γ-inducible protein-10 release in human intestinal subepithelial myofibroblasts. *Journal of gastroenterology*. 2005;40(5):483-9.

[85] Vinolo, M. A., Rodrigues, H. G., Hatanaka, E., Sato, F. T., Sampaio, S. C., Curi, R. Suppressive effect of short-chain fatty acids on production of proinflammatory mediators by neutrophils. *The Journal of nutritional biochemistry*. 2011;22(9):849-55.

[86] Tedelind, S., Westberg, F., Kjerrulf, M., Vidal, A. Anti-inflammatory properties of the short-chain fatty acids acetate and propionate: a study with relevance to inflammatory bowel disease. *World Journal of Gastroenterology*. 2007;13(20):2826.

[87] Zapolska-Downar, D., Naruszewicz, M. Propionate reduces the cytokine-induced VCAM-1 and ICAM-1 expression by inhibiting nuclear factor-kappa B (NF-kappaB) activation. *J. Physiol. Pharmacol*. 2009;60(2):123-31.

[88] Menzel, T., Lührs, H., Zirlik, S., Schauber, J., Kudlich, T., Gerke, T., et al. Butyrate inhibits leukocyte adhesion to endothelial cells via modulation of VCAM-1. *Inflammatory bowel diseases*. 2004;10(2):122-8.

[89] Dianzani, C., Cavalli, R., Zara, G. P., Gallicchio, M., Lombardi, G., Gasco, M. R., et al. Cholesteryl butyrate solid lipid nanoparticles inhibit adhesion of human neutrophils to endothelial cells. *British journal of pharmacology*. 2006;148(5):648-56.

[90] Park, J.-S., Lee, E.-J., Lee, J.-C., Kim, W.-K., Kim, H.-S. Anti-inflammatory effects of short chain fatty acids in IFN-γ-stimulated RAW 264.7 murine macrophage cells:

Involvement of NF-κB and ERK signaling pathways. *International immunopharmacology*. 2007;7(1):70-7.

[91] Chakravortty, D., Koide, N., Kato, Y., Sugiyama, T., Mu, M. M., Yoshida, T., et al. The inhibitory action of butyrate on lipopolysaccharide-induced nitric oxide production in RAW 264.7 murine macrophage cells. *Journal of endotoxin research*. 2000;6(3):243-7.

[92] Böhmig, G., Krieger, P. M., Säemann, M., Wenhardt, C., Pohanka, E., Zlabinger, G. n-Butyrate downregulates the stimulatory function of peripheral blood-derived antigen-presenting cells: a potential mechanism for modulating T-cell responses by short-chain fatty acids. *Immunology*. 1997;92(2):234-43.

[93] Cox, M. A., Jackson, J., Stanton, M., Rojas-Triana, A., Bober, L., Laverty, M., et al. Short-chain fatty acids act as antiinflammatory mediators by regulating prostaglandin E2 and cytokines. *World journal of gastroenterology: WJG*. 2009;15(44):5549.

[94] Usami, M., Kishimoto, K., Ohata, A., Miyoshi, M., Aoyama, M., Fueda, Y., et al. Butyrate and trichostatin A attenuate nuclear factor< i> κ</i> B activation and tumor necrosis factor< i> α</i> secretion and increase prostaglandin E< sub> 2</sub> secretion in human peripheral blood mononuclear cells. *Nutrition Research*. 2008; 28 (5):321-8.

[95] Perez, R., Stevenson, F., Johnson, J., Morgan, M., Erickson, K., Hubbard, N. E., et al. Sodium Butyrate Upregulates Kupffer Cell PGE< sub> 2</sub> Production and Modulates Immune Function. *Journal of Surgical Research*. 1998;78(1):1-6.

[96] Harris, S. G., Padilla, J., Koumas, L., Ray, D., Phipps, R. P. Prostaglandins as modulators of immunity. *Trends in immunology*. 2002;23(3):144-50.

[97] Vinolo, M. A., Hatanaka, E., Lambertucci, R. H., Newsholme, P., Curi, R. Effects of short chain fatty acids on effector mechanisms of neutrophils. *Cell biochemistry and function*. 2009;27(1):48-55.

[98] L Millard A., Mertes, P., Ittelet, D., Villard, F., Jeannesson, P., Bernard, J. Butyrate affects differentiation, maturation and function of human monocyte-derived dendritic cells and macrophages. *Clinical and Experimental Immunology*. 2002;130(2):245-55.

[99] Mills, S. W., Montgomery, S. H., Morck, D. W. Evaluation of the effects of short-chain fatty acids and extracellular pH on bovine neutrophil function in vitro. *American journal of veterinary research*. 2006;67(11):1901-7.

[100] Eftimiadi, C., Tonetti, M., Cavallero, A., Sacco, O., Rossi, G. Short-chain fatty acids produced by anaerobic bacteria inhibit phagocytosis by human lung phagocytes. *Journal of Infectious Diseases*. 1990;161(1):138-42.

[101] Liu, Q., Shimoyama, T., Suzuki, K., Umeda, T., Nakaji, S., Sugawara, K. Effect of sodium butyrate on reactive oxygen species generation by human neutrophils. *Scandinavian journal of gastroenterology*. 2001;36(7):744-50.

[102] Stringer, R., Hart, C., Edwards, S. Sodium butyrate delays neutrophil apoptosis: role of protein biosynthesis in neutrophil survival. *British journal of haematology*. 1996;92 (1): 169-75.

[103] Nakao, S., Moriya, Y., Furuyama, S., Niederman, R., Sugiya, H. Propionic acid stimulates superoxide generation in human neutrophils. *Cell biology international*. 1998; 22(5):331-7.

[104] Cavaglieri, C. R., Nishiyama, A., Fernandes, L. C., Curi, R., Miles, E. A., Calder, P. C. Differential effects of short-chain fatty acids on proliferation and production of pro-and

anti-inflammatory cytokines by cultured lymphocytes. *Life sciences*. 2003;73(13):1683-90.

[105] Tao, R., de Zoeten, E. F., Özkaynak, E., Chen, C., Wang, L., Porrett, P. M., et al. Deacetylase inhibition promotes the generation and function of regulatory T cells. *Nature medicine*. 2007;13(11):1299-307.

[106] Dagtas, A. S., Edens, R. E., Gilbert, K. M. Histone deacetylase inhibitor uses p21< sup> Cip1</sup> to maintain anergy in CD4< sup>+</sup> T cells. *International immunopharmacology*. 2009;9(11):1289-97.

[107] Smith, P. M., Howitt, M. R., Panikov, N., Michaud, M., Gallini, C. A., Bohlooly-Y. M., et al. The microbial metabolites, short-chain fatty acids, regulate colonic Treg cell homeostasis. *Science*. 2013;341(6145):569-73.

[108] Arpaia, N., Campbell, C., Fan, X., Dikiy, S., van der Veeken, J., deRoos, P., et al. Metabolites produced by commensal bacteria promote peripheral regulatory T-cell generation. *Nature*. 2013;504(7480):451-5.

[109] Furusawa, Y., Obata, Y., Fukuda, S., Endo, T. A., Nakato, G., Takahashi, D., et al. Commensal microbe-derived butyrate induces the differentiation of colonic regulatory T cells. *Nature*. 2013;504(7480):446-50.

[110] Kim, Y. I. Short-chain fatty acids in ulcerative colitis. *Nutr. Rev*. 1998;56(1 Pt 1):17-24.

[111] Vernia, P., Gnaedinger, A., Hauck, W., Breuer, R. I. Organic anions and the diarrhea of inflammatory bowel disease. *Dig. Dis. Sci*. 1988;33(11):1353-8.

[112] Den Hond, E., Hiele, M., Evenepoel, P., Peeters, M., Ghoos, Y., Rutgeerts, P. In vivo butyrate metabolism and colonic permeability in extensive ulcerative colitis. *Gastro-enterology*. 1998;115(3):584-90.

[113] Simpson, E. J., Chapman, M. A., Dawson, J., Berry, D., Macdonald, I. A., Cole, A. In vivo measurement of colonic butyrate metabolism in patients with quiescent ulcerative colitis. *Gut*. 2000;46(1):73-7.

[114] Butzner, J., Parmar, R., Bell, C., Dalal, V. Butyrate enema therapy stimulates mucosal repair in experimental colitis in the rat. *Gut*. 1996;38(4):568-73.

[115] Hamer, H. M., Jonkers, D. M., Vanhoutvin, S. A., Troost, F. J., Rijkers, G., de Bruïne, A., et al. Effect of butyrate enemas on inflammation and antioxidant status in the colonic mucosa of patients with ulcerative colitis in remission. *Clinical nutrition*. 2010; 29(6):738-44.

[116] Vieira, E. L., Leonel, A. J., Sad, A. P., Beltrão, N. R., Costa, T. F., Ferreira, T. M., et al. Oral administration of sodium butyrate attenuates inflammation and mucosal lesion in experimental acute ulcerative colitis. *The Journal of nutritional biochemistry*. 2012;23 (5):430-6.

[117] Harig, J. M., Soergel, K. H., Komorowski, R. A., Wood, C. M. Treatment of diversion colitis with short-chain-fatty acid irrigation. *N Engl. J. Med*. 1989;320(1):23-8.

[118] Scheppach, W., Sommer, H., Kirchner, T., Paganelli, G. M., Bartram, P., Christl, S., et al. Effect of butyrate enemas on the colonic mucosa in distal ulcerative colitis. *Gastro-enterology*. 1992;103(1):51-6.

[119] Tarrerias, A. L., Millecamps, M., Alloui, A., Beaughard, C., Kemeny, J. L., Bourdu, S., et al. Short-chain fatty acid enemas fail to decrease colonic hypersensitivity and inflammation in TNBS-induced colonic inflammation in rats. *Pain*. 2002;100(1-2):91-7.

[120] Guillemot, F., Colombel, J. F., Neut, C., Verplanck, N., Lecomte, M., Romond, C., et al. Treatment of diversion colitis by short-chain fatty acids. Prospective and double-blind study. *Diseases of the colon and rectum*. 1991;34(10):861-4.

[121] Masui, R., Sasaki, M., Funaki, Y., Ogasawara, N., Mizuno, M., Iida, A., et al. G Protein-Coupled Receptor 43 Moderates Gut Inflammation Through Cytokine Regulation from Mononuclear Cells. *Inflammatory bowel diseases*. 2013.

[122] Fernandez-Banares, F., Hinojosa, J., Sanchez-Lombrana, J. L., Navarro, E., Martinez-Salmeron, J. F., Garcia-Puges, A., et al. Randomized clinical trial of Plantago ovata seeds (dietary fiber) as compared with mesalamine in maintaining remission in ulcerative colitis. Spanish Group for the Study of Crohn's Disease and Ulcerative Colitis (GETECCU). *Am. J. Gastroenterol.* 1999;94(2):427-33.

[123] Kuo, S. M. The interplay between fiber and the intestinal microbiome in the inflammatory response. *Adv. Nutr.* 2013;4(1):16-28.

[124] Hallert, C., Kaldma, M., Petersson, B. G. Ispaghula husk may relieve gastrointestinal symptoms in ulcerative colitis in remission. *Scand. J. Gastroenterol.* 1991;26(7):747-50.

[125] Kanauchi, O., Nakamura, T., Agata, K., Mitsuyama, K., Iwanaga, T. Effects of germinated barley foodstuff on dextran sulfate sodium-induced colitis in rats. *J. Gastroenterol.* 1998;33(2):179-88.

[126] Jacobasch, G., Schmiedl, D., Kruschewski, M., Schmehl, K. Dietary resistant starch and chronic inflammatory bowel diseases. *International journal of colorectal disease*. 1999; 14(4-5):201-11.

[127] Nishimura, T., Andoh, A., Hashimoto, T., Kobori, A., Tsujikawa, T., Fujiyama, Y. Cellobiose prevents the development of dextran sulfate sodium (DSS)-induced experimental colitis. *Journal of clinical biochemistry and nutrition*. 2010;46(2):105.

[128] Rodríguez-Cabezas, M. E., Galvez, J., Lorente, M. D., Concha, A., Camuesco, D., Azzouz, S., et al. Dietary fiber down-regulates colonic tumor necrosis factor α and nitric oxide production in trinitrobenzenesulfonic acid-induced colitic rats. *The Journal of nutrition*. 2002;132(11):3263-71.

[129] McIntyre, A., Gibson, P., Young, G. Butyrate production from dietary fibre and protection against large bowel cancer in a rat model. *Gut*. 1993;34(3):386-91.

[130] Medina, V., Afonso, J., Alvarez-Arguelles, H., Hernandez, C., Gonzalez, F. Sodium butyrate inhibits carcinoma development in a 1, 2-dimethylhydrazine-induced rat colon cancer. *Journal of Parenteral and Enteral Nutrition*. 1998;22(1):14-7.

[131] Wong, C. S., Sengupta, S., Tjandra, J. J., Gibson, P. R. The influence of specific luminal factors on the colonic epithelium: high-dose butyrate and physical changes suppress early carcinogenic events in rats. *Diseases of the colon and rectum*. 2005;48 (3):549-59.

In: Butyrate: Food Sources, Functions and Health Benefits
Editor: Cong-Jun Li
ISBN: 978-1-63117-657-9
© 2014 Nova Science Publishers, Inc.

Chapter 7

BIOLOGICAL EFFECTS OF SODIUM BUTYRATE IN THE REGULATION OF GENE EXPRESSION ON ASTROCYTOMA CELL LINES AND IMPROVEMENT OF THERAPIES

***Monika Garrido-Armas*[1] *and Francisco Arenas-Huertero*[1,2,*]**
[1]Laboratory of Experimental Pathology. Hospital Infantil de México Federico Gómez, México City, Mexico
[2]Facultad de Ciencia y Tecnología, Universidad Simón Bolívar, México

ABSTRACT

Sodium Butyrate (NaBu), is a short chain fatty acid synthesized by proximal intestinal microbiota during fermentation of several types of fibers, for example the flour of whole grain cereals, inulin and *Psyllum*, among other natural fibers. The benefits of NaBu produced by fermentation are both intestinal and extra-intestinal. Other applications derive from *in vitro* assays on cancer cells. Results from these assays have potential applications *in vivo*. NaBu and such analogs as sodium phenylbutyrate prolong their effects from 12 hours for NaBu to 48 hours for sodium phenylbutyrate, which enhances the therapeutic effects of radiotherapy and chemotherapy in combined applications. Higher degree astrocytoma cells are more diverse in their responses to therapy and the resistant phenotype is a challenge in oncology. Analyses of the effects of NaBu on *in vitro* systems reveal important results. For example, in astrocytoma cell lines, NaBu induces important cellular changes after 12 h of exposition, including chromatin decondensation and the presence of several vesicles positive to acridine orange, which confirms their acidic nature. Viability assays *in vitro* reveal reduction and autophagic cell death. Ultrastructural analysis shows the presence of autophagic vesicles with mitochondrial remains and other cellular debris. NaBu at 8 mM for 24 h can induce re-expression of several genes in human astrocytoma cell lines, such as histone deacetylases

[*] Corresponding author: Francisco Arenas-Huertero. Laboratory of Experimental Pathology. Hospital Infantil de México Federico Gómez. Dr. Márquez 162. Colonia Doctores. 06920. México, D. F. E-mail: farenashuertero@yahoo.com.mx.

(HDAC3), histone acetylases (p300), pro-apoptotic genes (BAX), and anti-apoptotic genes (BCL2). One of the important applications of NaBu is enhancing cell death induced by photodynamic therapy. Also, NaBu increases the expression of genes of heme biosynthesis *in vitro*. Due to its epigenetic effects, NaBu has been proven to have benefits in treating several malign tumors, including those of the colon, prostate and central nervous system, such as astrocytoma, which is the first cause of death in children. In the future, NaBu must be used and applied not only in neoplastic malignant human diseases, but also in other chronic degenerative diseases, such as β-thalassemia, chronic ulcerative colon inflammation and other inflammatory processes.

Keywords: Central nervous system tumors, Astrocytoma, autophagy, HDAC, Sodium Butyrate

1. Introduction: Sodium Butyrate: Structure, Natural Biosynthesis and Effects on Cells and the Organism

Sodium butyrate (NaBu) is a small-chain fatty acid (SCFA) whose chemical formula is CH_3-CH_2-CH_2-COONa (Figure 1). It is synthesized metabolically in small amounts by the proximal intestinal microbiota during fermentation of the fiber produced by the digestion of whole grain flour in cereals, inulin, and *Psyllium*, among other foods. Its principal producer is the commensal bacteria *Faecalibacterium prausnitzii*.

SCFAs are absorbed by each intestinal segment. Colonocytes absorb them through different mechanisms of the apical membrane, including non-ionic diffusion, SCFA/HCO_3 exchange, and active transport by SCFA carriers. The absorption of these fatty acids signify-cantly affects absorption of NaCl and the overall electrolyte balance, thus maintaining intestinal homeostasis [1]. For obvious reasons, the first effects were described initially in the colon, so it is important to review them. The intestinal effects of NaBu are:

1 Stimulating production of mucin (defense of the intestinal mucosa) by increasing the expression of the genes of MUC 2.
2 Proliferation of normal enterocytes.
3 Inhibiting the expression of NF-kB and various cytokines, such as IL1B, IL2, IL6, and IL8.

The anti-inflammatory benefit of NaBu has been utilized in therapies for inflammatory diseases of the intestine and radiation-induced proctitis. In the case of ulcerative colitis, NaBu has been administered mainly by enema, but when delivered in conjunction with mesalazine it improves the anti-inflammatory results, as clinical data, endoscopic observation and histologi cal analysis have corroborated.

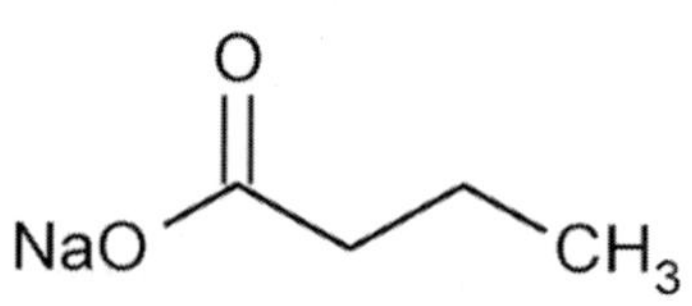

Figure 1. Structure of NaBu.

Today we know that the use of NaBu can prevent colorectal cancer, thanks to the results of studies with mice and humans [2].

1.1. Extra-Intestinal Benefits of NaBu

1.1.1. Anti-Inflammatory

As mentioned above, NaBu modulates expression of IL8 and other cytokines. With respect to its mechanism, NaBu controls ROS mediated NF-κB activation, which is a powerful regulator of the inflammatory response [3].

Also, it negatively regulates production of the tumor necrosis factor α, interferon gamma, and increases prostaglandin E_2, which are inflammatory mediators [4].

Cathelicidin, for example, is an antimicrobial protein that plays an important role in defense against bacterial infections. Many studies show that NaBu induces the expression of cathelicidin genes in the EBC-1 epithelial cell line of the lung, and is both the mRNA of cathelicidin and the expression of the protein [5].

1.1.2. Antioxidant/Regulation of Oxidative Stress

Oxidative stress results from an imbalance between the generation of reactive oxygen and nitrogen and the mechanisms of antioxidant defense. The most important source of reactive oxygen in normal conditions in aerobic organisms is probably the loss of activated oxygen (superoxide anion) from the mitochondria during the functioning of oxidative respiration. Hydrogen peroxide, another oxidant, is formed by such enzymes as the mono-oxygenases and oxidases. Pre-incubation of rat and human colonocytes with NaBu produced a significant reduction of DNA damage caused by hydrogen peroxide. It reduces the species of reactive oxygen by increasing the amount of reduced glutathione [2]. In this same environment, oxidative stress plays a very important role in the pathogenesis of certain illnesses, such as inflammatory intestinal disease, including Crohn's disease. High concentrations of species of reactive oxygen induce the activation of transcription factor NF-κB that, in turn, triggers the inflammation mediators. NaBu reduces the expression of NF-κB through the mechanism described above, effectuated by the mononuclear cells of the basal lamina in the lesions of patients affected by this illness.

1.1.3. Obesity

NaBu can lower the expression of genes that participate in the biosynthesis of cholesterol, triglycerides and apolipoproteins, in addition to modulating the biogenesis of lipoproteins.

Obese individuals have a lower amount of species of bacteroides and more firmicutes in the intestine. NaBu binds to receptors, including those coupled to the GPR41 protein, for example, which are present on the surface of the intestinal cells and can stimulate peptides that, in turn, inhibit intestinal motility and increase satiety. Studies with laboratory animals demonstrate that NaBu and sodium propionate can reduce obesity and resistance to insulin in mice with GPR41 deficiency as an independent mechanism [6].

It has been shown that NaBu provides direct protection in cardiovascular diseases, since it is atheroprotective with antiatherogenic potential through G1-specific altering of proteins and the cell cycle achieved by means of the remodeling of chromatin activity to arrest cell proliferation in the smooth vascular muscle, a critical cellular component of the blood vessel that plays a key role in the development of atherosclerosis [5].

1.1.4. Neuroprotective Effect

Animal studies with rats reveal that NaBu can stimulate neuronal proliferation in zones that have suffered cerebral ischemia, can markedly reduce cell death and neuroinflammation, and can generate better neurological performance in rats subjected to occlusion of the medial cerebral artery. These affects may be associated with cell proliferation and regulation of the neural progenitor cells after a brain lesion induced by apoplexy [7].

1.1.5. Anticarcinogenic Effect

NaBu is also an important substance in epigenetic regulation that offers benefits at the genetic level, as it can induce re-expression of diverse genes, including HDACs (Section 5), histone acetylases (Section 5), and pro-apoptotic (Section 5 and 6), anti-apoptotic (Section 5), and differentiation genes (Section 5).

In this context, NaBu has the potential to exert an effect in quimioprevention secondary to treatment with antineoplastic drugs, and in the control of other types of diseases, by decreasing growth and activating apoptosis in, for example, colon cancer cells.

But it can also act in primary chemoprevention; that is, in the early stages of damage and dysplastic lesions in the epithelia caused by contaminants like cigarette smoke, among others.

The mechanism proposed involves the transcriptional regulation of disintoxication enzymes, like glutathione-sulfhydryl-transferase (GST), as mentioned above. Modulation of the gene GST can protect cells from genotoxic carcinogens, such as H_2O_2 and 4-hydroxynonenal, among others [5]

2. Butyrate and Analogues

After the discovery of the biological properties of butyrate, and once it was demonstrated that high concentrations are required for it to achieve its effect (in the order of mM, and to sustain its effect for more time, minimum 24 hours) other SCFA were analyzed.

Also, a substitute was bound to the original molecule –NaBu– to prolong its effects and reduce the concentrations required. Some of these analogues are described below.

2.1. Valproic Acid

Valproic acid (VPA), or 2-n-propylpentanoic acid, is a small-chain ramified fatty acid that was discovered –by accident– to act as an anticonvulsive while it was being utilized as a dissolvent (Figure 2).

Today, VPA is used to treat psychiatric diseases such as bipolar syndrome, convulsive disorders, migraine and neuropathic pain. It functions as an HDAC inhibitor, has cytotoxic effects *in vitro* and antitumor potency in *in vivo* systems, either alone or when combined with other chemical and/or cytotoxic agents. It is generally effective in neurological diseases and psychiatric disorders [8].

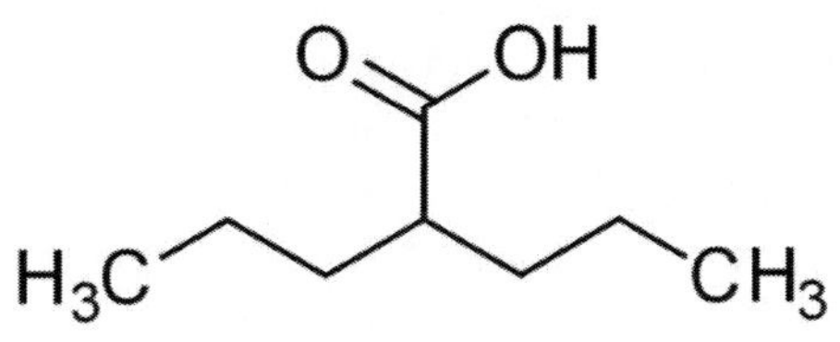

Figure 2. Structure of VPA.

Though usually well tolerated, use of VPA early in pregnancy is associated with a higher risk for congenital deformities, including spina bifida in 1 to 2% of cases.

Deformities appear to be related to the decrease in the degree of DNA methylation (DNMT) that normally DNMTs recruits HDAC and its inhibition of HDAC affects DNMTs interaction. When inhibited, the HDAC could alter the methylation pattern and, as a result, generate this congenital malformation. VPA functions as a potent HDAC inhibitor.

Since HDACs may be over-expressed in malignant tissue, HDAC inhibitors can produce re-expression of the tumor suppressor genes that are silenced in tumor cells and, potentially, lead to cell differentiation and apoptosis.

As in the case of other biological effects, we know that the primary mechanism of VPA toxicity is interference with mitochondrial β-oxidation, due to its structural similarity to a simple fatty acid. VPA has a powerful effect on acute myeloid leukemia cells, where it demonstrates its ability to induce differentiation and exert antiproliferative and pro-apoptotic effects. However, the responses of patients with this disease are markedly heterogeneous [9].

Children who suffer from it show a reduction of verbal intelligence, and there is an association between exposure to VPA *in utero* and autism in children [10].

Among other therapeutic effects, VPA promotes locomotor recuperation in the posterior members in models of spinal cord injuries, and significantly preserves damaged tissue in rats with sectional spinal trauma [11].

2.2. 4-Phenylbutyrate

This is a phenyl group bound to NaBu, so it is named 4-phenylbutyrate (4-PB) and its structure is shown in Figure 3. This compound has been used in treating disorders of the urea cycle and in some cancers, where it reduces phosphorylation of the E1a factor. It has also been utilized in the management of prostate cancer and, at therapeutic concentrations, has reduced toxicity levels. Also, it has antibacterial effects, confirmed in relation to *Helicobacter pylori* [12].

In addition, 4-PB improves morphological, locomotor and biochemical abnormalities in a zebra fish model with deficiency in the pyruvate dehydrogenase complex, and prevents systemic lactic acidosis induced in mice with partial hepatectomy.

This drug has been approved for use in humans with clearly-marked profiles of deficiency in this enzyme complex with lactic acidosis. 4-PB has demonstrated benefits in treating different types of cancer.

Our current understanding is that it acts as an HDAC action inhibitor by increasing hyper-methylation of the histones, opening chromatin contexts and allowing gene transcription.

Hence, it could be an option for managing patients who are receiving chemotherapy for different types of tumors [13]. Oral administration of 4-PB helps the innate immune response of the pulmonary mucosa, as it increases expression of innate defense proteins.

Mutations in the gene that codifies the surfactant-C protein are associated with interstitial pulmonary disease in children and adults. It is believed that pathogenesis is related to an accumulation of cytotoxic aggregates of a surfactant-C with a modified conformation.

Treatment with 4-PB is used to rescue at least one mutant from degradation of the proteasome, restore traffic in the endolysosomal pathway, and thus convert the protein into the mature peptide. Therefore, the use of 4-PB may be an option for treating some patients with mutations in this gene [14].

3. Morphological Effects of NaBu in Astrocytoma Cell Lines

3.1. Effects on Cell Morphology

Because it is a 4-carbon organic acid, NaBu has been the subject of study and evaluation, together with other organic acids with 2-to-6 carbon atoms, to compare their effects. Results show that the acids that do not have 4 carbon atoms fail to exert the same effects as NaBu, because the other organic acids can be metabolized more easily, thus allowing them to exercise their biological effects [15]. Findings clearly indicate that NaBu has the greatest effect in inducing expression of alkaline phosphatase as a protein of a rapid evaluation gene in HeLa cells, while also inhibiting the deacetylated state of histones in nuclei of calf thymus.

Moreover, it has proven to be the most effective acid in inducing arrest of proliferation, at least in normal fibroblasts [16]. The arrest of cell proliferation is accompanied by morphological changes, first described by Ginsburg and cols. in 1973 in HeLa cells treated with 5 mM of NaBu. Those cells are normally semicircular in morphology with borders only loosely adhered to the culture surface, but after exposure to 5 mM of NaBu they show significant changes that appear as filaments and protrusions in the form of spines, and an appearance that is more polygonal than semicircular. Also, the cells adhere firmly to the substrate. This effect appears after 7-8 h of exposure and disappears 2 h after washing and transfer of the cells to a medium alone [17]. This change is due to the significant effect on the microtubules of the cytoskeleton, as described below.

In 1978, Macher and cols. also demonstrated the dramatic change in the morphology of the KB cells of epidermoid carcinoma: at low concentrations of 2-4 mM of NaBu the cells change from small polygons to elongated fibroblastoid forms with the formation of membrane processes such as laminae.

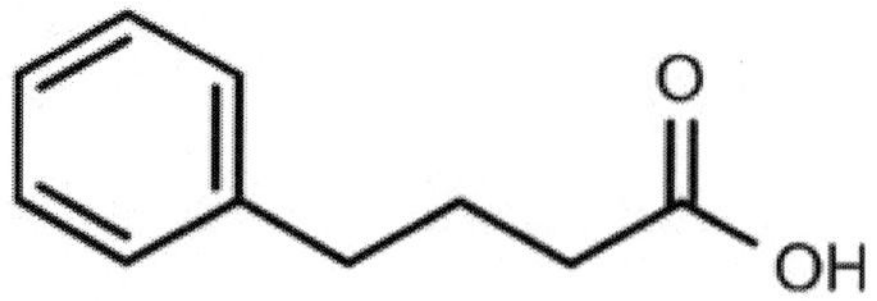

Figure 3. Structure of 4-PB.

Also, their morphological appearance is homogenized with cytoplasmic bridges of cellular connection. This effect is reversible after 24 hours when the cells are returned to the medium alone [18].

3.2. Effects on the Cytoskeleton

In general, all the cells cultivated pertained to cell lines of transformed cells with characteristics that distinguish them from normal ones, including a rounder morphology with smooth borders that are highly refractive to light under clear-field microscopy. Cell-substrate adhesion decreases, as does intercellular communication. In almost all cases with tumor cell lines, NaBu suppresses many of these characteristics of transformed cells and induces a morphology more similar to that of normal cells.

These results may be due to the effect of NaBu on elements of the cytoskeleton [15], since this is one of its most important targets.

Outside the cell, NaBu organizes the glycoprotein fibronectin that NRK kidney cells transformed by the Kisten sarcoma virus normally lack. NaBu also induces secretion of the soluble form of fibronectin in a way similar to its production by normal kidney cells [19].

This explains why in tumor cells in general – that show growth regardless of anchoring– NaBu produces, among other changes, high adhesion efficiency and clonal growth that, moreover, are reversible [20].

3.3. Other Effects of NaBu on Different Types of Cell Lines

Some effects of NaBu are more general on different cell types and depend on activation of the p21 gene with its inhibitor effect on cell proliferation.

However, many other effects are dependent on cell type. Additional effects of NaBu reported are induction of proteins including enzymes, hormones and hemoglobin, reversion of the phenotype of cells transformed to normal morphological and biochemical patterns, higher interferon levels and, with that, greater efficiency of its antiviral action even against integrated viruses.

3.4. Effects on Astrocytoma Cells

With regard to glioma cells, Weingarten and De Vellis [21] demonstrated that in the C6 glioma cell line of rats, hydrocortisone increases the glycerol-phosphate-dehydrogenase enzyme 2-to-3.4-fold.

Simultaneously, epinephrine increases twofold dehydrogenase activity. NaBu interferes completely with the effect produced by hydrocortisone, but without affecting induction by epinephrine.

We now know that NaBu acts at the level of nuclear-type receptors by recruiting co-repressors through a mechanism similar to that achieved by the estradiol receptor in different cell types [22].

3.5. Effects on the Expression of the Glial Fibrillary Acidic Protein in the Morphology of Astrocytoma Cell Lines

In 1997, Engelhards and col. showed that exposure to 2 mM of NaBu for 72 h can increase expression of the glial fibrillary acidic protein (GFAP) by as much as 420%, as a differentiation marker [23].

Later, that working group extended its analysis of the effects of NaBu on 4 astrocytoma cell lines and 2 lines of primary isolates, also during 72h. Their results revealed morphological changes compatible with differentiation and an increase in GFAP expression [24]. In the case of astrocytoma cells, GFAP – an intermediate filament of the cytoskeleton– has been considered a specific marker of astrocytoma differentiation, though in reality it is a protein that can be induced by differentiation inducers like NaBu through a form of induction that depends on the origin of the primary tumor.

Indeed, the WHO's classification of astrocytomas is based on histopathological criteria, including GFAP. Thus, grade I and II astrocytomas conserve morphological characteristics of the tissue that caused them. Here, Chen and cols. (1998) demonstrated that NaBu significantly induces GFAP only in astrocytoma cell lines isolated from low-degree tumors.

Thus, when evaluating NaBu's effect on inducing differentiation as a significant morphological change, it is important to take into account the context of the tumor grade from which the cell lines were isolated [25].

3.6. Morphological Effects on Astrocytoma Cell Lines: Intercellular Bonds, Reduction of the Nucleus/Cytoplasm Ratio and the Presence of Autophagic Vacuoles

Evidence has shown that exposure to 8 mM of NaBu during 24 h can induce important changes in astrocytoma cell lines. For example, the D54-MG cell line has a polygonal morphology with the presence of vacuoles (Figure 4A). After 24 h of exposure to 8 mM of NaBu, these cells reduce the nucleus/cytoplasm ratio but with a significant increase of large vesicles, and an increase in firm intercellular bonds (Figure 4C). When grown in the culture medium alone cells are not positive for cytochemical staining of GFAP with ammoniacal silver (Figure 4D); though it is induced by NaBu despite the fact that it is a line isolated from a glioblastoma multiforme (grade IV), (Figure 4E). This increase in the number of large vesicles in the cytoplasm is significantly similar to that induced by 100 μM of curcumin after 24 h, in this and 3 other astrocytoma cell lines [26]. The U373-MG cell line, in contrast, has a more astrocytic morphology with a high nucleus/cytoplasm ratio and intercellular bonds that are less firm (Figure 4F**).

After exposure to 8 mM of NaBu, these cells change morphologically with firmer bonds and a significant increase in the number of small vacuoles in the cytoplasm (Figure 4H).

Previously, Hernández-Romero and cols. (2013) demonstrated that this cell line is positive for the presence of acidic vacuoles when grown in culture alone; which suggests that the vacuoles correspond to autophagic vesicles.

This, in turn, strongly suggests induction of autophagy by NaBu at 8 mM.

On the other hand, in the presence of curcumin, a low proportion of these autophagic vacuoles of the U373-MG cell line continue to evidence autophagy and appear in numerous large vesicles, which are compatible with the form of cell death known as methuosis [27]. When grown in culture medium alone, this cell line is positive for cytochemical staining with ammoniacal silver (Figure 4L), which proves the presence of GFAP. This cell line was isolated from an anaplastic astrocytoma (GIII), so cytochemical staining increased after exposure to NaBu (Figure 4J). Finally, the T98G cell line presented nuclear pleomorphism and some polyploid cells, which means they show different-sized nuclei (Figure 4K).

Exposure to 8 mM of NaBu standardizes the aspect of the cells (Figure 4L), with nuclei that are less pyknotic and the emergence of large vesicles (Figure 4M). These cells are positive for the cytochemical reaction that reveals GFAP (Figure 4N), which increase in number in the presence of NaBu, which better organizes them (Figure 4O).

4. Ultrastructural Changes Induced by NaBu in Cells

4.1. Electronic Transmission Microscopy Analysis of Melanoma Cells

One of the classic studies describing the effect of NaBu at the ultrastructural level was conducted by Nordenberg and cols. [28] in 1987. They described how a membrane enzyme like gamma-glutamyl-transpeptidase increases due to the effect of a higher concentration of NaBu, from 0.5 to 2 mM. Also, activity of the NADPH-cytochrome C reductase enzyme, one characteristic of the endoplasmic reticulum, increased.

Ultrastructurally, under electronic transmission microscopy, this group described an increase of the endoplasmic reticulum. Another of their important findings was the presence of drops of free lipids in the cytoplasm of melanoma cells, which they also reported for fibroblasts. In this case, treatment with NaBu induced higher activity of the enzyme glycerol-phosphate dehydrogenase, a key enzyme in adipocyte differentiation [29].

4.2. Electronic Transmission Microscopy Analysis of the Effects of NaBu on Astrocytoma Cell

Evidence has shown that when the U373-MG and T98G human astrocytoma cell lines are treated for 24 h with 8 mM of NaBu, cellular proliferation decreases [29]. Analysis of microphotographs identified important changes, such as the presence of looser chromatin in the nuclei of the treated cells (Figures 5C, 5D, 5G), and "naked" nucleoli mainly in the U373-MG line (Figures 5C-5D). This cell line has a peculiarity in that it contains autophagic vacuoles described previously by Romero-Hernández and cols. [26] that become visible in the ultrastructure (Figures 5A, 5B) and persist even after exposure to NaBu (Figures 5C, 5D).

The T98G cell line has numerous mitochondria at baseline (Figures 5E, 5F), but after exposure to NaBu the quantity decreases significantly and autophagic vacuoles are visible (Figures 5G, 5H). The nuclei of the T98G cells treated with NaBu also present loose chromatin and, in some cases, "naked" nucleoli that are also loose (Figure 5H).

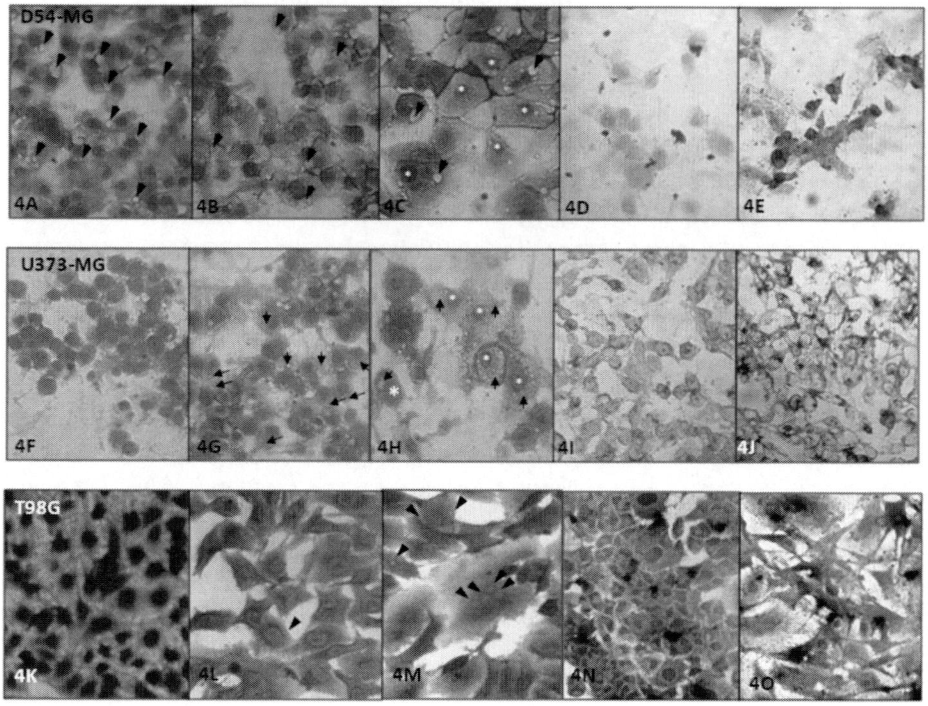

Figure 4. Morphological effects of NaBu on astrocytoma cell lines. D54-MG (4A to 4E), U373-MG (4F to 4J) and T98G (4K to 4O) were exposed to NaBu 8 mM (4B, 4C, 4E, 4G, 4H, 4J, 4L, 4M, 4O). An increase of vesicles with different sizes (arrow head) are evident by violet crystal. Histochemistry by ammoniacal silver (4D, 4E, 4I, 4J, 4N, 4O) was performed to reveal intermediate filaments and glial fibrilar acidic protein. Only D54-MG cells were positive after BuNa exposure (4E). U373-MG and T98G cells were positive in control conditions (medium alone) (4I, 4N) and maintained the signal after NaBu (4J, 4O). All 20X magnification except 4C, 4H, 4M were 40X.

Finally, they reveal an increase of the endoplasmic reticulum, apparently smooth, similar to what occurs in the U373-MG line cell, as reported in mice melanoma cells by Nordenberg and cols. [28].

5. Effects of Sodium Butyrate at the Level of Gene Expresion in Astrocytoma Cells

5.1. Earliest Evidence of the Effect of Sodium Butyrate in Regulating Gene Expression

The first studies conducted to evaluate various effects of sodium butyrate revealed that in addition to finding that this compound arrests cell proliferation and modifies morphology, as described above, it can also induce or repress the expression of different genes [31].

In 1977, Rigs and cols. used HeLa cells and Friend erythroleukemia cells to demonstrate that NaBu increases acetylated histones [32]. Later, it was shown that NaBu can also inhibit HDACs, and that this is its mechanism of action. Therefore, it can favorably affect the appearance of sites sensitive to the action of DNasa I, and a better chromatin digest [33-35].

As a result of histone acetylation, the conformation and folding of the chromatin are modified [36]. Thus, the reduced electrostatic interaction between the phosphate residues of the DNA and the lysine residues in the histones improves chromatin solubility to pH and physiological ionic forces [37].

In relation to the degree of histone acetylation in the nucleosomes, they should not be totally modified to prevent compacting in the nucleus. Early evidence showed that a 46% degree of histone acetylation is sufficient to prevent the organization, folding and closure of the chromatin and to induce transcription by RNApol III [38]. Histone acetylation in the lysine residues of the amino terminal domains interferes with interactions with other proteins or with the DNA itself, thus propitiating the break-up of highly-organized, folded chromatin.

These combined effects, produced by histone acetylation upon generating destabilization of the chromatin and its aperture, facilitate access to RNApol II and gene transcription [39].

Modification of the histones through the action of histone deacetylase inhibitors (*i.e.*, acetylation in lysine residues) is reinforced by the fact that the transcription factors in general recruit histone acetylases that further increase the level of acetylation and, as a result, the transcriptional activity of the gene [40].

The process of histone acetylation in mammal cells normally has 2 dynamics: one fast – $t_{1/2}$ of 3-to-7 min– that generates 10-to-15% of the acetylated histones [41]; the other slower – with a $t_{1/2}$ of 30 min– that modifies 60-to-70% of the remaining histones [42]. The rest of the histones remain unmodified [40].

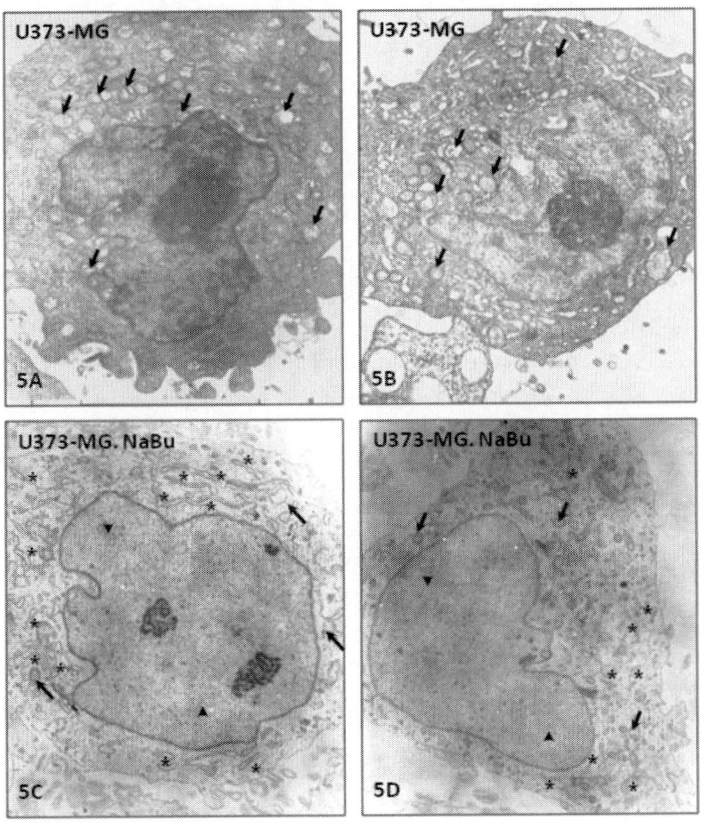

Figure 5. (Continued).

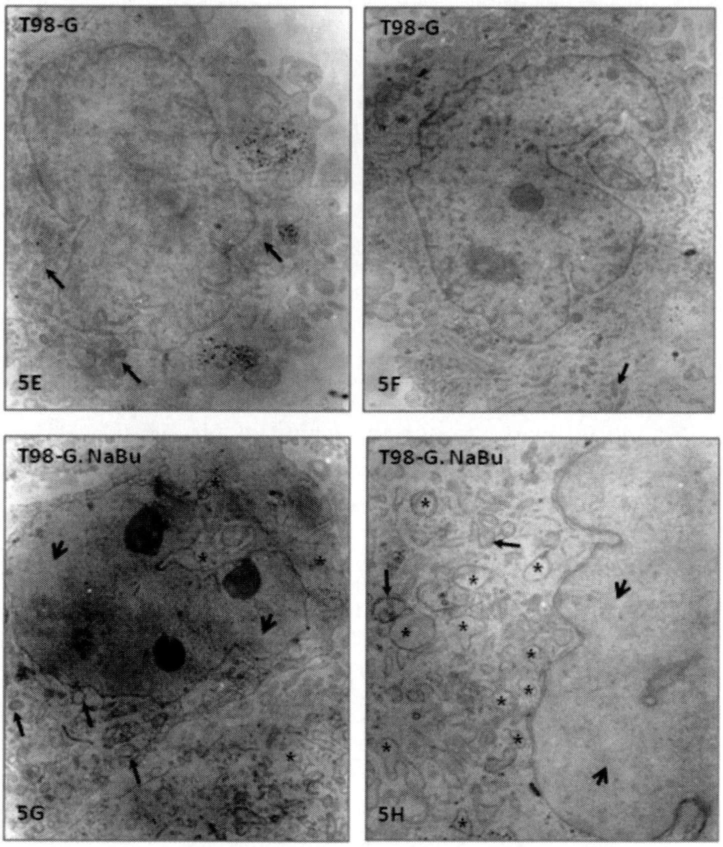

Figure 5. Ultrastructural analysis of NaBu 8 mM effects on astrocytoma cells. U373-MG cells (5A to 5D) and T98G cells (5E to 5H) were anlyzed in fine sections. U373-MG cells in control conditions (medium alone) were characterized with prominent nucleoli and heterochromatin/euchromatin into the nucleous and some autophagyc vesicles (5A, 5B; arrows), but they decreased after NaBu exposure, and cells have hyperplasia of endoplasmic reticulum (asterisk) and a more euchromatinic nuclei (5C, 5D). T98G cells in control conditions have mitochondria (5E, 5F; arrows), they decreased after NaBu exposure but there is an increase of reticulum endoplasmic cysternae dilated (5G, 5H; asterisks). Magnified 5000X. Transmission Electronic Microscopy.

5.2. Response Elements, or *Cis* Sequences of the Response Genes to NaBu

Studies based on analyses of gene expression and response elements to NaBu reveal that this specific organic acid is the most effective one in stimulating or repressing gene transcripttion [44]. Within the sequence of the promoters of the response genes to NaBu there is a response element or sequence to this acid. This response element can be divided into different groups depending on the DNA sequence of the gene involved [45-48].

One group of genes that can be induced or repressed by NaBu shares a DNA sequence in the response element, suggesting that they may have a common transcription factor to this site that could depend on their post-traductional modification, which decides whether to activate or repress gene expression.

The other group shares the promoter binding sites to Sp1/Sp3 in the response elements to NaBu.

Table 1. DNA sequence of the NaBu response element and the corresponding repression/induction effect

EFFECT	SEQUENCE
Repression	AGCCACCTCCA
Repression	. . . . .TO G . . . . .
Induction	. . . . TO .G . . . . .
Induction	. . . . .C. .T. . . . .
Induction	Sp1/Sp3 binding site

The Sp1 and Sp3 transcription factors are expressed in numerous cells in mammals and have a ubiquitous action that can trigger either the activation or repression of gene transcription [49]. The Sp1 factor exerts an action similar to that of the multimers, and thus presents various interactions with other proteins or transcriptional activators, such as histone acetylase p300/CBP, histone 1 deacetylase (HDAC1), E2F1 and the estrogen receptor [50-53]. Whether these factors act to promote or inhibit transcription depends on the abundance and life span of the components that interact with the Sp1multimer. The best example of interacttion among these factors in regulating gene expression is seen in breast cancer tumor lines [54]. One report shows that Sp1 associates with HDAC1 to induce inhibition of gene expression [51]. Both Sp1 and Sp3 are associated with the activity of histone deacetylase in breast cancer cells [54].

5.3. The p21 Gene As an Example of a Target Gene Regulated by NaBu

Analysis of the promoter of gene p21 reveals the presence of 6 binding sites to Sp1/Sp3 as response sites to NaBu. Later, it was shown that factor Sp3 is the one that binds to this gene promoter [55]. Also, the protein with fingers of zinc 89 (ZBP-89) is associated with one or more of these Sp1/Sp3 sites. The mode of action for activating gene expression through the effect of this protein, ZBP-89, involves its capacity to recruit the histone acetylase p300, a co-activator (26). In this way, the differential effect of expressing or repressing gene expression occurs as follows: the ZBP-89 protein could activate the gene by recruiting histone acetylases that open the chromatin context, and if Sp3 expression is induced it could recruit histone deacetylases 1, HDAC1, and inhibit expression of the genes between them to p21 [56, 57].

Then, inhibition of the histone deacetylase activity by NaBu would foster the activity of histone acetylases like p300, thus raising the levels of histone acetylation to that of promoter [57].

Initially, there is an increase in p21 expression to regulate and maintain the cells in interfase in the G1 condition. The p21 protein inhibits activity of the cyclin-dependent kinase E-Cdk2 complex [58] and promotes formation of the cyclin D1-Cdk4/6 complex. Later, expression of p21 is repressed, the levels of its protein decrease and the cyclin E-Cdk2 complex is activated which, in turn, phosphorylates to the protein Rb and is released. The transcription factor E2F then acts to induce expression of the genes that will participate in the S phase of the cell cycle and activate replication [58, 59]. NaBu induces expression of p21 by recruiting the protein ZBP-89 and histone acetylases in the Sp1/Sp3 regions of the gene promoter.

In this way, formation of the cyclin E-Cdk2 complex is reduced and cell division is arrested. As a result, the cells may differentiate or suffer cell death [49]. Since the p21 protein is a generalized regulator of the transition from the G1 phase to the S phase, treatment with NaBu and its effects are observed quite clearly in most of the cells so treated. Finally, NaBu induces all the morphological and ultrastructural effects described previously.

Other effects of NaBu on different cells include DNA repair and genomic recombination, as well as protein synthesis [60, 61], which explains there is an increase of the cisternae in the endoplasmic reticulum as an ultrastructural effect described above (Figure 6).

5.4. Effect of NaBu on the Expression of Genes of Histone Acetylases, Histone Deacetylases and Cell Death in Human Astrocytoma Cell Lines

Since NaBu exerts a significant effect in controlling the expression of proliferation genes, among others, in addition to inducing cell differentiation, this and other histone deacetylase inhibitor compounds have potential therapeutic applications and are already being applied in some cases of the management and control of malignant tumors and in some cases of leukemia. The effect of NaBu on the expression of different types of genes, including the histone deacetylases HDAC1, HDAC3 and HDAC9, the histone acetylases p300 and PCAF, and genes related to cell death, such as BCL2, BAK1, BAX, CASP3 and CASP9, in human astrocytoma cell lines was evaluated. The cell lines used were D54-MG, U373-MG and T98G. A summary of the pattern of gene expression demonstrated that at baseline the D54-MG cell line expressed 8 of the 10 genes evaluated; while the U373-MG and T98G lines expressed only 2 and 3 genes, respectively. After treatment with 12 μm of 5´azacytidine for 24h it was possible to achieve expression of the genes HDAC9 and BAK1, two additional genes of the D54-MG cell line. On the basis of these results it can be concluded that these 2 genes do not seem to contain response elements to NaBu, and that DNA methylation is the key mechanism for repressing their expression. It is important to mention that the D54-MG cell line is made up of a group of cells that lack differentiation markers under cytochemical staining of intermediate filaments of the glial fibrillary acidic protein (Figure 6), when compared to the 2 remaining cell lines that do show differentiation markers.

After treatment with NaBu as a histone deacetylase inhibitor in the U373-MG cell line, 6 additional genes were re-expressed, and re-expression of the remaining one –BAK1– was achieved by the effect of 12 μM of 5´azacytidine. In this way, it became possible to achieve expression of 9 of the 10 genes evaluated. The evidence shows that the genes HDAC1, HDAC3, BCL-2, BAK-1, BAX-1 and CASP3 definitely include among their promoters response elements to NaBu. Only one gene –HDAC9– clearly has another code or response element distinct from that of NaBu. It is possible that mechanisms of histone methylation, among others, form part of this type of regulation. For the case of the T98G cell line, re-expression of 4 of the remaining genes was achieved through the effect of NaBu, thus integrating the expression of 7 of the 10 genes evaluated (Figure 6).

These genes were HDAC1, p300, BCL2, and CASP3; virtually the same ones regulated by NaBu in the U373-MG cell line. Finally, for this cell line (T98G) re-expression of the 3 remaining genes was achieved through treatment with 12 μm of 5´azacytidine, proving that its regulation takes place through DNA methylation.

The evidence has shown that each one of these cell lines could represent a different patient, and is characterized by a unique program of epigenetic modification.

Moreover, on some occasions the degree of differentiation correlates with the global pattern of gene expression.

The potential medical applications are imminent; primarily reducing cell proliferation, inducing differentiation (Figure 6), and regulating and re-expressing important genes such as the HDACs, pro-apoptotic genes and caspases, among others.

Finally, the evidence has shown that treatment of diverse pediatric tumor explants with NaBu can reduce the secretion of pro-MMP-9 alone 0.62-fold [62].

6. Applications of Sodium Butyrate in Inducing Cell Death by Photodynamic Therapy

6.1. Applications: The Principle of Photodynamic Therapy

Photodynamic therapy is another non-invasive form of management and control used in Oncology and Dermatology, as it permits treatment of certain solid superficial tumors and benign lesions such as hemangiomas, among others [63].

The principle behind it is administration of a photosensibilizer (FS); *i.e.*, a chemical compound with certain properties that is allowed a certain time to extend and accumulate in the lesion. Later, the FS-enriched lesion is exposed to light at a wavelength that excites the FS through absorption of the energy of photons. This activation energy then triggers a photo-chemical reaction that normally leads to the formation of reactive oxygen species [64], thus inducing oxidative damage in some cell components, such as the membrane lipids, which produces a cytotoxic effect, followed by cell death.

Together with the lipids, DNA may also be among the target components of the oxidative stress generated by the photodynamic effect and evaluated as a toxic effect [65].

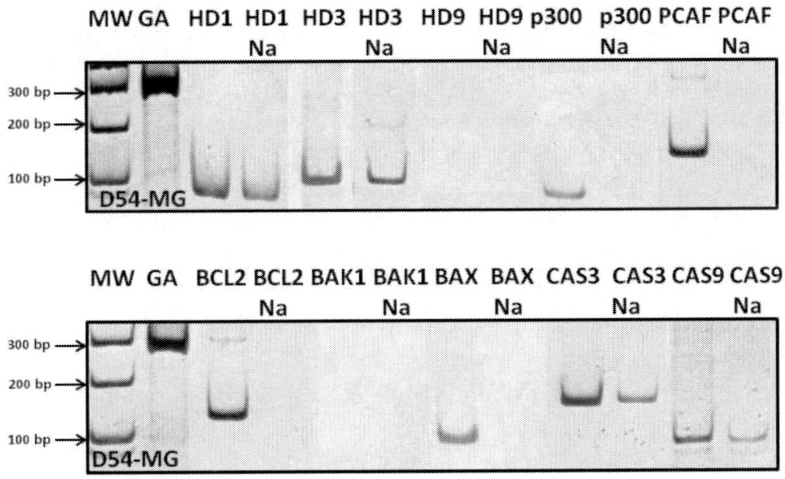

Figure 6. (Continued).

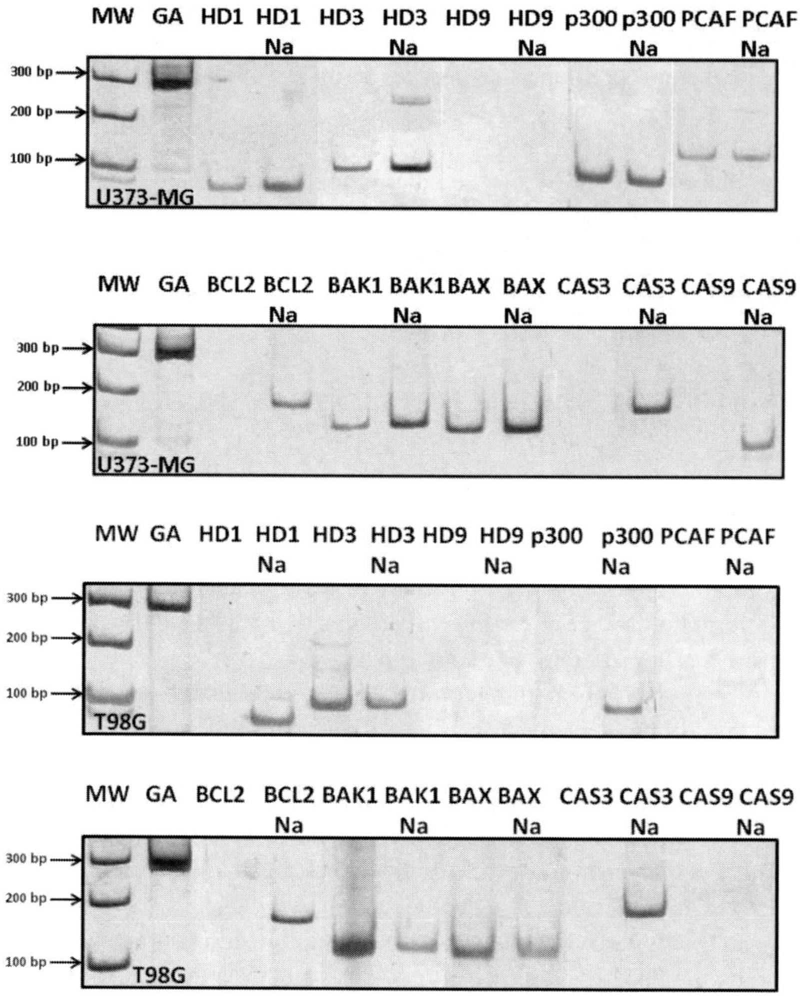

Figure 6. Pattern of expression of several genes in D54-MG (6A), U373-MG (6B) and T98G (6C) cell lines, and the effect of NaBu 8 mM (Na) in each line is illustrated. Expression of the constitutive gene, glyceraldehyde phospate dehydrogenase (GA) is shown in second lane. Markers of molecular weight are in the first lane (MW). The genes were HD1, HDAC1; HD3, HDAC3; HD9, HDAC9; CAS3, CASPASE 3; CAS9, CASPASE 9. Electrophoresis in acrylamide at 10% with silver stain.

6.2. Effect of NaBu in Improving Response to Photodynamic Therapy in Astrocytoma Cell Lines

The evidence has shown that NaBu exerts 2 principal effects:

1. Increasing histone acetylation in the treated cells while loosening the chromatin [64]; and,
2. Modulating the differential gene expression of different classes of genes, from histone acetylase inhibitors and, histone acetylases, p21, to genes related to apoptosis [66].

The principle of photodynamic therapy is based on the accumulation of the FS molecule in the cells [67]. An endogenous FS molecule exists which is represented as protoporphyrin IX (PpIX). We know that tumor cells have deficient ferrochelatase activity, the enzyme that incorporates the iron atom into the center of the heme group of the PpIX, which is required for accumulation [66].

The evidence has shown that accumulation of PpIX in the presence of the precursor, δ-aminolevulinic acid, is different between the D54-MG and U373-MG cell lines. The former has higher concentrations of 0.36 ± 0.10 μg/2.5X10^6 cells compared to 0.12 ± 0.04 μg/2.5 X10^6 for the latter. In these conditions they were exposed to 80 J/cm^2 with a laser at a wavelength of 488 nm. Cell death was evaluated at 24 h, and results showed 4.45% and 0.06% of cell death in the D54-MG and U373-MG cell lines, respectively.

Given an exposure to 8 mM of NaBu for 24 h, followed by exposure to 80 μM of δ-aminolevulinic acid, δ-ALA, the PpIX precursor. In effect, results revealed a significant increase in cell death of 96.70% and 70.62% in these conditions for the D54-MG and U373-MG cell lines, respectively. These findings corroborated the notion that the increase in induction of cell death depends on the change in the chromatin, which increases acetylation of the H4 histone, and not on the increase in FS levels, since cell death in the presence of the precursor alone, δ-ALA, only reached 28.89% and 16.67%, respectively, for the D54-MG and U373-MG cell lines. These results confirm that the first effect of NaBu in inducing chromatin loosening is important and allows a significant increase in cell death induced by photodynamic therapy [64].

Another aspect that is reinforced is the capacity to express genes related to cell death in these cell lines through the effect of NaBu. The U373-MG cell line does not normally express the CASP3 and CASP9 genes, but NaBu induces their expression by 0.43 and 0.40 times, respectively. Also, the BAX and BAK1 genes increase expression by 0.23 and 0.16 times, respectively, due to the effect of NaBu [31].

This may also explain, at least in part, why cell death increased in this cell line. Finally, for the D54-MG cell line, no regulation effect of NaBu was observed on the increase in the expression of these genes, a finding that also supports the result obtained of a high percentage of cell death in this cell line, described above: from 4.45% in control conditions to 96.70% under previous exposure for 24h to NaBu, followed by exposure to δ-ALA [64].

These results are important because they reinforce the idea that NaBu significantly increases cell death induced by Photodynamic Therapy.

This result is similar to the one described Kim et al. (2006) who obtained an increase in cell death after treatment with radiotherapy [68].

7. Future Perspectives

The profile that arises at first sight is that management and treatment of many chronic-degenerative diseases must be modified by incorporating schemes that combine medications already protocolized on the basis of many years of experience and applying compounds in which cells respond and that, in turn, modify the structure of the chromatin, thus fostering histone acetylation, which is the net effect of NaBu as a histone acetylase inhibitor. In some pathologies, such as certain leukemias, NaBu induces differentiation.

In other tumors, like astrocytic ones, differentiation can be induced to give them more regular borders that would facilitate more complete surgical resection, or lower the indexes of tumor proliferation. The use of antineoplastic drugs for many years also selects for chemo-resistant tumors that represent an ongoing challenge for Oncology.

The use of such modifiers as NaBu thus opens new doors for the control and management of tumors, based on the principle of chromatin organization and modification of the principle components, such as histone hyperacetylation.

This represents an example of the application of the basic principles of DNA organization as a means of managing and controlling cells with alterations in different processes, such as proliferation, differentiation, cell death, and other biochemical processes.

Finally, it is important to recognize that simple compounds like NaBu –an organic acid produced by fermentation of whole grain fiber– can exert biological effects as powerful as those described in this chapter; which at the tissue level have more marked effects in terms of chromatin organization as packed by the DNA in the nucleus, which is one of the most elemental and basic functions in Biology.

Conclusion

After analyzing the different effects of NaBu, we must recognize in general two important effects that this compound produces in the cells:

1. Modifying the chromatin towards a looser conformation that can enhance interaction of antineoplastic compounds and other intermediate radiotherapy reagents, among others, with the DNA and damage it; and,
2. Regulation of gene expression, mainly of the negative regulators of the cell cycle, such as p21, and inducers of differentiation and/or cell death and/or chromatin modifiers genes.

Finally, we should mention the effects that this substance has on the cytoplasm, including hyperplasia of the endoplasmic reticulum, which reflect a more active metabolic condition and increased protein synthesis activity and/or store some kind of lipids (hyperplasia of smooth endoplasmic reticulum). These effects are practically unique to this 4-carbon-atom organic acid, because other acids with more, or fewer, than 4 carbon atoms do not present these effects, which are therefore unique to NaBu, a molecule that is selected in some way by the histone deacetylases, HDACs, and propitiates non-competitive, but effective, inhibition at such high concentrations as 8 mM applied for short periods due to its activity that, though less sustained, is still effective, unlike many chemical agents.

Finally, this substance has the additional advantage of being a molecule that is not foreign to the organism and has important biological activities.

ACKNOWLEDGMENTS

To Dirección de Investigación of the Hospital Infantil de México Federico Gómez and to Coordinación de Investigación of the Universidad Simón Bolívar to support the expenses of production of this chapter.

REFERENCES

[1] Canani, R. B., Di Costanzo, M. D., Leone, L., Pedata, M., Meli, R., Calignano, A. Potencial beneficial effects of butyrate in intestinal and extraintestinal diseases. *Worl J. Gastroenterol*. 2011;17(12):1519-1528.

[2] Sossai, P. Butyric acid: what is the future for this old substance?. *Swiss Med. Wkly*. 2012;142:w13596.

[3] Russo, I., Luciani, A., De Cicco, P., Troncone, E., Ciacci, C. Butyrate attenuates lipopolysaccharide-induced inflammation in intestinal cells and Crohn´s mucosa through modulation of antioxidant defense machinery. *PLos ONE*. 2012;7(3):e32841.

[4] Ohira, H., Fujioka, Y., Katagiri, C., Mamoto, R., Aoyama-Ishikawa, M., Amako, K., Izumi, Y., Nishiumi, S., Yoshida, M., Usami, M., Ikeda, M. Butyrate attenuates inflammation and lipolysis generated by the interaction of adipocytes and macrophages. *J. Atheroscler. Thromb*. 2013;(20):425-442.

[5] Canani, B., Di Costanzo, M., Leone, L. The epigenetic effects of butyrate: potential therapeutic implications for clinical practice. *Clin. Epigenetics*. 2012;4(1):4.

[6] Lin, H. V., Frassetto, A., Kowalik, E. J. Jr, Nawrocki, A. R., Lu, M. M., Kosinsky, J. R., Hubert, J. A., Szeto, D., Yao, X., Forrest, G., Marsh, D. J. Butyrate and propionate protect against diet-induced obesity and regulate gut hormones via free fatty acid receptor 3-indipendent mechanisms. *PloS One*. 2012;7(4):e35240.

[7] Kim, H. J., Leeds, P., Chuang, D. M. The HDCA inhibitor, sodium butyrate, stimulates neurogenesis in the ischemic brain. *J. Neurochem*. 2009;110:1226-1240.

[8] Zhang, L., Ma, N., Liu, Q., Ma, Y. Genome-Wide Screening for genes associated with valproic acid sensitivity in fission yeast. *PLoS ONE*. 2013;8(7): e68738.

[9] Fredly, H., Gjertsen, B. T., Bruserud, O. Histone deacetylase inhibition in the treatment of acute myeloid leukemia: the effects of valproic acid on leukemic cells, and the clinical and experimental evidence for combining valproic acid with other antileukemic agents. *Clin. Epigenetics*. 2013;5:12.

[10] Favre, M. R., Barkat, T. R., Lamendola, D., Khazen, G., Markram, H., Markram, K. General developmental health in the VPA- rat model of autism. *Front Behav. Neurosci*. 2013;7:88.

[11] Lu, W. H., Wang, C. Y., Chen, P. S., Wang, J. W., Chuang, D. M., Yang, C. S., Tzeng, S. F. Valproic acid attenuates microgliosis in injured spinal cord and purinergic P2X4 receptor expression in activated microglia. *J. Neurosci. Res*. 2013;91(5):694-705.

[12] Lo, C. Y., Cheng, H. L., Hsu, J. L., Liao, M. H., Yen, R. L., Chen, Y. C. The antimicrobial activities of phenylbutyrates against Helicobacter pylori. *Chem. Pharm. Bull*. 2013;61(6):604-610.

[13] Ferriero, R., Brunetti-Pierri, N. Phenylbutyrate increases activity of pyruvate dehydrogenase complex. *Oncotarget*. 2013;4(6):804-805.

[14] Stewart, G. A., Ridsdale, R., Martin, E. P., Na, C. L., Xu, Y., Mandapaka, K., Weaver, T. E. 4-Phenylbutyric acid treatment rescues trafficking and processing of a mutant surfactant protein-C. *Am. J. Respir. Cell Mol. Biol*. 2012;47(3):324-331.

[15] Kruh, J. Effects of sodium butyrate, a new pharmacologic agent, on cells in culture. *Mol. Cell. Biochem*. 1982;42(2):65-82.

[16] Davie, J. R. Inhibition of histone deacetylase activity by butyrate. *J. Nutr*. 2003;2485S-2493S.

[17] Ginsburg, E., Salomon, D., Sreevalsan, T., Freese, E. Growth inhibition and morphological changes caused by lipophilic acids in mammalian cells. *Proc. Natl. Acad. Sci.* 1973;70(8):2457-2461.

[18] Macher, B. A., Lockney, M., Moskal, J. R., Fung, Y. K., Sweeley, C. C. Studies on the mechanism of butyrate-induced morphological changes in KB cell. *Exp. Cell Res*. 1978; 117(1):95-102.

[19] Hayman, E. G., Engvall, E., Ruoslahti, E. Butyrate restores fibronectin at surface of transformed cells. *Exp. Cell. Res*. 1980;127(2):478-481.

[20] Leavitt, J., Barrett, J. C., Crawford, B. D., Ts'O, P. O. Butyric acid suppression of the in vitro neoplastic state of Syrian hamster cells. *Nature*.1978;271(5642):262-265.

[21] Weingarten, D., de Vellis, J. Selective inhibition bye sodium butyrate of the flucocorticoid induction of glycerol phosphate dehydrogenase in glial cultures. *Biochem. Biophys. Res. Commun*. 1980;93(4):1297-1304.

[22] Ropero, S., Esteller, M. The role of histone deacetylases (HDACs) in human cancer. *Mol. Oncol*. 2007;1(1):19-25.

[23] Engelhard, H. H., Duncan, H. A., Dal Canto, M. Molecular characterization of glioblastoma cell differentiation. *Neurosurgery*. 1997;41(4):886-896.

[24] Engelhard, H. H., Duncan, H. A., Kim, S., Criswell, P. S., Van Eldrik, L. Therapeutic effects of sodium butyrate on glioma cells in vitro and in the rat C6 glioma model. *Neurosurgery*. 2001;48(3):616-624.

[25] Chen, M. H., Yang, W. K., Whang-Peng, J., Lee, L. S., Huang, T. S. Differential inducibilities of GFAP expression, cytostasis and apoptosis in primary cultures of human astrocytic tumours. *Apoptosis*. 1998;3(3):171-182.

[26] Romero-Hernández, M. A., Eguía Aguilar, P., Perézpeña-Diaz, C., Rodríguez-Leviz, A., Sadowinski-Pine, S., Velasco-Rodríguez, L. A., Cáceres Cortés, J. C., Arenas-Huertero, F. Toxic effects induced by curcumin in human astrocytoma cell lines. *Toxicol. Mech. Methods*. 2013;23(9):650-659.

[27] Robinson, M. W., Overmeyer, J. H., Young, A. M., Erhardt, Pw, Maltese, W. A. Syntesis and evaluation of indole-based chalcones as inducers of methuosis, a novel type of nonapoptotic cell death. *J. Med. Chem*. 2012;55(5):1940-1956.

[28] Nordenberg, J., Wasserman, L., Peledl, A., Malik, Z., Stenzel, K. H., Novogrodsky, A. Biochemical and ultrastructural alterations accompany the anti-proliferative effect of butyrate on melanoma cells. *Br. J. Cancer*. 1987;55(5):493-497.

[29] Wawra, E. Long-term effects of sodium butyrate on mouse fibroblasts: A model for differentiation. *Cell. Mol. Biol*. 1986;32(2):121-129.

[30] Solís-Paredes, M., Eguía-Aguilar, P., Chico-Ponce de León, F., Sadowinski-Pine, S., Pérezpeña-Diazconti, M., Arenas-Huertero, F. Epigenetic modifications in cell lines of

human astrocytoma differentially regulate expression of apoptotic genes. *Childs Nerv. Syst.* 2013; Aug.

[31] Prasad, K. N., Sinha, P. K. Effect of sodium butyrate on mammalian cells in culture: a review. *In Vitro*. 1976;12(2):125–132.

[32] Riggs, M. G., Whittaker, R. G., Neumann, J. R., Ingram, V. M. n-Butyrate causes histone modification in HeLa and Friend erythroleukaemia cells. *Nature*. 1977; 268 (5619):462–464.

[33] Candido, E. P., Reeves, R., Davie, J. R. Sodium butyrate inhibits histone deacetylation in cultured cells. *Cell*. 1978;14(1):105–113.

[34] Boffa, L. C., Vidali, G., Mann, R. S., Allfrey, V. G. Suppression of histone deacetylation in vivo and in vitro by sodium butyrate. *J. Biol. Chem.* 1978;253(10): 3364–3366.

[35] Vidali, G., Boffa, L. C., Bradbury, E. M., Allfrey, V. G. Butyrate suppression of histone deacetylation leads to accumulation of multiacetylated forms of histones H3 and H4 and increased DNase I-sensitivity of the associated DNA sequences. *Proc. Natl. Acad. Sci. US.* 1978;75(5):2239–2243.

[36] Garcia-Ramirez, M., Rocchini, C., Ausio, J. Modulation of chromatin folding by histone acetylation. *J. Biol. Chem*. 1995; 270(30):17923–17928.

[37] Wang, X., He, C., Moore, S. C., Ausio, J. Effects of histone acetylation on the solubility and folding of the chromatin fiber. *J. Biol. Chem.* 2001;276(16):12764–12768.

[38] Tse, C., Sera, T., Wolffe, A. P., Hansen, J. C. Disruption of higher-order folding by core histone acetylation dramatically enhances transcription of nucleosomal arrays by RNA polymerase III. *Mol. Cell. Biol.* 1998;18(8):4629–4638.

[39] Nightingale, K. P., Wellinger, R. E., Sogo, J. M., Becker, P. B. Histone acetylation facilitates RNA polymerase II transcription of the Drosophila hsp26 gene in chromatin. *EMBO J*. 1998;17(10):2865–2876.

[40] Davie, J. R., Moniwa, M. Control of chromatin remodeling. *Crit. Rev. Eukaryot. Gene Expr*. 2000;10(3-4):303–325.

[41] Sun, J. M., Chen, H. Y., Davie, J. R. Effect of estradiol on histone acetylation dynamics in human breast cancer cells. *J. Biol. Chem*. 2001;276(52):49435–49442.

[42] Davie, J. R. Nuclear matrix, dynamic histone acetylation and transcriptionally active chromatin. *Mol. Biol. Rep*. 1997;24(3):197–207.

[43] Kruh, J. Effects of sodium butyrate, a new pharmacological agent, on cells in culture. *Mol. Cell. Biochem*. 1982;42(2):65–82.

[44] Yang, J., Kawai, Y., Hanson, R. W., Arinze, I. J. Sodium butyrate induces transcription from the G alpha(i2) gene promoter through multiple Sp1 sites in the promoter and by activating the MEK-ERK signal transduction pathway. *J. Biol. Chem*. 2001;276(28): 25742–25752.

[45] Siavoshian, S., Segain, J. P., Kornprobst, M., Bonnet, C., Cherbut, C., Galmiche, J. P., Blottiere, H. M. Butyrate and trichostatin A effects on the proliferation/differentiation of human intestinal epithelial cells: induction of cyclin D3 and p21 expression. *Gut*. 2000;46(4):507–514.

[46] Tran, C. P., Familari, M., Parker, L. M., Whitehead, R. H., Giraud, A. S. Short-chain fatty acids inhibit intestinal trefoil factor gene expression in colon cancer cells. *Am. J. Physiol*. 1998;275:G85–G94.

[47] Lu, Y., Lotan, R. Transcriptional regulation by butyrate of mouse galectin-1 gene in embryonal carcinoma cells. *Biochim. Biophys. Acta*. 1999;1444(1):85–91.

[48] Walker, G. E., Wilson, E. M., Powell, D., Oh, Y. Butyrate, a histone deacetylase inhibitor, activates the human IGF binding protein-3promoter in breast cancer cells: molecular mechanism involves an Spl/Sp3 multiprotein complex. *Endocrinology.* 2001:142(9):3817–3827.

[49] Davie, J. R. Inhibition of histone deacetylase activity by butyrate. *J. Nut.* 2003; 133: 24 85S-2493S.

[50] Ryu, S., Zhou, S., Ladurner, A. G., Tjian, R. The transcriptional cofactor complex CRSP is required for activity of the enhancer-binding protein Sp1. *Nature.* 1999;397 (6718):446–450.

[51] Doetzlhofer, A., Rotheneder, H., Lagger, G., Koranda, M., Kurtev, V., Brosch, G., Wintersberger, E., Seiser, C. Histone deacetylase 1 can repress transcription by binding to Sp1. *Mol. Cell. Biol.* 1999;19(8):5504–5511.

[52] Xiao, H., Hasegawa, T., Isobe, K. p300 collaborates with Spl and Sp3 in p21 (wafl/ cipl) promoter activation induced by histone deacetylase inhibitor. *J. Biol. Chem.* 2000; 275(2):1371–1376.

[53] Porter, W., Saville, B., Hoivik, D., Safe, S. Functional synergy between the transcripttion factor Spl and the estrogen receptor. *Mol. Endocrinol.* 1997;11(11):1569–1580.

[54] Sun, J. M., Chen, H. Y., Moniwa, M., Litchfield, D. W., Seto, E., Davie, J. R. The transcriptional repressor Sp3 is associated with CK2-phosphorylated histone deacetylase 2. *J. Biol. Chem.* 2002;277(39):35783–35786.

[55] Sowa, Y., Orita, T., Minamikawa-Hiranabe, S., Mizuno, T., Nomura, H., Sakai, T. Sp3, but not Spl, mediates the transcriptional activation of the p21/WAF1/Cipl gene promoter by histone deacetylase inhibitor. *Cancer Res.* 1999;59(17):4266–4270.

[56] Bai, L., Merchant, J. L. Transcription factor ZBP-89 cooperates with histone acetyltransferase p300 during butyrate activation of p21wafl transcription in human cells. *J. Biol. Chem.* 2000;275(39):30725–30733.

[57] Richon, V. M., Sandhoff, T. W., Rifkind, R. A., Marks, P. A. Histone deacetylase inhibitor selectively induces p21WAF1 expression and gene-associated histone acetylation. *Proc. Natl. Acad. Sci. US.* 2000;97(18):10014–10019.

[58] Cheng, M., Olivier, P., Diehl, J. A., Fero, M., Roussel, M. F., Roberts, J. M., Sherr, C. J. The p21(Cip1) and p27(Kip1) CDK "inhibitors" are essential activators of cyclin D-dependent kinases in murine fibroblasts. *EMBO J.* 1999;18(6):1571–1583.

[59] Roovers, K., Assoian, R. K. Integrating the MAP kinase signal into the G1 phase cell cycle machinery. *Bioessays.* 2000;22(9):818–826.

[60] Polo, S. E., Almouzni, G. Histone metabolic pathways and chromatin assembly factors as proliferation markers. *Cancer Lett.* 2005;220(1):1–9.

[61] Vidanes, G. M., Bonilla, C. Y., Toczyski, D. P. Complicated tails: histone modifications and the DNA damage response. *Cell.* 2005;121(7):973–976.

[62] Rodríguez-Salvador, J., Armas-Pineda, C., Pérezpeña-Diazconti, M., Chico-Ponce de León, F., Sosa-Sáinz, G., Lezama, P., Recillas-Targa, F., Arenas-Huertero, F. Effect of sodium butyrate on the pro-matrix metalloproteinase-9 and -2 differential secretion in pediatric tumors and cell lines. *J. Exp. Clin. Cancer Res.* 2005;24(3):463-473.

[63] Schmidt-Erfurth, U., Diddens, H., Birngruber, R., Hasan, T. Photodynamic targeting of human retinoblastoma cells using covalent low-density lipoprotein conjugates. *Br. J. Cancer.* 1997;75(1):54–61.

[64] Flores-Ancona, R. M., García-Gómez, F. Y., Jiménez-Betanzos, A. M., Solís-Paredes, M., Castro-Leyva, V., Cruz-Orea, A., Arenas-Huertero, F., Ramón-Gallegos, E. Effects of sodium butyrate on cell death induced by photodynamic therapy in U373-MG and D54-MG astrocytoma cell lines. *Photochem. Photobiol.* 2009; 85(5):1182-1188.

[65] Oleinick, N. L., Morris, R. L., Belichenko, I. The role of apoptosis in response to photodynamic therapy: What, where, why and how. *Photochem. Photobiol. Sci.* 2002;1 (1):1–21.

[66] Bueno-Carrazco, J., Castro-Leyva, V., García-Gomez, F., Solís-Paredes, M., Ramón-Gallegos, E., Cruz-Orea, A., Eguía-Aguilar, P., Arenas-Huertero, F. Sodium butyrate increases the effect of the photodynamic therapy: a mechanism that involves modulation of gene expression and differentiation in astrocytoma cells. *Childs Nerv. Syst.* 2012;28(10):1723-1730.

[67] Kessel, D., Woodburn, K. Biodistribution of photosensitizing agents. *Int. J. Biochem.* 1993;25(10):1377–1383.

[68] Kim, I. A., Shin, J. H., Kim, I. H., Kim, J. H., Kim, J. S., Wu, H. G., Chie, E. K., Ha, S. W., Park, C. I., Kao, G. D. Histone deacetylases inhibitor-mediated radiosensitization of human cancer cells: class differences and the potential influence of p53. *Clin. Cancer Res.* 2006;12:940-949.

In: Butyrate: Food Sources, Functions and Health Benefits ISBN: 978-1-63117-657-9
Editor: Cong-Jun Li © 2014 Nova Science Publishers, Inc.

Chapter 8

BUTYRATE, WNT SIGNALING AND COLORECTAL CANCER

Michael Bordonaro * ***and Darina L. Lazarova***

Department of Basic Sciences, The Commonwealth Medical College, Scranton, PA, US

ABSTRACT

Diet modulates colorectal cancer (CRC) incidence; for example, dietary fiber intake reduces the risk of this malignancy. Treatment of CRC cells *in vitro* with the histone deacetylase inhibitor (HDACi) butyrate, a fermentation product of dietary fiber, modulates WNT/beta-catenin signaling, a pathway which is constitutively activated in the majority of CRCs, and induces apoptosis. Analyses of CRC cell lines exposed to butyrate have established that the levels of apoptosis are dependent upon the fold induction of WNT/beta-catenin transcriptional activity. Therefore, fiber, a major source of butyrate in the colon, may reduce CRC risk through butyrate-mediated hyperactivation of WNT/beta-catenin signaling in neoplastic cells and their consequent apoptosis. One factor that determines the preventive role of fiber-derived butyrate against CRC is the stage at which the colonic neoplasm is exposed to the agent. Early stage neoplasms are likely the main target of butyrate, since microadenoma cells *in vitro* are more sensitive to the agent than colonic carcinoma cells. Interestingly, epidemiological studies indicate that individuals with fiber intake that is relatively high for a Western type diet (35g/day) are still at risk of developing CRC, albeit that risk is reduced by 40% compared to individuals consuming 15g of fiber/day. These statistics could be explained by the existence of subtypes of colonic neoplasms and the development of butyrate resistance in transformed colonic cells. The existence of CRC subtypes with varying degrees of butyrate sensitivity is suggested by the variability in the levels of induced WNT/beta-catenin activity and apoptosis in butyrate-treated CRC cell lines *in vitro*.

The likelihood that butyrate-resistance develops *in vivo* is supported by the *in vitro* development of butyrate-resistant CRC cells. Since such cells are cross-resistant to clinically relevant HDACis, dissecting the mechanisms underlying the phenomenon is of significance for both CRC prevention and therapy.

* Corresponding author: Michael Bordonaro. Department of Basic Sciences, The Commonwealth Medical College, 525 Pine Street, Scranton, PA 18509. E-mail: mbordonaro@tcmedc.org.

Butyrate resistance might be based upon alterations in WNT/catenin signaling through a partial switch to noncanonical WNT signaling that does not rely on beta-catenin, and modified activity of the remaining beta-catenin – based WNT transcriptional complexes. For example, the extent of association between beta-catenin and the transcriptional coactivators CREB-binding protein (CBP) and p300 influences WNT signaling, and the ability of butyrate to modulate this pathway and apoptosis in a cell-type specific manner. Paradoxically, our increased knowledge about the mechanisms by which butyrate affects CRC cells has multiplied the unanswered questions. We discuss how these questions will shape future studies on butyrate, fiber, and CRC.

Keywords: Butyrate, fiber, WNT/catenin, CBP, p300

Introduction

Overview of Studies on Fiber and Butyrate

Colorectal cancers (CRCs) are amenable to a high degree of prevention through diet [1-3]. In 1971, Burkitt [4] reported an association between high dietary fiber intake (e.g., more than 50 g of fiber/day, [5]) and a low incidence of colon cancer (CC) in African populations. In 2003, two large clinical studies confirmed this relationship [6, 7]. One of them, a large prospective study that included 519,978 individuals from ten European countries (the EPIC study), reported that when the total fiber intake of 15 g/day is increased to 35 g/day, there is a 40% decrease in colon cancer (CC), but not in rectal cancer, incidence [6]. In contrast to these reports, several epidemiological studies have found no relationship between fiber intake and CC incidence [8], even when proper assessment of potential confounders (e.g., dietary factors other than butyrate) was performed [9, 10]. In 2011, based upon more comprehensive meta-analyses of accumulating new studies, the World Cancer Research Fund and the American Institute for Cancer Research upgraded the protective effect of fiber against CC from "probable" to "convincing" [11].

The most recent update of the EPIC study, based upon a longer follow-up time (mean 11 years) and an increased number of CRC cases (4,517), concluded that total dietary fiber is inversely associated with both colon and rectal cancer incidence [12].

The effects of dietary fiber on the incidence of CC have been attributed to several factors, including a decreased exposure of the colonic epithelium to carcinogens, and the fermentation of fiber by colonic anaerobic bacteria to produce acetate, propionate, and butyrate [13, 14]. Of the three short-chain fatty acids, butyrate is of particular interest since it functions as an inhibitor of histone deacetylases (HDACis) and at physiologically relevant concentrations it produces cell cycle arrest, differentiation, and/or apoptosis of CRC cells *in vitro* [15-18].

Concentrations of butyrate in the human colon have been reported based upon analyses of subjects who died suddenly from coronary heart disease or violent death [19]. These analyses indicated that colonic butyrate is present at the highest levels in the caecum (26.1 mM /kg contents), and this concentration decreases to 24.5 mM in the ascending colon, 24.4 mM in the transverse colon, 14.7 mM in the descending colon, and 17.9 mM in the sigmoid colon. The concentration of butyrate in human feces ranges from 11 to 27 mM [20, 21].

Similar to the results from fiber studies, analyses of the effects of butyrate on intestinal cancer have reached controversial conclusions.

Some *in vivo* studies have reported no effect of butyrate on colonic tumorigenesis [22-24]; whereas, others have demonstrated the opposite. Thus, oral administration of the butyrate-producing bacteria *Butyrivibrio fibrisolvens* enhances the rate of butyrate production, and reduces the formation of aberrant crypt foci, an early colonic lesion, in the colon and rectum of mice treated with 1,2-dimethylhydrazine [25].

Kameue *et al.* [26] have reported that in rats with intestinal tumors induced by azoxymethane and deoxycholic acid, dietary sodium gluconate increases the levels of butyrate and decreases the numbers of tumors in the large bowel. A diet supplemented with high-amylose maize starch and butyrate that results in high luminal butyrate is also associated with reduced tumor incidence (number and size) in a rat model of CRC [27]. The inverse relation between intestinal cancer in rats and intake of butyrylated starch is due to augmented apoptosis in the colonic epithelium, and this apoptotic effect of the increased luminal butyrate levels is most prominent in the base and the proliferative zone of the crypts [28]. It is likely that the protective effect of butyrate is due to the removal (via apoptosis) of colonocytes with damaged DNA [29-31].

Lupton has suggested several reasons for the equivocal results from studies on the CC-protective effects of fiber and butyrate: (a) differences between *in vitro* and *in vivo* experimental conditions, (b) stage of neoplastic development versus timing of butyrate application, (c) variable amounts of butyrate achieved in each experiment, (d) effects of fiber that are independent of butyrate production (e.g., transit time of the colonic digesta, fecal bulk, additional bioactive agents present in the fiber), and (e) the effect of other dietary components on the activity of dietary fiber [32]. We have also proposed that the existence of CC subtypes, individual variations in the butyrate-producing colonic microflora, and the time, at which the colorectal lesions are exposed to fiber/butyrate (early vs. late stages) are factors that might influence the protective role of fiber against CC [33].

Relationship between WNT/ Beta-Catenin Signaling and Apoptosis

A common characteristic of the majority of CRCs is the constitutive activation of the canonical WNT signaling pathway due to mutations in the *APC*, *beta-catenin* and *axin* genes [34-42]. The aberrant activation of this signaling is believed to be the initiating event in colonic tumorigenesis [43, 44]. Canonical WNT signaling (also referred to as WNT/catenin signaling) is induced by the binding of WNT ligands to their cell surface receptors and the consequent inhibition of glycogen synthase kinase-3 beta (GSK-3beta) activity [45, 46].

Active GSK-3beta, in complex with adenomatous polyposis coli (APC) and Axin, promotes the phosphorylation and degradation of beta-catenin [34-36].

However, when GSK-3beta activity is inhibited, dephosphorylated beta-catenin accumulates and interacts with TCF/LEF DNA binding proteins [37-41, 47].

Beta-catenin-TCF (BCT) transcriptional complexes can be detected by their ability to drive transcription from TCF/LEF binding site-containing promoter constructs [39, 40].

We have discovered that butyrate hyperinduces WNT/catenin transcriptional activity in SW620 CRC cells [48], a finding that was unexpected since, prior to our analyses, only the downregulation of WNT activity has been associated with CRC cell apoptosis.

However, subsequent analyses of ten human CRC cell lines exposed to butyrate have confirmed this initial finding, and have established a linear causative relationship between the fold induction of WNT/catenin transcriptional activity and the level of apoptosis [49]. Butyrate induces low levels of apoptosis and reversible growth arrest in CRC cells with no, or low, levels of induced WNT/catenin signaling; whereas, CRC cells that respond to butyrate with high levels of induced WNT signaling exhibit a strong apoptotic response [49].

Suppression of the butyrate-induced increase in WNT/catenin activity through the use of dominant negative TCF4 [39] decreases apoptosis of CRC cells, demonstrating a causative connection between the hyperactivation of WNT/catenin signaling and apoptosis [49]. Both hyperactivation of WNT/catenin signaling and apoptosis are insignificant in RKO CRC cells that do not have mutations in the WNT/beta-catenin pathway [49].

A number of *in vivo* studies support the causal association between enhanced WNT/catenin activity and apoptosis. Thus, (a) homozygous mutation in the *Drosophila* homolog of *APC* results in neuronal cell apoptosis in the *Drosophila* retina [50]; (b) expression of stable, amino-terminally truncated beta-catenin results in a 3- to 4-fold higher apoptotic level in the intestinal villi of transgenic mice [51]; (c) conditional targeting of *Apc* in murine neural crest cells results in massive apoptosis of cephalic and cardiac neural crest cells at 11.5 days post coitum [52]; (d) expression of constitutively active beta-catenin in 129/Sv cells of chimeric mice results in apoptosis of these cells [53], and (e) WNT transcriptional activity upregu-lates the expression of the two pro-apoptotic genes *BAX* and *BOK* [54].

How can these findings be reconciled with the known ability of WNT/catenin signaling to promote cell proliferation? We propose that canonical WNT/catenin activity exists as a gradient, within which absence of WNT signaling corresponds to terminal differentiation and apoptosis, relatively low levels lead to controlled self-renewal, moderate levels promote uncontrolled cell proliferation (as in cancer), and relatively high levels result in apoptosis [55]. This concept is consistent with the "just right hypothesis" for CRC formation, which is derived from the observation that, in colorectal adenomas of patients with familial adenomatous polyposis, there is a selection for *APC* mutants that retain some ability to downregulate WNT/catenin activity [56]. According to this model, complete inactivation of APC leading to high levels of WNT/catenin signaling is not advantageous for tumor formation. Cells with *APC* mutations that result in moderate levels of WNT/catenin signaling proliferate and give rise to tumors; whereas, cells with relatively high levels of WNT/catenin activity due to different *APC* mutations are eliminated by apoptosis. This interpretation is supported by murine studies, in which two types of *Apc* mutations were compared: of the two analyzed mutations, the one that resulted in lower levels of nuclear beta-catenin (Apc^{1322T}) led to more severe polyps, with earlier onset, and more numerous adenomas [57].

The Existence of CC Subtypes May Influence the Association between High Fiber Intake and Lowered Risk for CC

The hyperactivation of WNT/catenin signaling by butyrate takes place only in colonic neoplastic cells with mutations in the pathway, and such mutations are detected in 80% of sporadic colon cancers [39, 58].

Based upon our *in vitro* findings [48, 49, 59] we have proposed that at sufficiently high levels, dietary butyrate hyperinduces WNT/catenin signaling, which is already constitutively activated by mutations in CC cells, and this spike in WNT/catenin activity augments apoptosis [55]. Therefore, aberrant WNT/catenin signaling, which initiates the tumorigenic process in colonic cells, also makes the cells vulnerable to the pro-apoptotic action of butyrate. In contrast, in normal colonic epithelial cells, for which butyrate is a main energy source [60], it is likely that the short-chain fatty acid supports proliferation by maintaining low to moderate levels of WNT/catenin signaling [55]. Human studies have revealed the effect of butyrate on the homeostasis of healthy colonic cells; thus, a two-week long series of daily butyrate enemas increased transcriptional regulation of pathways affecting fatty acid metabolism, electron transport and oxidative stress [61].

The differential effect of butyrate on normal and neoplastic colonic cells constitutes the "butyrate paradox", and based upon our data, we propose that only CRC cells with mutations in the WNT/catenin pathway, which are able to hyperactivate this signaling, respond to butyrate with apoptosis [49, 59]. There are alternative explanations for the butyrate paradox, and some of these hypothetical mechanisms could also be linked to the constitutive activation of WNT/catenin signaling in most CRCs. Thus, it has been proposed that a change in the preferred energy source (e.g., glucose instead of butyrate) accounts for the different response of normal and neoplastic colonic cells to butyrate [62, 63]. Singh *et al.* have observed that under standard culture conditions (25 mM glucose), butyrate inhibits growth and induces apoptosis in CRC cells [62]. The cells also exhibit increased apoptosis in absence of glucose; however, low butyrate concentrations (0.5 to 2 mM) reduce the apoptosis induced by glucose deprivation, and maintain cell proliferation [62]. Thus, whether butyrate is growth-stimulatory or growth-inhibitory may depend upon the availability of other energy sources.

Interestingly, a switch from mitochondrial oxidative respiration to aerobic glycolysis (Warburg effect) is common in cancer cells, and more recently, it has been proposed that the Warburg effect combined with the histone acetylation changes induced by butyrate explain the butyrate paradox [64]. The possibility that in CRC cells butyrate functions mostly as a HDACi rather than as an energy source could account for the differential effects of the short-chain fatty acid in normal and malignant colonic cells. This explanation is supported by the observation that synthetic HDACis, structurally unrelated to butyrate, mimic the activity of butyrate on CRC cells [59, 65].

Interestingly, in addition to butyrate [49, 59], glucose also augments, albeit to a limited extent, WNT/beta-catenin transcriptional activity [66]. The upregulation of WNT/catenin signaling by nutrients could have a physiological relevance in normal colonocytes. In such cells, WNT/catenin signaling maintains cell proliferation, and it should be activated in the presence of nutrients (e.g., butyrate, glucose).

However, in the absence of nutrients, proliferation should slow down, and this would be mediated by lower levels of WNT/beta-catenin activity. The increase of WNT/catenin activity in the presence of glucose may contribute to the Warburg effect in cancer cells, as it has been reported that WNT signaling induces a glycolytic switch via increased levels of glycolytic enzymes and glucose consumption [67-69].

Signaling mechanisms other than WNT/catenin activity have also been proposed to explain the differential effect of butyrate on normal and neoplastic colonic cells. Klampfer *et al.*, have reported that the targeted deletion of a mutant k-*ras* allele in CC cells is sufficient to protect the cells from butyrate-induced apoptosis [70].

Further, the authors presented evidence that the *k-ras* activating mutation promotes apoptosis, at least in part, through its ability to downregulate the expression of gelsolin, an actin-binding protein that protects cells from butyrate-induced apoptosis. There might be additional factors and/or other members of the KRAS signaling pathway that modulate the apoptosis of human CRC cells by butyrate, as in the analyses of 10 CRC cell lines we have observed that cells with differential response to butyrate have similar mutation status of *KRAS,* and/or its downstream mediator *BRAF* [49]. For example, among the CRC cells that commit to high levels of apoptosis are: COLO201 (*KRAS* wild type, *BRAF* mutant), HCT-116 (*KRAS* mutant type, *BRAF* wild), LS174T (*KRAS* mutant, *BRAF* wild type). CC cell lines that are relatively resistant to the apoptotic effect of butyrate are SW48 (*KRAS* wild type, *BRAF* wild), HT29 (*KRAS* wild type, *BRAF* mutant), LoVo (*KRAS* mutant, *BRAF* wild type), and SW480 (*KRAS* mutant, *BRAF* wild type).

In conclusion, differential effects of butyrate are detected not only in normal versus neoplastic colonic cells, but also within a panel of CRC cells [49]. These findings support the existence of colonic neoplasms with differential sensitivity to the apoptotic effect of butyrate.

Levels of Dietary Fiber Intake and Variations in Colonic Microflora May Modulate the Effects of Fiber on Colon Cancer

The ambiguous findings of *in vivo* studies investigating the effects of butyrate and fiber on intestinal tumorigenesis could be due to the variable levels of intestinal butyrate achieved by different experimental protocols [32]. This interpretation is in agreement with our *in vitro* findings that higher levels of butyrate (5 versus 1-2 mM) result in stronger hyperactivation of WNT/catenin transcriptional signaling and apoptosis in CRC cells [49]. Bingham et al., who reported a strong protective role for fiber against colon cancer, proposed that a previous study reached an opposite conclusion due to lower daily intake of dietary fiber in the analyzed cohort [6]. Thus, the levels of butyrate produced by different amounts of dietary fiber intake may partially explain the variable findings from epidemiological studies [6-12]. Such studies should take into account what constitutes a high fiber-diet; for example, it has been indicated that the daily intake of dietary fiber among the African tribes in which Dr. Denis Burkitt recorded lower incidence of CRC was more than 50 g [4, 5].

The concentration of butyrate in the colonic lumen depends not only upon the amount/ type of consumed fiber, but also on the presence of specific intestinal microorganisms that ferment fiber [19]. Inter-individual variations in the composition of intestinal microbiota, as well as differences in the bacterial species based upon age, gender, and geographic region have been documented and discussed [71-73]. In infants as young as six weeks, in addition to the country/region of birth, even delivery mode and feeding method influence the fecal microbiota [74]. With so many factors affecting the composition of colonic microbiota, it is plausible that the same type of dietary fiber intake results in varying levels of colonic butyrate levels in different individuals. However, there is also evidence that the microbiota profile is dynamic, and changes quickly in response to dietary adjustments. For example, Walker et al. reported that 320 phylotypes of human colonic microbiota cluster stronger by individual than by diet; however, qPCR time course analyses revealed reversible 'blooms' in specific bacterial groups upon a dietary change [75]. Therefore, while the inter-individual variations in colonic microbiota may be due to age, gender, and country of origin, there is still a possibility for targeted change in the intestinal bacterial species by dietary modifications [76].

Time of Exposure of Colorectal Lesions to Fiber/Butyrate Influences the Effect of Fiber on CC Incidence

While it is difficult to assess whether fiber and butyrate affect the formation of adenomas or the subsequent progression to carcinomas, several studies suggest that relatively early colonic lesions are more susceptible to the protective role of fiber and butyrate. The timing of butyrate administration with respect to tumor development has already been discussed as a factor influencing the protective role of butyrate against CC [33, 55]. The likelihood that a high fiber intake specifically affects early tumor development in the colon is supported by the report of Peters and colleagues [7], who demonstrated that the association between fiber and adenoma risk does not differ significantly between advanced and non-advanced adenomas.

Therefore, dietary fiber intake may not affect the progression to advanced adenomas (and, subsequently, to carcinomas). These conclusions are consistent with the view that modulation of WNT/catenin activity by butyrate may underlie the protective role of fiber against CRC, as mutations in the WNT/beta-catenin signaling pathway are the earliest events in colonic tumorigenesis [43, 44].

We have found that prolonged *in vitro* exposure of CC cells to relatively low levels of butyrate selects for cell populations that are resistant to the effects of the agent on WNT/catenin activity and apoptosis [59]. The butyrate-resistant cells exhibit cross-resistance to the apoptotic action of structurally unrelated HDACis, suggesting that increased butyrate metabolism is not the mechanism by which resistance is established [59, 109].

Thus, it is plausible that for early stage adenomas, a relatively low intake of dietary fiber, resulting in low levels of colonic butyrate, selects for malignant cells unresponsive to the apoptotic effects of fiber-derived butyrate.

Therefore, later-stage, more advanced adenomas may consist mostly of butyrate-resistant cells. The growth and progression of such colonic lesions to carcinomas would not be affected by increased fiber intake. Our *in vitro* findings therefore suggest that only the continuous intake of relatively high levels of dietary fiber, resulting in high concentrations of colonic butyrate, induce substantial fold induction of WNT/beta-catenin activity, and subsequent apoptosis of neoplastic colonic cells. In agreement with this hypothesis, the Health Professionals Follow-up Study [77] found that the inverse association of fiber intake with adenoma risk is strongest in men who had a negative endoscopy at some point before the study. These findings imply that fiber has a stronger effect in suppressing the development of new adenomas compared to effects on inhibiting the growth of pre-existing colonic lesions. The same research group also reported [77] an earlier finding that the intake of total fiber was inversely associated with small and incident polyps; whereas, there was no such association for large and prevalent polyps.

Thus, fiber might be most effective at reducing CRC risk by suppressing the early stages of colonic tumorigenesis and least effective in inhibiting subsequent progression.

Despite the likelihood that butyrate is most effective against early stage colonic neoplasia, *in vitro* studies with butyrate have utilized CRC cell lines that correspond to later stages of colonic tumorigenesis, and thus likely not fully representative of the neoplastic colonic cells on which butyrate exercises its effects *in vivo*. Therefore, it would be useful to evaluate the effects of butyrate on early adenoma, rather than carcinoma, cells. The LT97 human cell line was isolated from a colonic microadenoma of a patient with hereditary familial adenomatous polyposis [78]. Therefore, LT97 cells are characterized by the presence of C-terminus truncated APC protein and a lack of full length, wild-type protein [78, 79].

Unlike colon carcinoma cells, LT97 cells are incapable of growing in soft agar, and therefore exhibit an early premalignant phenotype that is distinct from that of typical carcinoma cells [78].

Interestingly, microadenoma LT97 cells are more sensitive to the growth-suppressing effects of butyrate than are HT-29 CRC cells [79], consistent with the hypothesis that butyrate exercises stronger effect on early stage colonic neoplasia. LT97 cells are also highly sensitive to the effects of butyrate on WNT/beta catenin signaling levels and apoptosis (manuscript in preparation). Likewise, the non-metastatic SW480 CRC cell line exhibits greater sensitivity to the effects of butyrate on WNT/catenin activity and apoptosis than the metastatic CRC cell line SW620, derived from the same patient [49, 59]. This further confirms that earlier-stage neoplastic colonic cells are more sensitive to HDACis than their later-stage counterparts.

These findings may explain the results reported by Bonithon-Kopp *et al.*, who observed that supplementation with low levels of fermentable ispaghula husk fiber increased the risk of adenoma recurrence in patients who had previously undergone polypectomy [80]. First, the levels of fiber utilized in that study were lower than those later shown to reduce CRC risk [2, 3, 5], suggesting that insufficient levels of butyrate were produced. Second, the fact that these patients had a prior positive endoscopy (i.e., polyps) suggests that some of these individuals may have already had established microadenomas at commencement of treatment, likely too late for butyrate to exert significant protective activity. Finally, as explained above, this cohort of patients may have been characterized by a heterogeneous population of neoplasms, some of which are resistant to butyrate.

The Role of CBP/p300 Activity in the Effects of Butyrate in CRC Cells

The association between beta-catenin and the transcriptional coactivators CREB-binding protein (CBP) and p300 has been shown to influence WNT/catenin signaling [81-86]. CBP and p300 are histone acetyl transferases (HATs) that can up- or downregulate WNT/catenin signaling in different vertebrate cell lines [81-90]. The interaction between CBP and WNT/catenin signaling is optimally evaluated with the small molecule inhibitor ICG-001, which binds to CBP but not to p300; treatment of CRC cells with ICG-001 suppresses the association between CBP and beta-catenin without blocking p300/beta-catenin association [81]. ICG-001 downregulates basal WNT/catenin reporter activity, inhibits proliferation, and enhances apoptosis in CRC cells [81]. In addition, a water soluble version of ICG-001 reduces the formation of intestinal neoplasms in the APC^{Min} mouse model of CRC [81], and currently, an ICG-001 analog has advanced to stage one clinical trials [91].

Modulation of CBP/p300 activity in CRC cells influences the ability of butyrate to upregulate WNT/catenin activity, and has cell type-specific effects on cell physiology, such as cell proliferation and the induction of apoptosis [92, 93]. Butyrate and ICG-001 cooperate in the suppression of CRC cell growth, but combinations of these agents have different cell-type specific effects on CRC cell apoptosis. Thus, in certain CRC cell lines, butyrate, which enhances WNT/catenin activity, and ICG-001, which represses WNT/catenin activity, interfere with each other's ability to induce apoptosis; however, in other CRC cells, this interference does not occur. Based on these findings, it is likely that the combination of butyrate and ICG-001-like agents would effectively suppress CRC cell growth *in vivo*; however, while growth suppression is of therapeutic utility, apoptosis is generally preferable to cytostasis. Since ICG-001-like agents and butyrate can counteract each other's effect on apoptosis, butyrate/ICG-001 co-treatment should be avoided at least in some cases of CRC [92, 93].

Since butyrate is produced by dietary fiber, animal studies should be conducted to determine the interaction of a fiber-rich diet with the anti-tumor activity of ICG-001-like agents. If diet-derived butyrate interferes with the therapeutic activity of ICG-001-like agents in mouse models of CRC, then a subset of CRC patients should be treated with ICG-001-like agents in a fasting state, or with a diet that does not increase colonic butyrate levels.

Further, we hypothesize [92, 93] that ICG-001-like agents would be particularly effective in inducing apoptosis in colon cancers that are resistant to the effects of butyrate and other HDACis [49, 59]. Right-sided colonic tumors may exhibit such resistance, since in patients with high dietary fiber intake, such neoplasms develop despite the high levels of butyrate in the proximal colon [94].

In resistant CRCs in which butyrate does not hyperinduce WNT/catenin signaling and apoptosis, ICG-001-like agents would likely enhance apoptosis through the suppression of WNT/catenin activity. The therapeutic choice of hyperactivating or suppressing WNT/catenin activity could be based upon assays of WNT/catenin signaling in cells obtained through biopsy.

Other possible approaches to evaluate the suitability of WNT/catenin-suppressing vs. WNT/catenin-enhancing therapeutic options include identification of the mutational profile of HDACi-resistant and HDACi-sensitive phenotypes, and/or determination of the expression levels of CBP and p300 [92, 93].

CRC cell populations are heterogeneous in terms of WNT/catenin signaling levels. The existence of high and low WNT/catenin activity fractions in CRC cell populations *in vitro* is well documented, and the relative proportions of each fraction are altered by physiologically relevant concentrations of butyrate [49, 59].

The modulation of WNT/catenin signaling heterogeneity by butyrate is likely of physiological and clinical relevance, since tumor cell fractions with sustained WNT/catenin activity represent a more stem cell-like and tumorigenic phenotype [95]. HCT-116 CRC cell lines stably transfected with TOP-EGFP (in which WNT/catenin sensitive promoter drives the expression of EGFP) or FOP-EGFP (in which WNT/catenin-non responsive promoter drives the expression of EGFP) were utilized to ascertain the relative number of cells with detectable WNT/catenin activity in a CRC cell population. Butyrate enhances the proportion of cells positive for WNT/catenin activity, and the fold change in the number of these cells correlates with augmented apoptosis [49]. This butyrate-induced increase of WNT/catenin-positive CRC cells is completely eliminated by ICG-001 treatment [92], demonstrating that CBP-mediated WNT/catenin activity is required for this effect of butyrate.

Therefore, the combined effect of ICG-001-like agents and butyrate should be taken into account when designing anti-CRC therapies.

Since CBP/p300-mediated WNT/catenin activity mediates the effects of butyrate, differences in CBP/p300 levels may explain changes in cell signaling and cell physiology that occur in the transition of colonic cells along the neoplastic continuum. We hypothesize that early stage microadenoma cells would be sensitive to the effects of modulation of CBP/p300 activity in the context of butyrate treatment. Indeed, preliminary data suggest that treatment of colonic microadenoma LT97 cells with ICG-001 markedly suppresses the heightened sensitivity of these cells to the effects of butyrate (manuscript in preparation). We believe that CBP/p300-mediated WNT/catenin activity will prove to be an important preventive and therapeutic target for inhibiting colonic neoplasia at its earliest stages.

BUTYRATE RESISTANCE IN CRC CELLS *IN VITRO*

Epidemiological studies indicate that individuals with fiber intake that is relatively high for a Western type diet (35g/day) are still at risk of developing CRC, albeit that risk is reduced by 40% compared to individuals consuming 15g of fiber/day [6]. This suggests that colonic neoplasms can develop resistance to the effects of butyrate. To model the development of such resistance, we have developed a butyrate-resistant cell line (HCT-R) which exhibits repressed WNT/catenin activity and apoptosis upon exposure to butyrate [59]. This cell line is cross-resistant to structurally distinct, clinically relevant HDACis (e.g., SAHA, MS279, LBH589) [59, 96]. Overexpression of Tcf3 was identified as being partially responsible for the butyrate-resistant phenotype of HCT-R cells, as this DNA-binding protein suppresses the hyperinduction of WNT/catenin activity by butyrate [97]. Accordingly, siRNA-mediated Tcf3 knockdown restores sensitivity of HCT-R cells to the effects of butyrate on WNT/catenin activity and clonal cell growth [97].

Although exogenously expressed Tcf3 reduces proliferation of butyrate-sensitive CRC cells, butyrate-resistant HCT-R cells are able to proliferate in the presence of high levels of Tcf3, due to increased expression of cell cycle factors, particularly those driving the G_1 to S transition (e.g., cyclin D2) [97].

Microarray analyses comparing butyrate-sensitive and butyrate-resistant cells also revealed a significant shift from beta-catenin-dependent WNT activity to noncanonical WNT signaling based upon increased WNT5A, WNT11, and ROR2 expression in HCT-R cells [96]. Suppressed expression of ROR2, the receptor for WNT5A, allows for a partial reversal of the butyrate resistance in HCT-R cells [96].

Finally, in comparison with butyrate-sensitive HCT-116 cells, butyrate-resistant HCT-R cells exhibit a markedly decreased expression of p300, as confirmed by western blot analyses [93]. Further, HCT-R cells show an increased sensitivity to the pro-apoptotic effects of ICG-001 compared to parental HCT-116 cells [92, 93]. CBP-mediated WNT/catenin activity has been associated with enhanced CRC cell proliferation, while p300-mediated WNT/catenin activity has been associated with differentiation [81-86].

Therefore, our hypothesis is that one mechanism by which HCT-R cells develop resistance to butyrate is through downregulation of p300 and p300-mediated WNT/catenin activity, coupled to maintenance of pro-proliferative CBP-mediated WNT/catenin activity.

Consistent with this, CBP-mediated WNT/catenin signaling promotes the acquisition of a drug-resistant, highly tumorigenic cell phenotype that exhibits characteristics of cancer stem cells [98]. Thus, resistance to butyrate and other HDACis may be associated with a shift of cancer cells from canonical (beta-catenin associated) to noncanonical WNT activity, and a shift from p300-mediated WNT/catenin signaling to CBP-mediated WNT/catenin signaling.

CONCLUSION

The increased knowledge about the mechanisms by which butyrate affects CRC cell physiology suggests new strategies for CRC prevention and therapeutics. Therefore, we conclude this chapter with several questions that may guide future studies.

1. Is the hyperinduction of WNT/catenin signaling or any other oncogenic function deregulated in cancer a therapeutic strategy? We have reported that butyrate hyperactivates the "oncogenic" WNT/catenin signaling in CRC cells with mutations in this pathway, and the fold increase in WNT activity associates causally with high levels of apoptosis.

This observation is likely to be a manifestation of a general phenomenon: thus, whereas moderate levels of oncogene activity support cancer development, hyperactivation of oncogenic functions results in cell death and senescence [99, 100].

This conclusion is based upon numerous reports that hyperactivation of signaling through RAS, MYC, RAF, and other oncogenes results in cancer cell senescence and/or apoptosis. For example, the hyperactivation of *RAS*, the most commonly mutated gene in human neoplasms [101], results in cell death in different experimental models [102-105].

Similarly, activation of ERK signaling contributes to programmed cell death [106, 107], and hyperinduction of the signal propagated through the epidermal growth factor receptor (EGFR) may facilitate apoptosis [108]. The phenomenon of hyperactivated oncogene inducing apoptosis has also been observed in Bcr-Abl overexpressing cells: when such cells are cultured in the presence of the kinase inhibitor imatinib, and then deprived of the drug, they commit to programmed death due to the increased Bcr-Abl activity, and the stimulation of its downstream pathways [109].

What is the mechanistic explanation of these observations? It is likely that the fold changes, rather than the absolute levels, of the oncogenic signaling trigger apoptosis of the neoplastic cells. Thus, Goentoro and Kirschner have reported that the physiologically significant cell response is dictated by the fold changes in a signaling pathway such as the WNT/beta-catenin pathway [110]. The authors concluded that the transcriptional activity of beta-catenin depends not only on its levels, but also on the fold-changes in these levels.

The hyperactivation of WNT/catenin signaling and apoptosis by butyrate in CRC cells is mimicked by synthetic HDACis, some of which are in the clinic [59]. Therefore, our results suggest a novel approach to anti-CRC therapy based upon the hyperinduction of the already deregulated WNT/beta-catenin pathway. Thus, the HDACis suberoylanilide hydroxamic acid, (SAHA, vorinostat), LBH589, and MS-275 hyperinduce WNT/beta-catenin signaling in CRC cells via the same mechanisms as butyrate [59, 96]. In recent years, HDACis have emerged as potent anti-cancer agents. SAHA (Merck's product, traded under the name of Zolinza), the first HDACi to reach the market, has been approved by the FDA for treatment of cutaneous T-cell lymphoma, and is being tested for treatment of other malignancies, including CRC.

Some additional HDACis in the clinic or clinical trials are LAQ-824, LBH-589 (both from Novartis), the natural product depsipeptide (FK-228, from Gloucester, FDA approved for cutaneous T-cell lymphoma), the benzamide SYND 275, and PCI-24781 (from Pharmacyclics). Potentially, all of these compounds can hyperactivate WNT/catenin activity in cells with mutations in the pathway. It would be of interest to ascertain whether the same compounds hyperactivate other mutation-induced oncogenic pathways, and thus, lead to apoptosis. Such studies may result in a novel anti-cancer therapeutic approach that relies upon the hyperactivation, rather than the suppression, of oncogenic activity. Exposed to such treatment, normal cells without mutations in the targeted oncogene will not hyperactivate its function, and, therefore, should be spared the apoptotic fate.

On the other hand, the suppression of oncogenic pathways (as in currently developed therapies) is sometimes detrimental since it may (a) decrease the viability of adult stem cells, and (b) impede the function of more specialized differentiated cells. For example, WNT/beta-catenin signaling is deregulated by mutations in different types of cancer, and developing inhibitors of the pathway has been a major endeavor. However, functional WNT/catenin signaling is essential for the survival of stem cells, and even for the function of highly differentiated cells, such as hippocampal neurons [111].

2. How does the colonic milieu affect the ability of butyrate to modulate WNT/catenin signaling and apoptosis of neoplastic colonic cells *in vivo*? The intake of fiber, the major source of butyrate in the colon, is accompanied by that of other bioactive ingredients, such as polyphenols and fats. Polyphenols have been reported to either upregulate or downregulate WNT/catenin signaling [112-115]; therefore, the question arises whether the effects of butyrate on WNT/catenin activity and apoptosis are modified by other dietary metabolites in the colon. If butyrate synergizes with other diet-derived compounds in hyperinducing WNT/catenin signaling and apoptosis, we can design diets and dietary supplements that decrease the risk of CRC. Preliminary studies have shown that caffeic acid phethyl ester (CAPE) and CAPE-containing propolis augment the apoptotic response of CRC cells to butyrate [96, 116]. Future studies that analyze complete diets and account for the complex interactions between colinic bioactives will facilitate the formulation of CRC-protective dietary regimens. One example for such analytical approach is the artificial human gastrointestinal tract developed by TNO in the Netherlands [117].

3. Do dietary habits (e.g., grazing behavior versus. fasting or fewer meals a day) modulate the effects of butyrate on WNT/catenin signaling and apoptosis? Epidemiological data suggest that a lesser number of eating episodes a day are associated with lower risk of CRC [118, 119]. Rodent studies also support the association between longer intervals of fasting and lower incidence of cancer [120, 121]. Combined with the observations that WNT/beta-catenin signaling fluctuates significantly in absence and presence of nutrients [49, 59, 66], these reports suggest that fewer eating episodes a day (without a change in total caloric intake) may protect against CRC through supporting high fold changes in WNT/catenin signaling. This interpretation is concordant with the finding that not the absolute level, but the fold induction, of WNT/catenin signaling correlates with the apoptotic outcome in ten CRC cell lines [49, 94]. The association between the fold change in WNT/catenin transcriptional activity and the apoptotic response of the neoplastic cells is reminiscent of Weber's physiology law, according to which sensations are perceived not based upon the absolute levels of the stimuli, but upon the fold change in the stimuli.

Several research reports support the notion that Weber's law applies at the individual cell level, as cells respond to fold changes, rather than to absolute levels, of signaling pathways [110, 122, 123] The preliminary conclusion from these findings is that grazing behavior does not allow for significant fluctuations in WNT/catenin activity, and therefore, may counteract the CRC preventive effect of fiber-derived butyrate. Carefully planned studies with animal models of intestinal cancer and prospective epidemiological studies could address this hypothesis.

4. Are the dietary history (e.g., fiber intake) of the patient and the anatomic location of colonic neoplasms (e.g., proximal versus distal) predictive of the response of CRCs to HDACi-based therapy? Following dietary fiber intake, the levels of butyrate are highest in the right colon, and decrease in the left colon [124-126].

Therefore, individuals with relatively high dietary fiber intake may develop right-sided CRCs only if the neoplastic cells become resistant to the apoptotic effect of the diet-derived butyrate. In such patients, HDACi-based therapies may not be appropriate since butyrate-resistant CRC cells are cross-resistant to synthetic HDACis [59].

In patients with low fiber intake, both left and right colonic neoplasms might be sensitive to synthetic HDACis, as in such individuals diet-derived butyrate may have been at low levels that do not induce apoptosis. This hypothesis could be addressed by analyses of the dietary history of the patients and the response the patients' colonic neoplastic cells to HDACis in *in vitro* assays.

Alternatively, the selective pressure of high butyrate levels may result in a specific genetic profile of the colonic lesions, and this common mutational profile could be identified with next generation sequencing, as this technology becomes cheaper and easier to access.

5. Obesity has become a worldwide epidemic, and it contributes to approximately 20% of all cancer cases, and at least 11% of the CRC cases [127, 128]. The mechanisms via which obesity predisposes to CRC are not well understood. Since butyrate induces apoptosis in CRC cells via hyperactivation of WNT/catenin signaling, it is plausible that obesity-associated cytokines counteract butyrate-induced apoptosis by suppressing WNT/beta-catenin activity. Addressing this possibility may suggest novel approaches that lower the risk of CRC in obese individuals.

6. Is the increased risk of CRC among populations with low socioeconomic status (SES) [129] mediated in part by their low-fiber intake? Is the shift from left-sided to right-sided CRCs in part due to the decreased intake of dietary fiber? An epidemiological necropsy study of 3,558 autopsies at Johns Hopkins Hospital revealed that for African Americans the ratio of right/left colonic adenomas is 6.4 for age 20-49 and 1.43 for age 50-89; however, for European Americans the ratio was 0.54 and 0.65 for the two age groups [130].

The prevalence of right-sided adenomas in African Americans is in agreement with the increasing rate of right-sided tumors in this population: for example, these tumors were detected at a rate of 36% in 1959-1970, and at 60% in 2001-2006 [131-133]. The increase of right-sided neoplasms has been a 50-year trend observed not only among African Americans, but in some European and Asian populations [131]. Whereas the right-sided shift of colonic carcinomas is attributed to both westernized lifestyle and diet [134, 135], and to increased screening for left-sided neoplasms (by sigmoidoscopy), the higher ratio of right- to left-sided adenomas in African Americans [130] can be attributed mostly to socioeconomic status (SES)-associated factors such as lifestyle and diet.

The 2009 *Policy and Action for Cancer Prevention*, a report published by the World Cancer Research Fund and the American Institute for Cancer Research (AICR), states that about 45% of all colon cancers are preventable through lifestyle and dietary changes. Therefore, the AICR report recommends physical activity, limited consumption of energy-dense foods and meat, and increased intake of fiber from fresh vegetables and fruit. Observing these recommendations is costly, and sometimes impossible for groups of low SES. It has been documented that lower quality diets based upon energy-dense foods tend to be consumed by groups of lower SES and more limited economic means [136, 137]. The disparities in fruit and vegetables consumption among groups of different SES are currently increasing [138]. Some of the reasons are (a) the faster increase in the price of vegetables and fruit relative to high-density foods, (b) the increased availability/marketing of the low-cost energy-dense foods [136, 139], and the decreased physical access of low-income families without cars to stores with fresh produce [140-142]. Future epidemiological studies on colonic adenoma and CRC incidence should account for indexes of SES that reflect on diet.

7. Does suppression of compensatory proliferation synergize with the apoptotic effect of butyrate on CRC cells? *In vitro* studies with butyrate-resistant CRC cells have revealed that one mechanism via which cells avoid programmed death in the presence of butyrate is through suppression of WNT/beta-catenin activity. The decrease in beta-catenin–dependent transcriptional activity is achieved by the increased expression of mediators of noncanonical WNT activity: WNT5A, WNT11, and ROR2, the receptor of WNT5A [109]. The noncanonical WNT pathway may induce pathways known to contribute to compensatory proliferation in apoptotic cell populations. For example, WNT5A induces downstream the cell survival AKT and JNK signaling [143-145]. Therefore, inhibition of the noncanonical WNT pathway or its downstream signaling pathways (e.g., AKT signaling) may allow for the formulation of preventive CRC strategies that account for the mechanisms of butyrate resistance [116].

8. CBP/p300-mediated WNT/catenin signaling plays an important role in mediating the effects of butyrate in CRC cells. Can the modulation of CBP/p300 activity influence neoplastic progression in patients? In addition, can butyrate/HDACi resistance be prevented or even reversed through alteration in the relative levels of CBP- vs. p300-mediated WNT/catenin activity? Will ICG-001-like agents show greater efficacy against colonic neoplasms arising in specific areas of the large bowel (e.g., right vs. left) due to differences in butyrate levels in these colonic segments and the probability that neoplasms arising in the right colon are butyrate resistant?

REFERENCES

[1] Huxley, R. R., Ansary-Moghaddam, A., Clifton, P., Czernichow, S., Parr, C. L., Woodward, M. The impact of dietary and lifestyle risk factors on risk of colorectal cancer: a quantitative overview of the epidemiological evidence. *Int. J. Cancer.* 2009; 125:171-180.

[2] Aune, D., Chan, D. S., Lau, R., Vieira, R., Greenwood, D. C., Kampman, E., Norat, T. Dietary fibre, whole grains, and risk of colorectal cancer: systematic review and dose-response meta-analysis of prospective studies. *BMJ.* 2011; 343:d6617. doi: 10.1136/bmj.d6617. Review.

[3] Derry, M. M., Raina, K., Agarwal, C., Agarwal, R. Identifying molecular targets of lifestyle modifications in colon cancer prevention. *Front Oncol*. 2013; 3:119.

[4] Burkitt, D. P. Epidemiology of cancer of the colon and rectum. *Cancer*. 1971; 28:3-13.

[5] Wolever, T. M., Jenkins, D. J. What is a high fiber diet? *Adv. Exp. Med. Biol*. 1997;427: 35-42. Review.

[6] Bingham, S. A., Day, N. E., Luben, R., Ferrari, P., Slimani, N., Norat, T., Clavel-Chapelon, F., Kesse, E., Nieters, A., Boeing, H., Tjonneland, A., Overvad, K., Martinzez, C., Dorronsoro, M., Gonzalez, C. A., Key, T. J., Trichopolou, A., Naska, A., Vineis, P., Tumino, R., Krogh, V., Bueno-de-Mesquita, H. B., Peeters, P. H., Berglund, G., Hallmans, G., Lund, E., Skeie, G., Kaaks, R., Riboli, E. Dietary fibre in food and protection against colorectal cancer in the European Prospective Investigation into Cancer and Nutrition (EPIC): an observational study. *Lancet*. 2003; 361:1496-1501.

[7] Peters, U., Sinha, R., Chaterjee, N., Subar, A. F., Ziegler, R. G., Kuldorff, M., Bresalier, R., Weissfeld, J. L., Flood, A., Schtzkin, A., Hayes, R. B. Dietary fibre and colorectal adenoma in a colorectal cancer early detection programme. *Lancet*. 2003; 361:1491-1495.

[8] Fuchs, C. S., Giovannucci, E., Colditz, G. A., Hunter, D. J., Stampfer, M. J., Rosner, B., Speizer, F. E., Willett, W. C. Dietary fiber and the risk of colorectal cancer and adenoma in women. *N Engl. J. Med*. 1999; 340:169-176.

[9] Park, Y., Hunter, D. J., Spiegelman, D., Bergkvist, L., Berrino, F., van den Brandt, P. A., Buring, J. E., Colditz, G. A., Freudenheim, J. L., Fuchs, C. S., Giovannucci, E., Goldbohm, R. A., Graham, S., Harnack, L., Hartman, A. M., Jacobs, D. R. Jr, Kato, I., Krogh, V., Leitzmann, M. F., McCullough, M. L., Miller, A. B., Pietinen, P., Rohan, T. E., Schatzkin, A., Willet, W. C., Wolk, A., Zeleniuch-Jacquotte, A., Zhang, S. M., Smith-Warner, S. A. Dietary fiber intake and risk of colorectal cancer: a pooled analysis of prospective cohort studies. *JAMA*. 2005; 294:2849-2857.

[10] Bingham, S. A., Norat, T., Moskal, A., Ferrari, P., Slimani, N., Chavel-Chapelon, F., Kesse, E., Nieters, A., Boeing, H., Tjonneland, A., Overvad, K., Martinzez, C., Dorronsoro, M., Gonzalez, C. A., Ardanaz, E., Navarro, C., Quiros, J. R., Key, T. J., Day, N. E., Trichopoulo, A., Naska, A., Krogh, V., Tumino, R., Palli, D., Panico, S., Vineis, P., Bueno-de-Mesquita, H. B., Ocke, M. C., Peeters, P. H. M., Berglund, G., Hallmans, G., Lund, E., Skeie, G., Kaaks, R., Riboli, E. Is the association with fiber from foods in colorectal cancer confounded by folate intake? *Cancer Epid. Biom. Prev*. 2005; 14:1552-1556.

[11] World Cancer Research Fund/American Institute for Cancer Research (2011) Continuous Update Project Report Summary. Food, Nutrition, Physical Activity, and the Prevention of Colorectal Cancer.

[12] Murphy, N., Norat, T., Ferrari, P., Jenab, M., Bueno-de-Mesquita, B., Skeie, G., Dahm, C. C., Overvad, K., Olsen, A., Tjønneland, A., Clavel-Chapelon, F., Boutron-Ruault, M. C., Racine, A., Kaaks, R., Teucher, B., Boeing, H., Bergmann, M. M., Trichopoulou, A., Trichopoulos, D., Lagiou, P., Palli, D., Pala, V., Panico, S., Tumino, R., Vineis, P., Siersema, P., van Duijnhoven, F., Peeters, P. H., Hjartaker, A., Engeset, D., González, C. A., Sánchez, M. J., Dorronsoro, M., Navarro, C., Ardanaz, E., Quirós, J. R., Sonestedt, E., Ericson, U., Nilsson, L., Palmqvist, R., Khaw, K. T., Wareham, N., Key, T. J., Crowe, F. L., Fedirko, V., Wark, P. A., Chuang, S. C., Riboli, E. Dietary

fibre intake and risks of cancers of the colon and rectum in the European prospective investigation into cancer and nutrition (EPIC). *PLoS One*. 2012;7:e39361.

[13] Bingham, S. Mechanisms and experimental evidence relating dietary fibre and starch to protection against large bowel cancer. *Proc. Nutr. Soc.* 1990; 49:153-171.

[14] Young, G. P., Hu, Y., Le Leu, R. K., Nyskohus, L. Dietary fibre and colorectal cancer: A model for environment-gene interactions. *Mol. Nutr. Food Res.* 2005; 49: 571–584.

[15] Boffa, L. C., Luption, J. R., Mariani, M. R., Ceppi, M., Newmark, H. L., Scalmati, A., Lipkin, M. Modulation of colonic epithelial cell proliferation, histone acetylation, and luminal short chain fatty acids by variation of dietary fiber (wheat bran) in rats. *Cancer Res.* 1992; 52:5906-5912.

[16] Heerdt, B. G., Houston, M. A., Augenlicht, L. H. Potentiation by specific short-chain fatty acids of differentiation and apoptosis in human colonic carcinoma cell lines. *Cancer Res.* 1994; 54:3288-3294.

[17] Hague, A., Elder, D. J., Hicks, D. J., Paraskeva, G. Apoptosis in colorectal tumor cells: induction by the short chain fatty acids butyrate, propionate and acetate and by the bile salt deoxycholate. *Int. J. Cancer.* 1995; 60:400-406.

[18] Medina, V., Young, G. P., Edmonds, B., James, R., Appleton, S., Zalewski, P. D. Induction of caspase-3 protease activity and apoptosis by butyrate and another inhibitor of histone deacetylase: dependence on protein synthesis and synergy with a mitochondrial/cytochrome c-dependent pathway. *Cancer Res.* 1997; 57:3697-3707.

[19] Cummings, J. H., Pomare, E. W., Branch, W. J., Naylor, C. P., Macfarlane, G. T. Short chain fatty acids in human large intestine, portal, hepatic and venous blood. *Gut.* 1987; 28: 1221-1227.

[20] Weaver, G. A., Tangel, C. T., Krause, J. A., Parfitt, M. M., Jenkins, P. L., Rader, J. M., Lewis, B. A., Miller, T. L., Wolin, M. J. Acarbose enhances human colonic butyrate production. *J. Nutr.* 1997; 127:717-723.

[21] Hallert, C., Björck, I., Nyman, M., Pousette, A., Grännö, C., Svensson, H. Increasing fecal butyrate in ulcerative colitis patients by diet: controlled pilot study. *Inflamm. Bowel Dis.* 2003; 9:116-121.

[22] Freeman, H. J. Effects of differing concentrations of sodium butyrate on 1,2-dimethylhydrazine-induced rat intestinal neoplasia. *Gastroenterology*. 1986; 91:596-602.

[23] Deschner, E. E., Ruperto, J. F., Lupton, J. R., Newmark, H. L. Dietary butyrate (tributyrine) does not enhance AOM-induced colon tumorigenesis. *Cancer Lett.* 1990; 52: 79-82.

[24] Caderni, G., Luceri, C., De Filippo, C., Salvadori, M., Giannini, A., Tessitore, L., Dolara, P. Slow-release pellets of sodium butyrate do not modify azoxymethane (AOM)-induced intestinal carcinogenesis in F344 rats. *Carcinogenesis*. 2001; 22:525-527.

[25] Ohkawara, S., Furuya, H., Nagashima, K., Asanuma, N., Hino, T. Oral administration of Butyrivibrio fibrisolvens, a butyrate-producing bacterium, decreases the formation of aberrant crypt foci in the colon and rectum of mice. *J. Nutr.* 2005; 135:2878-2883.

[26] Kameue, C., Tsukahara, T., Yamada, Y., Koyama, H., Iwasaki, Y., Nakayama, K., Ushida, K. Dietary sodium gluconate protects rats from large bowel cancer by stimulating butyrate production. *J. Nutr.* 2004; 134:940-944.

[27] Clarke, J. M., Topping, D. L., Bird, A. R., Young, G. P., Cobiac, L. Effects of high-amylose maize starch and butyrylated high-amylose maize starch on azoxymethane-induced intestinal cancer in rats. *Carcinogenesis*. 2008; 29:2190-2194.

[28] Clarke, J. M., Young, G. P., Topping, D. L., Bird, A. R., Cobiac, L., Scherer, B. L., Winkler, J. G., Lockett, T. J. Butyrate delivered by butyrylated starch increases distal colonic epithelial apoptosis in carcinogen-treated rats. *Carcinogenesis*. 2012; 33:197-202.

[29] Bajka, B. H., Clarke, J. M., Cobiac, L., Topping, D. L. Butyrylated starch protects colonocyte DNA against dietary protein-induced damage in rats. *Carcinogenesis*. 2008; 29:2169-2174.

[30] Conlon, M. A., Kerr, C. A., McSweeney, C. S., Dunne, R. A., Shaw, J. M., Kang, S., Bird, A. R., Morell, M. K., Lockett, T. J., Molloy, P. L., Regina, A., Toden, S., Clarke, J. M., Topping, D. L. Resistant starches protect against colonic DNA damage and alter microbiota and gene expression in rats fed a Western diet. *J. Nutr*. 2012; 142:832-840.

[31] Toden, S., Bird, A. R., Topping, D. L., Conlon, M. A. Resistant starch attenuates colonic DNA damage induced by higher dietary protein in rats. *Nutr. Cancer*. 2005; 51: 45-51.

[32] Lupton, J. R. Microbial degradation products influence colon cancer risk: the butyrate controversy. *J. Nutr*. 2004; 134:479-482.

[33] Bordonaro, M., Lazarova, D. L., Sartorelli, A. C. Butyrate and Wnt signaling: a possible solution to the puzzle of dietary fiber and colon cancer risk? *Cell Cycle*. 2008; 7:1178-1183.

[34] Rubinfeld, B., Souza, B., Albert, I., Muller, O., Chamberlain, S. H., Masiarz, F. R., Munimetsu, S., Polakis, P. Association of the APC gene product with ß-catenin. *Science*. 1993; 262:1731-1734.

[35] Su, L. K., Vogelstein, B., Kinzler, K. W. Association of the APC tumor suppresser protein with catenins. *Science*. 1993; 262:1734-1737.

[36] Munemitsu, S., Albert, I., Souza, B., Rubinfeld, B., Polakis, P. Regulation of intracellular ß-catenin levels by the adenomatous polyposis coli (APC) tumor-suppressor protein. *Proc. Natl. Acad. Sci. US*. 1995; 92:3046-3050.

[37] Behrens, J., Von Kries, J. P., Kuhl, M., Bruhn, L., Wedlich, D., Grosschedl, R., Birchmeier, W. Functional interaction of ß-catenin with the transcriptional factor LEF-1. *Nature*. 1996; 382:638-642.

[38] Molenaar, M., Van De Wetering, M., Osterwegel, M. XTcf-3 transcription factor mediates ß-catenin-induced axis formation in Xenopus embryos. *Cell*. 1996; 86:391-399.

[39] Korinek, V., Barker, N., Morin, P. J., Van Wichen, D., De Weger, R., Kinzler, K. W., Vogelstein, B., Clevers, H. Constitutive transcriptional activation by a beta-catenin-Tcf complex in APC-/- colon carcinoma. *Science*. 1997;275:1784-1787.

[40] Morin, J., Sparks, A. B., Korinek, V., Barker, N., Clevers, H., Vogelstein, B., Kinzler, K. W. Activation of beta-catenin-Tcf signaling in colon cancer by mutations in beta-catenin or APC. *Science*. 1997; 275:1787-1790.

[41] Miyaki, M., Iijima, T., Kimura, J., Yasuno, M., Mori, T., Hayashi, Y., Koike, M., Shitara, N., Iwama, T., Kuroki, T. Frequent mutation of ß-catenin and APC genes in primary colorectal tumors from patients with hereditary nonpolyposis colorectal cancer. *Cancer Res*. 1999; 59:4506-4509.

[42] Webster, M. T., Rozycka, M., Sara, E., Davis, E., Smalley, M., Young, N., Dale, T. C., Wooster, R. Sequence variants of the axin gene in breast, colon, and other cancers: an analysis of mutations that interfere with GSK3 binding. *Genes Chrom. Cancer*. 2000: 28:443-453.

[43] Kinzler, K. W., Vogelstein, B. Lessons from hereditary colorectal cancer. *Cell*. 1996; 87:159-170.

[44] Bienz, M., Clevers, H. Linking colorectal cancer to Wnt signaling. *Cell*. 2000; 103:311-320.

[45] Woodgett, J. Regulation and functions of the glycogen synthase kinase-3 subfamily. *Sem. Cancer Biol*. 1994; 5:269-275.

[46] Cook, D., Fry, M., Hughes, K., Sumathipala, R., Woodgett, J., Dale, T. Wingless inactivates glycogen synthase kinase-3 via an intracellular signaling pathway which involves a protein kinase C. *EMBO J*. 1996; 15:4526-4536.

[47] Roose, J., Clevers, H. Tcf transcription factors: molecular switches in carcinogenesis. *Biochim. Biophys. Acta*. 1999; 87456:23-27.

[48] Bordonaro, M., Mariadason, J. M., Aslam, F., Heerdt, B. G., Augenlicht, L. H. Butyrate-induced apoptotic cascade in colonic carcinoma cells: modulation of the beta-catenin-Tcf pathway and concordance with effects of sulindac and trichostatin A but not curcumin. *Cell Growth and Differentiation*. 1999; 10:713-720.

[49] Lazarova, D. L., Bordonaro, M., Carbone, R., Sartorelli, A. C. Linear relationship between WNT activity levels and apoptosis in colorectal carcinoma cells exposed to butyrate. *Int. J. Cancer*. 2004; 110:523-531.

[50] Ahmed, Y., Hayashi, S., Levine, A., Wieschaus, E. Regulation of Armadillo by a Drosophila APC inhibits neuronal apoptosis during retinal development. *Cell*. 1998; 93: 1171-1182.

[51] Romagnolo, B., Berrebi, D., Saadi Keddoucci, S., Porteu, A., Pichard, A. I., Peuchmaur, M., Vandewalle, A., Kahn, A., Perret, C. Intestinal dysplasia and adenoma in transgenic mice after overexpression of an activated beta-catenin. *Cancer Res*. 1999; 59:3875-3879.

[52] Hasegawa, S., Sato, T., Akazawa, H., Okada, H., Maeno, A., Ito, M., Sugitani, Y., Shibata, H., Miyazaki, J., Katsuki, M., Yamauchi, Y., Yamamura Ki, K., Katamine, S., Noda, T. Apoptosis in neural crest cells by functional loss of APC tumor suppressor gene. *Proc. Natl. Acad. Sci. US*. 2002; 99:297-302.

[53] Wong, M. H., Huelsken, J., Birchmeier, W., Gordon, J. I. Selection of multipotent stem cells during morphogenesis of small intestinal crypts of Lieberkühn is perturbed by stimulation of Lef1/ß-catenin signaling. *J. Biol. Chem*. 2002; 277:15843-15850.

[54] Zeilstra, J., Joosten, S. P., Wensveen, F. M., Dessing, M. C., Schütze, D. M., Eldering, E., Spaargaren, M., Pals, S. T. WNT signaling controls expression of pro-apoptotic BOK and BAX in intestinal cancer. *Biochem. Biophys. Res. Commun*. 2011;406:1-6. doi: 10.1016/j.bbrc.2010.12.070.

[55] Bordonaro, M., Lazarova, D. L., Sartorelli, A. C. Hyper-induction of Wnt activity: a new paradigm for the treatment of colorectal cancer? *Oncology Res*. 2008; 17:1-9.

[56] Albuquerque, C., Breukel, C., van der Luijt, R., Fidalgo, P., Lage, P., Slors, F. G. M., Leitao, C. N., Fodde, R., Smits, R. The just-right signaling model: APC somatic mutations are selected based on a special level of activation of the beta-catenin signaling cascade. *Hum. Mol. Genet*. 2002; 11:1549-1560.

[57] Lewis, A., Segditsas, S., Deheragoda, M., Pollard, P., Jeffery, R., Nye, E., Lockstone, H., Davis, H., Clark, S., Stamp, G., Poulsom, R., Wright, N., Tomlinson, I. Severe polyposis in Apc(1322T) mice is associated with submaximal Wnt signalling and increased expression of the stem cell marker Lgr5. *Gut*. 2010;59:1680-1686.
[58] Polakis, P., Hart, M., Rubinfeld, B. Defects in the regulation of beta-catenin in colorectal cancer. *Adv. Exp. Med. Biol*. 1999;470:23-32.
[59] Bordonaro, M., Lazarova, D. L., Sartorelli, A. C. The activation of beta-catenin by Wnt signaling mediates the effects of histone deacetylase inhibitors. *Exp. Cell Res*. 2007; 313:1652-1666.
[60] Roediger, W. E. W. Role of anaerobic bacteria in the metabolic welfare of the colonic mucosa in man. *Gut*. 1980; 21:793-798.
[61] Vanhoutvin, S. A., Troost, F. J., Hamer, H. M., Lindsey, P. J., Koek, G. H., Jonkers, D. M., Kodde, A., Venema, K., Brummer, R. J. Butyrate-induced transcriptional changes in human colonic mucosa. *PLoS One*. 2009; 4:e6759.
[62] Singh, B., Halestrap, A. P., Paraskeva, C. Butyrate can act as a stimulator of growth or inducer of apoptosis in human colonic epithelial cell lines depending on the presence of alternative energy sources. *Carcinogenesis*. 1997;18:1265-1270.
[63] Jass, J. R. Diet, butyric acid and differentiation of gastrointestinal tract tumours. *Med. Hypotheses*. 1985;18:113-118.
[64] Donohoe, D. R., Collins, L. B., Wali, A., Bigler, R., Sun, W., Bultman, S. J. The Warburg effect dictates the mechanism of butyrate-mediated histone acetylation and cell proliferation. *Mol. Cell*. 2012; 48:612-626.
[65] Gibson, P. R., Rosella, O., Wilson, A. J., Mariadason, J. M., Rickard, K., Byron, K., Barkla, D. H. Colonic epithelial cell activation and the paradoxical effects of butyrate. *Carcinogenesis*. 1999; 4:39-44.
[66] Anagnostou, S. H. and Shepherd, P. R. Glucose induces an autocrine activation of the Wnt/beta-catenin pathway in macrophage cell lines. *Biochem. J*. 2008; 416: 211-218.
[67] Lee, S. Y., Jeon, H. M., Ju, M. K., Kim, C. H., Yoon, G., Han, S. I., Park, H. G., Kang, H. S. Wnt/Snail signaling regulates cytochrome C oxidase and glucose metabolism. *Cancer Res*. 2012;72:3607-3617.
[68] Esen, E., Chen, J., Karner, C. M., Okunade, A. L., Patterson, B. W., Long, F. WNT-LRP5 signaling induces Warburg effect through mTORC2 activation during osteoblast differentiation. *Cell Metab*. 2013;17: 745-755.
[69] Chocarro-Calvo, A., García-Martínez, J. M., Ardila-González, S., De la Vieja, A., García-Jiménez, C. Glucose-induced β-catenin acetylation enhances Wnt signaling in cancer. *Mol. Cell*. 2013; 49: 474-486.
[70] Klampfer, L., Huang, J., Sasazuki, T., Shirasawa, S., Augenlicht, L. Oncogenic Ras promotes butyrate-induced apoptosis through inhibition of gelsolin expression. *J. Biol. Chem*. 2004; 279: 36680-36688.
[71] Lay, C., Rigottier-Gois, L., Holmstrøm, K., Rajilic, M., Vaughan, E. E., de Vos, W. M., Collins, M. D., Thiel, R., Namsolleck, P., Blaut, M., Doré, J. Colonic microbiota signatures across five northern European countries. *Appl. Environ. Microbiol*. 2005; 71: 4153-4155.
[72] Mueller, S., Saunier, K., Hanisch, C., Norin, E., Alm, L., Midtvedt, T., Cresci, A., Silvi, S., Orpianesi, C., Verdenelli, M. C., Clavel, T., Koebnick, C., Zunft, H. J., Doré, J., Blaut, M. Differences in fecal microbiota in different European study populations in

relation to age, gender, and country: a cross-sectional study. *Appl. Environ. Microbiol.* 2006; 72:1027-1033.

[73] O'Toole, P. W., Cooney, J. C. Probiotic bacteria influence the composition and function of the intestinal microbiota. *Interdiscip. Perspect. Infect. Dis*. 2008; 2008:175285.

[74] Fallani, M., Young, D., Scott, J., Norin, E., Amarri, S., Adam, R., Aguilera, M., Khanna, S., Gil, A., Edwards, C. A., Doré, J.; Other Members of the INFABIO Team. Intestinal microbiota of 6-week-old infants across Europe: geographic influence beyond delivery mode, breast-feeding, and antibiotics. *J. Pediatr. Gastroenterol. Nutr.* 2010; 51:77-84.

[75] Walker, A. W., Ince, J., Duncan, S. H., Webster, L. M., Holtrop, G., Ze, X., Brown, D., Stares, M. D., Scott, P., Bergerat, A., Louis, P., McIntosh, F., Johnstone, A. M., Lobley, G. E., Parkhill, J., Flint, H. J. Dominant and diet-responsive groups of bacteria within the human colonic microbiota. *ISME J.* 2011; 5:220-230.

[76] Flint, H. J. The impact of nutrition on the human microbiome. *Nutr. Rev*. 2012; 70 Suppl. 1:S10-3.

[77] Platz, E. A., Giovannucci, E., Romm, E. B., Rockett, H. R. H., Stampfer, M. J., Colditz, G. A., Willett, W. C. Dietary fiber and distal colorectal adenomas in men. *Cancer Epidemiol. Biomarkers and Prevention* 1997; 6:661-670.

[78] Richter, M., Jurek, D., Wrba, F., Kaserer, K., Wurzer, G., Karner-Hanusch, J., Marian, B. Cells obtained from colorectal microadenomas mirror early premalignant growth patterns *in vitro*. *Euro. J. Cancer*. 2002; 38:1937-1945.

[79] Kautenberger, T., Beyer-Sehlmeyer, G., Festag, G., Haag, N., Kuhler, S., Kuchler, A., Weise, A., Marian, B., Peters, W. H. M., Liehr, T., Claussen, U., Pool-Zobel, B. L. The gut fermentation product butyrate, a chemopreventive agent, suppresses glutathione S-transferase theta (hGSTT1) and cell growth more in human colon adenoma cells (LT97) than tumor (HT29) cells. *J. Cancer Res. Clin. Oncol*. 2005; 131:692-700.

[80] Bonithon-Kopp, C., Kronberg, O., Giacosa, A., Rath, U., Faivre, J. Calcium and fibre supplementation in prevention of colorectal adenoma recurrence: a randomized intervention trial. European Cancer Prevention Organisation Study Group. *Lancet*. 2000; 356: 1300-1306.

[81] Emami, K. H., Nguyen, C., Ma, H., Kim, D. H., Jeong, K. W., Eguchi, M., Moon, R. T., Teo, J. L., Oh, S. W., Kim, H. Y., Moon, S. H., Ha, J. R., Kahn, M. A small molecule inhibitor of β-catenin/CREB-binding protein transcription. *Proc. Natl. Acad. Sci. US*. 2004; 101:12682-12687.

[82] McMillan, M., Kahn, M. Investigating WNT signaling: a chemogenomic safari. *Drug Disc. Today*. 2005; 10:1467-1474.

[83] Teo, J. L., Ma, H., Nguyen, C., Lam, C., Kahn, M. Specific inhibition of CBP/β-catenin interaction rescues defects in neuronal differentiation caused by presenilin-1 mutation. *Proc. Natl. Acad. Sci. US*. 2005; 102:12171-12176.

[84] Ma, H., Nguyen, C., Lee, K. S., Kahn, M. Differential roles for the coactivators CBP and p300 on TCF/β-catenin-mediated survivin gene expression. *Oncogene*. 2005; 24: 3619-3631.

[85] Miyabayashi, T., Teo, J. L., Yamamoto, M., McMillian, M., Nguyen, C., Kahn, M. WNT/β-catenin-catenin/CBP signaling maintains long-term murine stem cell pluripotency. *Proc. Natl. Acad. Sci. US*. 2007; 104:5668-5673.

[86] Teo, J. L., Kahn, M. The WNT signaling pathway in cellular proliferation and differentiation: a tale of two coactivators. *Adv. Drug Delivery Rev*. 2010; 62:1149-1155.

[87] Waltzer, L., Bienz, M. *Drosophila* CBP represses the transcription factor TCF to antagonize Wingless signaling. *Nature*. 1998; 395:521-525.

[88] Hecht, A., Vleminckx, K., Stemmler, M. P., van Roy, F., Kremler, R. The p300/CBP acetyltransferases function as transcriptional coactivators of beta-catenin in vertebrates. *EMBO J*. 2000; 19:1839-1850.

[89] Li, J., Sutter, C., Parker, D. S., Blauwkamp, T., Fang, M., Cadigan, K. M. CBP/p300 are bimodal regulators of WNT signaling. *EMBO J*. 2007; 26:2284-2294.

[90] Levy, L., Wei, Y., Labalette, C., Wu, Y., Renard, C. A., Buendia, M. A., Neuveut, C. Acetylation of beta-catenin by p300 regulates beta-catenin-Tcf4 interaction. *Mol. Cell. Biol*. 2004; 24:3404-3414.

[91] Takahashi-Yanaga, F., Kahn, M. Targeting WNT signaling: can we safely eradicate cancer stem cells? *Clin. Cancer Res*. 2010; 16:3153-3162.

[92] Lazarova, D. L., Chiaro, C., Wong, T., Drago, E., Rainey, A., O'Malley, S., Bordonaro, M. CBP activity mediates effects of the histone deacetylase inhibitor butyrate on WNT activity and apoptosis in colon cancer cells. *J. Cancer*. 2013; 4:481-490.

[93] Lazarova, D. L., Wong, T., Chiaro, C., Drago, E., Bordonaro, M. p300 influences butyrate-mediated WNT hyperactivation in colorectal cancer cells. *J. Cancer*. 2013; 4: 491-501.

[94] Lazarova, D. L., Bordonaro, M. Extreme fluctuations in Wnt/beta-catenin signaling as an approach for colon cancer prevention and therapy. *Adv. Studies in Biology*. 2012; 4:351-362.

[95] Fodde, R., Brabletz, T. WNT/beta-catenin signaling in cancer stemness and malignant behavior. *Curr. Opin. Cell Biol*. 2007; 19:150-158.

[96] Bordonaro, M., Tewari, S., Cicco, C. E., Atamna, W., Lazarova, D. L. A switch from canonical to noncanonical Wnt signaling mediates drug resistance in colon cancer cells. *PLoS One*. 2011; 6:e27308.

[97] Chiaro, C., Lazarova, D. L., Bordonaro, M. Tcf3 and cell cycle factors contribute to butyrate resistance in colorectal cancer cells. *Biochem. Biophys. Res. Commun*. 2012; 428:121-126.

[98] He, K., Xu, T., Xu, Y., Ring, A., Kahn, M., Goldkorn, A. Cancer cells acquire a drug resistant, highly tumorigenic, cancer stem-like phenotype through modulation of PI3K/ β-catenin/CBP pathway. *Int. J. Cancer*. 2013; [Epub. ahead of print] doi: 10.1002/ijc. 28341.

[99] Hanahan, D., Weinberg, R. A. Hallmarks of cancer: the next generation. *Cell*. 2011; 144:646-674.

[100] Pauklin, S., Kristjuhan, A., Maimets, T., Jaks, V. ARF and ATM/ATR cooperate in p53-mediated apoptosis upon oncogenic stress. *Biochem. Biophys. Res. Commun*. 2005; 334:386-394.

[101] Ayllón, V., Rebollo, A. Ras-induced cellular events. *Mol. Membr. Biol*. 2000;17:65–73.

[102] Gourlay, C. W., Ayscough, K. R. Actin-induced hyperactivation of the Ras signaling pathway leads to apoptosis in Saccharomyces cerevisiae. *Mol. Cell. Biol*. 2006;26: 6487-6501.

[103] An, H. J., Maeng, O., Kang, K. H., Lee, J. O., Kim, Y. S., Paik, S. G., Lee, H. Activation of Ras up-regulates pro-apoptotic BNIP3 in nitric oxide-induced cell death. *J. Biol. Chem.* 2006; 281:33939-33948.

[104] Huang, W. J., Tung, C. W., Ho, C., Yang, J. T., Chen, M. L., Chang, P. J., Lee, P. H., Lin, C. L., Wang, J. Y. Ras activation modulates methylglyoxal-induced mesangial cell apoptosis through superoxide production. *Ren. Fail.* 2007; 29:911-921.

[105] Zhao, Y., Chaiswing, L., Bakthavatchalu, V., Oberley, T. D., St Clair, D. K. Ras mutation promotes p53 activation and apoptosis of skin keratinocytes. *Carcinogenesis.* 2006; 27:1692-1698.

[106] Rutkowski, R., Dickinson, R., Stewart, G., Craig, A., Schimpl, M., Keyse, S. M., Gartner, A. Regulation of Caenorhabditis elegans p53/CEP-1-dependent germ cell apoptosis by Ras/MAPK signaling. *PLoS Genet.* 2011; 7:e1002238.

[107] Kim, H. S., Hwang, J. T., Yun, H., Chi, S. G., Lee, S. J., Kang, I., Yoon, K. S., Choe, W. J., Kim, S. S., Ha, J. Inhibition of AMP-activated protein kinase sensitizes cancer cells to cisplatin-induced apoptosis via hyper-induction of p53. *J. Biol. Chem.* 2008; 283: 3731-3742.

[108] Cuadrado, A., Garcia-Fernandez, L. F., Gonzalez, L., Suarez, Y., Losada, A., Alcaide, V., Martinez, T., Fernandez-Sousa, J. M., Sanchez-Puelles, J. M., Munoz, A. Aplidin induces apoptosis in human cancer cells via glutathione depletion and sustained activation of the epidermal growth factor receptor, Src, JNK, and p38 MAPK. *J. Biol. Chem.* 2003; 278:241-250.

[109] Dengler, M. A., Staiger, A. M., Gutekunst, M., Hofmann, U., Doszczak, M., Scheurich, P., Schwab, M., Aulitzky, W. E., van der Kuip, H. Oncogenic stress induced by acute hyper-activation of Bcr-Abl leads to cell death upon induction of excessive aerobic glycolysis. *PLoS One.* 2011; 6:e25139.

[110] Goentoro, L., Kirschner, M. W. Evidence that fold-change, and not absolute level, of beta-catenin dictates Wnt signaling. *Mol. Cell* 2009; 36:872-884.

[111] Kim, H., Won, S., Hwang, D. Y., Lee, J. S., Kim, M., Kim, R., Kim, W., Cha, B., Kim, T., Kim, D., Costantini, F., Jho, E. H. Downregulation of Wnt/β-catenin signaling causes degeneration of hippocampal neurons *in vivo*. *Neurobiol. Aging*. 2011; 32:2316. e1-15.

[112] Patel, R., Ingle, A., Maru, G. B. Polymeric black tea polyphenols inhibit 1,2-dimethyl-hydrazine induced colorectal carcinogenesis by inhibiting cell proliferation via Wnt/ beta-catenin pathway. *Toxicol. Appl. Pharmacol.* 2008; 227:136-146.

[113] Kim, J., Zhang, X., Rieger-Christ, K. M., Summerhaves, J. C., Wazer, D. E., Paulson, K. E., Yee, A. S. Suppression of Wnt signaling by the green tea compound [-]-epigallo-catechin 3-gallate [EGCG] in invasive breast cancer cells. Requirement of the transcrip-tional repressor HBP1. *J. Biol. Chem.* 2006; 281:10865-10875.

[114] Pahlke, G., Ngiewih, Y., Kern, M., Jakobs, S., Marko, D., Eisenbrand, G. Impact of quercetin and EGCG on key elements of the Wnt pathway in human colon carcinoma cells. *J. Agric. Food Chem.* 2006; 54:7075-7082.

[115] Kern, M., Pahlke, G., Ngiewih, Y., Marko, D. Modulation of key elements of the Wnt pathway by apple polyphenols. *J. Agric. Food Chem.* 2006; 54:7041-7046.

[116] Drago, E., Bordonaro, M., Lee, S., Atamna, W., and Lazarova, D. L. Propolis augments apoptosis induced by butyrate via targeting cell survival pathways. *PLoS One* 2013; 8:e 73151.

[117] Minekus, M., Smeets-Peeters, M., Bernalier, A., Marol-Bonnin, S., Havenaar, R., Marteau, P., Alric, M., Fonty, G., Huis in't Veld, J. H. A computer-controlled system to simulate conditions of the large intestine with peristaltic mixing, water absorption and absorption of feremntation products. *Appl. Microbiol. Biotechnol.* 1999; 53:108-114.

[118] De Verdier, M. G., Longnecker, M. P. Eating frequency-a neglected risk factor for colon cancer? *Cancer Causes Control.* 1992; 3:77-81.

[119] Wei, J. T., Connelly, A. E., Satia, J. A., Martin, C. F., Sandler, R. S. Eating frequency and colon cancer risk. *Nutr. Cancer.* 2004; 50:16-22.

[120] Mattson, M. P. The need for controlled studies of the effects of meal frequency on health. *Lancet.* 2005; 365:1978-1980.

[121] Varady, K. A., Hellerstein, M. K. Alternate-day fasting and chronic disease prevention: a review of human and animal trials. *Am. J. Clin. Nutr.* 2007;86:7-13.

[122] Goentoro, L., Shoval, O., Kirschner, M. W., Alon, U. The incoherent feedforward loop can provide fold-change detection in gene regulation. *Mol. Cell.* 2009; 36:894-899.

[123] Cohen-Saidon, C., Cohen, A. A., Sigal, A., Liron, Y., Alon, U. Dynamics and variability of ERK2 response to EGF in individual living cells. *Mol. Cell* 2009; 36:885–893.

[124] Macfarlane, G. T., Gibson, G. R., Cummings, J. H. Comparison of fermentation reactions in different regions of the human colon. *J. Appl. Bacteriol.* 1992; 72:57-64.

[125] Macfarlane, S., Macfarlane, G. T. Regulation of short-chain fatty acid production. *Proc. Nutr. Soc.* 2003; 62:67-72.

[126] Hijova, E., Chmelarova, A., Short chain fatty acids and colonic health. *Bratisl. Lek. Listy.* 2007; 108:354-358.

[127] James, P. T., Leach, R., Kalamara, E., Shayeghi, M., The Worldwide Obesity Epidemic, *Obesity Res.* 2001; 9:228S–233S.

[128] Wolin, K. Y., Carson, K., Colditz, G. A. Obesity and cancer. *Oncologist.* 2010;15:556-565.

[129] Doubeni, C. A., Laiyemo, A. O., Major, J. M., Schootman, M., Lian, M., Park, Y., Graubard, B. I., Hollenbeck, A. R., Sinha, R. Socioeconomic status and the risk of colorectal cancer: an analysis of more than a half million adults in the National Institutes of Health-AARP Diet and Health Study. *Cancer.* 2012; 118:3636-3644.

[130] Pendergrass, C., Edelstein, D. L., Hylind, L. M., Phillips, B. T., Iacobuzio-Donahue, C., Romans, K., Griffin, C. A., Cruz-Correa, M., Tersmette, A. C., Offerhaus, G. J., Giardiello, F. M. Occurrence of colorectal adenomas in younger adults: an epidemiologic necropsy study. *Clin. Gastroenterol. Hepatol.* 2008; 6:1011-1015.

[131] Ashktorab, H., Nouraie, M., Hosseinkhah, F., Lee, E., Rotimi, C., Smoot, D. A 50-Year Review of Colorectal Cancer in African Americans: Implications for Prevention and Treatment. *Dig. Dis. Sci.* 2009; 54:1985-1990.

[132] Cheng, X., Chen, V. W., Steele, B., Ruiz, B., Fulton, J., Liu, L., Carozza, S. E., Greenlee, R., Subsite-specific incidence rate and stage of disease in colorectal cancer by race, gender, and age group in the United States, 1992-1997. *Cancer* 2001; 92:2547-2554.

[133] Fairley, T. L., Cardinez, C. J., Martin, J., Alley, L., Friedman, C., Edwards, B., Jamison, P. Colorectal cancer in US adults younger than 50 years of age, 1998-2001. *Cancer* 2006; 107:1153-1161.

[134] Friedenreich, C., Norat, T., Steindorf, K., Boutron-Ruault, M. C., Pischon, T., Mazuir, M., Clavel-Chapelon, F., Linseisen, J., Boeing, H., Bergman, M., Johnsen, N. F.,

Tjønneland, A., Overvad, K., Mendez, M., Quirós, J. R., Martinez, C., Dorronsoro, M., Navarro, C., Gurrea, A. B., Bingham, S., Khaw, K. T., Allen, N., Key, T., Trichopoulou, A., Trichopoulos, D., Orfanou, N., Krogh, V., Palli, D., Tumino, R., Panico, S., Vineis, P., Bueno-de-Mesquita, H. B., Peeters, P. H., Monninkhof, E., Berglund, G., Manjer, J., Ferrari, P., Slimani, N., Kaaks, R., Riboli, E., Physical activity and risk of colon and rectal cancers: the European prospective investigation into cancer and nutrition. *Cancer Epidemiol. Biomarkers Prev*. 2006; 15:2398-2407.

[135] Lee, K. J., Inoue, M., Otani, T., Iwasaki, M., Sasazuki, S., Tsugane, S.; JPHC Study Group, Physical activity and risk of colorectal cancer in Japanese men and women: the Japan Public Health Center-based prospective study. *Cancer Causes Control*. 2007; 18: 199-209.

[136] Darmon, N., Drewnowski, A. Does social class predict diet quality? *Am. J. Clin. Nutr.* 2008; 87:1107-1117.

[137] Monsivais, P., Drewnowski, A., Lower-energy-density diets are associated with higher monetary costs per kilocalorie and are consumed by women of higher socioeconomic status. *J. Am. Diet. Assoc*. 2009; 109:814-822.

[138] Stables, G. J., Subar, A. F., Patterson, B. H., Dodd, K., Heimendinger, J., Van Duyn, M. A., Nebeling, L. Changes in vegetable and fruit consumption and awareness among US adults: results of the 1991 and 1997 5 A Day for Better Health Program surveys. *J. Am. Diet. Assoc*. 2002; 102:809–817.

[139] Drewnowski, A., Darmon, N. The economics of obesity: dietary energy density and energy cost. *Am. J. Clin. Nutr*. 2005; 82(suppl.):265S–273S.

[140] Rose, D., Richards, R. Food store access and household fruit and vegetable use among participants in the US Food Stamp Program. *Public Health Nutr*. 2004;7:1081-1088.

[141] Caraher, M., Dixon, P., Lang, T., Carr-Hill, R. Access to healthy foods: part I. Barriers to accessing healthy foods: differentials by gender, social class, income and mode of transport. *Health Educ. J*. 1998; 57:191–201.

[142] Kaufman, P. R. The rural poor's access to supermarkets and large grocery stores. *Fam. Econ. Nutr. Rev*. 1999;12:90-92.

[143] Kawasaki, A., Torii, K., Yamashita, Y., Nishizawa, K., Kanekura, K., Katada, M., Ito, M., Nishimoto, I., Terashita, K., Aiso, S., Matsuoka, M. Wnt5a promotes adhesion of human dermal fibroblasts by triggering a phosphatidylinositol-3 kinase/Akt signal. *Cell Signal*. 2007;19:2498-2506.

[144] Feike, A. C., Rachor, K., Gentzel, M., Schambony, A. Wnt5a/Ror2-induced upregulation of xPAPC requires xShcA. *Biochem. Biophys. Res. Commun*. 2010; 400: 500-506.

[145] Oishi, I., Suzuki, H., Onishi, N., Takada, R., Kani, S., Ohkawara, B., Koshida, I., Suzuki, K., Yamada, G., Schwabe, G. C., Mundlos, S., Shibuya, H., Takada, S., Minami, Y. The receptor tyrosine kinase Ror2 is involved in non-canonical Wnt5a/JNK signalling pathway. *Genes Cells*. 2003; 8:645-654.

In: Butyrate: Food Sources, Functions and Health Benefits ISBN: 978-1-63117-657-9
Editor: Cong-Jun Li © 2014 Nova Science Publishers, Inc.

Chapter 9

BUTYRATE-MEDIATED PROTECTION AGAINST COLONIC INFLAMMATION AND COLON CARCINOGENESIS: ROLE OF BUTYRATE TRANSPORTERS AND BUTYRATE RECEPTORS

Vadivel Ganapathy*[*], *Puttur D. Prasad, Muthusamy Thangaraju, Pamela M. Martin and Nagendra Singh

Department of Biochemistry and Molecular Biology, Medical College of Georgia, Georgia Regents University, Augusta, GA, US

ABSTRACT

Butyrate is a short-chain fatty acid generated at millimolar concentrations in colonic lumen by bacterial fermentation of dietary fiber. This bacterial metabolite elicits a plethora of biological effects on the host, influencing the function of not only the colonic epithelial cells but also that of the gut-associated immune cells and enteric neurons. In the past, most of the research on the role of butyrate in colon focused on its ability to inhibit histone deacetylases with consequent changes in gene expression. Recent studies have expanded the area of research on butyrate with the identification of specific transporters that facilitate the entry of butyrate into cells. This includes the low-affinity/high capacity transporters SLC16A1, SLC16A3 and SLC16A7, and the high-affinity/low-capacity transporter SLC5A8. These transporters are relevant to the ability of butyrate to inhibit histone deacetylases in colon cells, gut-associated immune cells, and enteric neurons. With optimal fiber intake, the luminal concentrations of butyrate are in the millimolar range, making the low-affinity transporters more relevant than the high-affinity transporters in colon cells. When the dietary fiber intake is low, the luminal concentrations of butyrate decrease, making the high-affinity transporter more relevant than the low-affinity transporters. The situation is different for the immune cells and neurons, which reside in the lamina propria beneath the epithelial cell layer. These cells are exposed only to micromolar concentrations of butyrate that cross the epithelial

[*] Corresponding Author: Department of Biochemistry and Molecular Biology, Medical College of Georgia, Georgia Regents University, Augusta, GA 30912, USA. Email: vganapat@gru.edu.

barrier; therefore, the high-affinity transporter is predominantly responsible for butyrate entry into these cells even when the dietary fiber intake is optimal. Butyrate elicits profound influence on mucosal immune cells and enteric neurons, and SLC5A8 is the transporter relevant to these biological effects of butyrate. The biological effects of butyrate are also mediated through three different G-protein-coupled receptors, namely GPR41, GPR43, and GPR109A. All three receptors are expressed on the apical membrane of colonic epithelial or enteroendocrine cells and are activated maximally by butyrate at concentrations found in the lumen. The signaling pathways associated with the activation of these receptors profoundly affect the biology of colon cells and mucosal immune cells. Butyrate provides significant protection against colonic inflammation and colon cancer, but little was known on the mechanisms responsible for these effects. The discovery of specific transporters and cell-surface receptors for butyrate in colon cells, mucosal immune cells, and enteric neurons provides a molecular basis for the beneficial effects of this bacterial metabolite in colon.

Keywords: Colonic bacteria; dietary fiber; fermentation; short-chain fatty acids; colonic epithelium; gut-associated immune cells; enteric neurons; histone deacetylases; monocarboxylate transporters; G-protein-coupled receptors; cyclic AMP

INTRODUCTION

Butyrate (a salt of butyric acid, systematic name: n-butanoic acid) is a short-chain monocarboxylic acid, first found in butter. It is present in milk in the form of triglycerides. Butyric acid is a colorless liquid, soluble in water. The carboxylic acid group in butyric acid has a pKa value of 4.8, meaning that in a solution of pH 4.8, the fraction of the protonated form (butyric acid) equals that of the unprotonated form (butyrate). The protonated form is easily permeable across biological membranes whereas the ionized form is not. The coenzyme A derivative of butyric acid (butyryl-CoA) is an intermediate in fatty acid metabolism (synthesis and degradation) in mammalian cells. The concentration of butyrate in systemic circulation is ~5 μM under normal physiologic conditions whereas the concentration in portal blood is several fold higher (10-60 μM) [1-3]. The levels in systemic blood are not dependent on the diet, suggesting endogenous generation as the primary source of butyrate in systemic circulation. Whether this is also true with butyrate in portal blood is not known. At physiological pH, butyrate exists in blood predominantly in the ionized form.

GENERATION OF BUTYRATE IN COLONIC LUMEN

Short-chain fatty acids (SCFAs), including butyrate, are produced at high concentrations in colonic lumen by bacterial fermentation of dietary fiber. Mammalian colon harbors trillions of bacteria, which have evolved for the most part a mutually beneficial symbiotic relationship with the host. Even though the term "commensal bacteria" is widely used to describe the colonic bacteria, the relationship between the bacteria and the host is mutualistic rather than commensal. Dietary fiber and undigested/unabsorbed carbohydrates constitute the primary nutritional source for these bacteria. Since most of the bacteria in mammalian colon are anaerobes, these organisms ferment carbohydrates to generate SCFAs as the major metabolic end products, with acetate, propionate and butyrate in an approximate molar ratio of 60:30:10 [4, 5]. The total concentration of all three SCFAs combined is ~150 mM in human colon, indicating that the levels of butyrate in the colonic lumen is ~15 mM. Gram-positive anaerobes are responsible for the generation of SCFAs, and the ability to produce butyrate as the fermentation product is distributed widely among these anaerobes. Glucose is the carbon source for butyrate production with acetyl-CoA, crotonoyl-CoA, and butyryl-CoA as the sequential intermediates [6]. Butyrate is generated from butyryl-CoA by two different pathways depending on the bacterial strain. In the first pathway, the enzyme phosphotransbutyrylase converts butyryl-CoA into butyrylphosphate in the presence of inorganic phosphate and then the enzyme butyrate kinase converts butyrylphosphate into butyrate coupled to the conversion of ADP into ATP [7, 8]. In the second pathway, which is more prevalent than the first, the enzyme butyryl-CoA:acetate CoA transferase converts butyryl-CoA into butyrate directly by transferring the CoA moiety from butyryl-CoA to acetate [7, 8].

PLASMA MEMBRANE TRANSPORTERS FOR BUTYRATE

The most widely recognized biological role of butyrate is the inhibition of histone deacetylases (HDACs) [9]. The ability of butyrate to modify the histone acetylation status implicates this bacterial metabolite as an important determinant of chromatin structure and transcriptome landscape in the colon. When selective lysine residues in histones are acetylated, the ε-amino group in the amino acid loses its positive charge and, as a result, the interaction between the histones and DNA is disrupted. This loosens the chromatin, consequently giving the transcriptional machinery access to selective genes. As such, the presence of histones in the acetylated form facilitates transcription. In contrast, when present in the deacetylated form, the histones interact with DNA strongly because of the positive charge on the ε-amino group of selective lysine residues; this causes compaction of the chromatin, reducing the accessibility of genes to transcriptional components, leading to silencing of the genes. As such, butyrate as an inhibitor of histone deacetylases facilitates gene transcription epigenetically. The histone acetylation status also influences recruitment of DNA methyltransferases to the genes, thus influencing the DNA methylation status [10]. Thus, butyrate also alters DNA methylation indirectly through inhibition of histone deacetylases. There are 11 histone deacetylases in mammalian cells, and butyrate is selective for HDAC1 and HDAC3 [11, 12]. For butyrate to act on its target HDACs inside the cells, it first has to traverse the plasma membrane. But, butyrate in its ionized form has low permeability across biological membranes, thus necessitating transport systems in the plasma membrane as an important component in the biological functions of butyrate as an HDAC inhibitor. The pH of the chyme in human colonic lumen is 5.5-6.0. With a pKa value of 4.8, about 10% of butyrate in the lumen exists in the unionized form, which can diffuse through the plasma membrane, and the remaining 90% is present in the deprotonated form, which depends on selective transport systems for passage through the plasma membrane.

There are multiple transporters in mammalian cells potentially involved in the transmembrane transfer of butyrate. These transporters fall into two gene families: *SLC16* and *SLC5*. There are four members in the SLC16 gene family, which transport butyrate and other monocarboxylates; these are MCT1 (monocarboxylate transporter 1), MCT2, MCT3, and MCT4. The Human Genome Organization identifies these transporters as SLC16A1, SLC16A7, SLC16A8, and SLC16A3, respectively [13]. In all cases, the transport is coupled to co-transport of H^+, which makes the process electroneutral. Among these MCTs, the mammalian intestinal tract expresses only MCT1, MCT2, and MCT4 [14-16]. MCT1 and MCT4 are expressed in intestinal and colonic epithelial cells as well as in immune cells whereas MCT2 is expressed only in enteric neurons. Since the epithelial cells of the intestinal tract are polarized, the location of the MCTs in the lumen-facing apical membrane versus the serosa-facing basolateral membrane dictates the physiological function of these transporters. The location of MCT1 in intestinal and colonic epithelial cells is controversial, but most studies have shown its expression to be restricted to the basolateral membrane [17-20]. However, it is possible that under certain conditions such as high fiber intake in the diet the expression of the transporter becomes evident in the apical membrane [20]. The rationale for this speculation is that when the luminal concentration of short-chain fatty acids, including butyrate, is high, there might be an upreglation of MCT1 expression with subsequent recruitment of the transporter to the apical membrane to promote the entry of these metabolites into the colon cells. With regard to the location of MCT4, there is a consensus; it is expressed predominantly in the basolateral membrane [14, 21].

Several reports in the literature have described the features of MCT1-mediated butyrate transport [22-24]. The Michaelis constant for the transport process is in the range of 2.5-10 mM. The affinities of MCT2 and MCT4 for butyrate have not been investigated; however, based on the affinities of these two transporters for butyrate analogs such as β-hydroxybutyrate, MCT2 is likely to have a higher affinity and MCT4 a lower affinity for butyrate than MCT1.

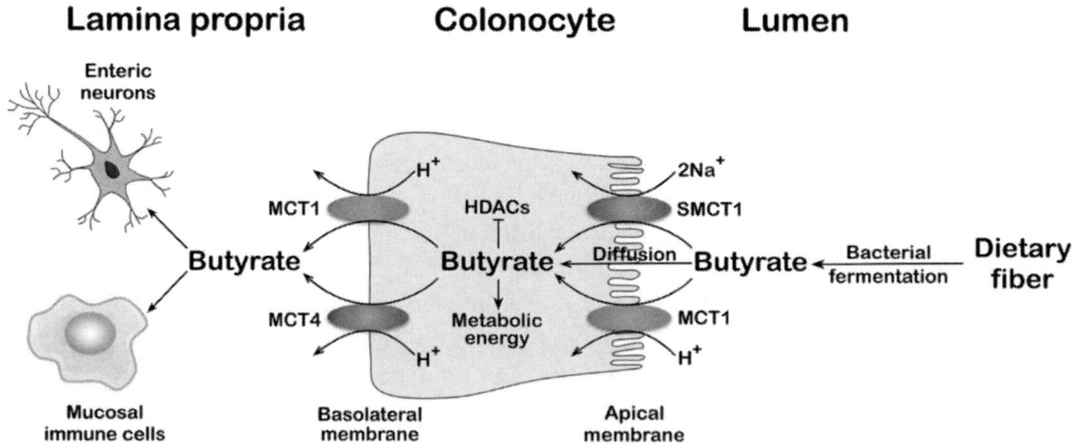

Figure 1. Carrier-mediated and diffusional pathways in colonic epithelial cells for the uptake and transcellular transfer of butyrate. SMCT1, sodium-coupled monocarboxylate transporter 1 (also known as SLC5A8); MCT1, H^+-coupled monocarboxylate transporter 1 (also known as SLC16A1), MCT4, H^+-coupled monocarboxylate transporter 4 (also known as SLC16A3); HDAC, histone deacetylases.

The *SLC5* gene family contains two transporters for monocarboxylates: SMCT1 and SMCT2 (sodium-coupled monocarboxylate transporters 1 and 2). The corresponding names according the Human Genome Nomenclature are SLC5A8 and SLC5A12 [25]. The transport mediated by SMCT1 involves co-transport with at least 2 Na^+, thus rendering the translocation of monocarboxylates an electrogenic process [26, 27]. SMCT2, though a Na^+-coupled transporter, mediates an electroneutral transport process, suggesting a Na^+:monocarboxylate molar ratio of 1:1 in the transport process [28]. SMCT1 is a high-affinity transporter for butyrate with a Michaelis constant (K_m) of ~100 μM; in contrast, SMCT2 is a low-affinity transporter with a K_m in the millimolar range. Both transporters are expressed in the small intestine whereas only SMCT1 is expressed in the colon [28-30]. As such, the low-affinity transporter SMCT2 does not seem to have any relevance to the uptake of butyrate by colonic epithelial cells. SMCT1 is expressed exclusively in the apical membrane of intestinal and colonic epithelial cells [30, 31]. SMCT1 is also expressed in immune cells, and butyrate influences the development of dendritic cells via SMCT1-dependent inhibition of histone deacetylases [32]. This high-affinity transporter is expressed in neurons [33], but whether or not the enteric neurons express the transporter has not been studied.

Since the mucosal immune cells and the enteric neurons are located on the serosal side of the intestinal and colonic epithelial cells, they would be exposed to bacterial metabolites only if the metabolites cross the epithelial monolayer. This is true also for butyrate. It has been known for a long time that the biology of the mucosal immune cells and enteric neurons is regulated by butyrate, leading to the conclusion that luminal bacteria constitute a critical determinant of the functions of the immune system and the nervous system in the intestinal tract. The assumption here is that the bacterial metabolite butyrate that is generated in the intestinal lumen gets across the epithelial cell layer, but little is known on the molecular mechanisms responsible for the transfer process. From what is known on the expression and location of various transporters for butyrate in the colonic epithelial cells, at least three routes are available for butyrate to traverse the apical membrane of the colonic epithelial cells: SMCT1, MCT1, and diffusion (Figure 1). Butyrate transport via SMCT1 is active, energized by the transmembrane Na^+ gradient and the membrane potential. However, since the Michaelis constant for the transporter is only ~100 μM, the transport process is saturated even at butyrate concentrations as low as 1 mM. Under conditions of optimal fiber intake in the diet, the luminal membrane expresses not only SMCT1 but also the low-affinity transporter MCT1. The latter is driven by the transmembrane H^+ gradient without the involvement of the membrane potential. The pH of the luminal contents is 5-6 and the concentration of butyrate is about 15 mM under these conditions, a situation ideal for maximal activity of MCT1, a H^+-coupled low-affinity transporter. Therefore, the contribution of MCT1 to butyrate transfer across the apical membrane is likely to be greater than that of SMCT1 when dietary fiber intake is optimal. In addition, diffusion would also contribute significantly to the process because the acidic pH of the colonic lumen would increase the proportion of butyric acid, the unionized form, which can traverse biological membranes independent of transport systems. Under conditions of low fiber intake, luminal concentrations of butyrate would decrease, the pH of luminal contents would increase, and the density of MCT1 in the apical membrane of colonic epithelial cells would decrease. The contribution of SMCT1 to the total butyrate transfer across the apical membrane would be greater than that of diffusion and MCT1 under these conditions. The bulk of butyrate that enters the colon cells would be metabolized as an energy source for the cells. It would also inhibit HDACs inside the cells. Only a small portion of butyrate would be available for the transfer across the basolateral membrane where MCT1 and MCT4 would be responsible for the exit process. The preferential utilization of butyrate by the colon cells as the source of biological energy explains the marked difference in butyrate levels between colonic lumen and the portal blood, which drains the colon. Thus, the immune cells and the enteric neurons that lie beneath the mucosal layer are exposed only to micromolar concentrations of butyrate irrespective of whether the dietary fiber content is high or low.

CELL-SURFACE RECEPTORS FOR BUTYRATE

GPR41 (also known as free fatty acid receptor FFAR3) and GPR43 (also called FFAR2) were the first to be identified as the receptors for SCFAs (acetate, propionate, and butyrate) [34, 35]. The concentration of butyrate necessary for half-maximal activation (EC_{50}) is in the range of 100-400 μM for both receptors. Several tissues, including colon, express these receptors [36-38]. In the intestinal tract, both receptors are expressed in enteroendocrine cells as well as in epithelial cells with preferential localization to the apical membrane, suggesting that both receptors are activated maximally by butyrate at concentrations normally found in the colonic lumen. Irrespective of the tissues in which these two receptors are expressed, SCFAs serve as the physiologic agonists. However, based on the EC_{50} values and the concentrations found locally at the site of the receptor expression, acetate and propionate are likely to be the physiologic agonists for these two receptors in non-colonic tissues. Butyrate is not found in systemic circulation at concentrations high enough to activate these receptors. In contrast, all three SCFAs, including butyrate, serve as the agonists in colon. Recently a third G-protein-coupled receptor, namely GPR109A (also known as HM74A or PUMA-G), has been identified as a butyrate receptor [31, 39]. Interestingly, unlike GPR41 and GPR43, GPR109A was not identified first as a SCFA receptor. It was originally described as a receptor for the B-complex vitamin niacin [40, 41]. But niacin is only a pharmacologic agonist because this vitamin is found in circulation under normal physiological conditions only at concentrations much lower than needed for the activation of the receptor. In latter studies, β-hydroxybutyrate was identified as the physiologic agonist for GPR109A [42]. Butyrate also activates the receptor but only at millimolar concentrations (EC_{50}, 1.6 mM), a condition never encountered in systemic circulation. However, since butyrate is found at high levels in the colonic lumen, this bacterial metabolite has relevance to activation of the receptor in this tissue. It has been shown recently that GPR109A is expressed in the colon, with its localization restricted to the apical membrane [31, 39]. As such, while β-hydroxybutyrate is the physiologic agonist for GPR109A in non-colonic tissues, butyrate is the physiologic agonist in the colon [43]. On the basis of its activation by β-hydroxybutyrate, GPR109A is currently identified as a member of the hydroxycarboxylic acid receptors or HCAs, which includes GPR81 (HCA1, a receptor for lactate), GPR109A (HCA2) and GPR109B (HCA3, a receptor for hydroxyoctanoic acid) [44].

GPR41, GPR43 as well as GPR109A are coupled to $G\alpha_{i/o}$; as a result, activation of these receptors leads to suppression of adenylate cyclase/cAMP signaling pathway [34, 35]. They are also coupled to $G\alpha_q$ resulting in activation of phospholipase C and increase in intracellular calcium levels [34, 35, 45-48]. In some cases, activation of MAP kinase and ERK pathways has also been demonstrated [35, 49, 50]. An interesting aspect of the signaling pathways associated with these receptors is the involvement of β-arrestin 1 (GPR109A), β-arrestin 2 (GPR43) and gustducin (GPR41 and GPR43) in differential modulation of selective pathways [50-52]. The various intracellular signals elicited by the activation of these three receptors in colonocyte or enteroendocrine cells are depicted schematically in Figure 2.

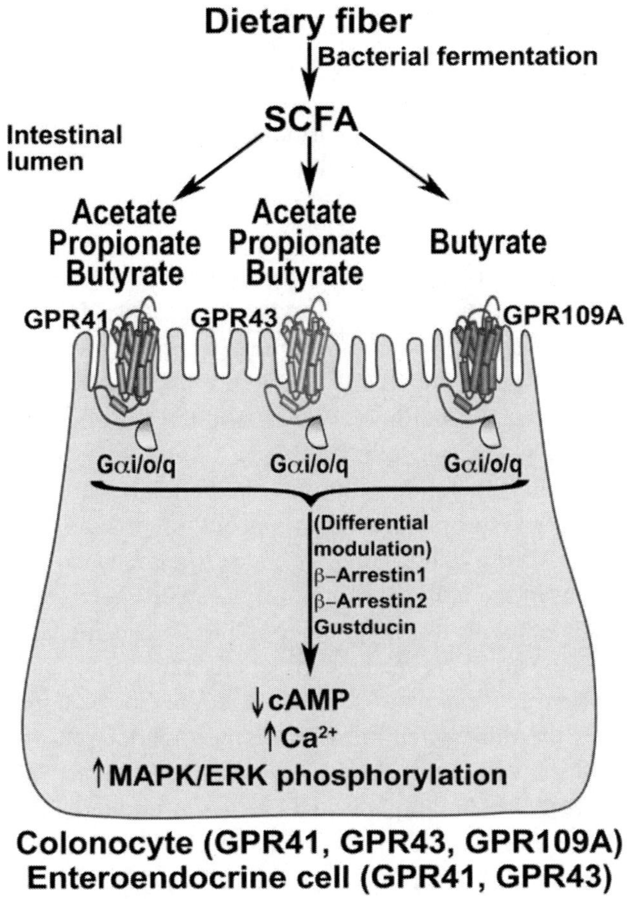

Figure 2. Cell-surface receptors that are activated by short-chain fatty acids in the colon: expression pattern and intracellular signaling. SCFA, short-chain fatty acids.

Biological Functions of Butyrate: Role of Butyrate Transporters

One of the perplexing paradoxes in biology is the presence of a massive number of bacteria in the colon coexisting with mucosal immune cells. The gut-associated immune cells constitute the largest immune system in the body; yet these cells tolerate the presence of bacteria in the colon. Bacterial metabolites arising from fermentation of dietary fiber have been implicated in the induction of the tolerogenic phenotype of the mucosal immune system. Butyrate as one of these metabolites is known to have a role in this phenomenon. In addition to the modulation of the gut-associated immune system, the bacterial fermentation products have also been implicated in a broad spectrum of beneficial effects on the colon, including supply of energy to epithelial cells, suppression of inflammation, protection against carcinogenesis, promotion of angiogenesis and gut perfusion, maintenance of the mucosal barrier, enhancement of intestinal motility, regulation of electrolyte and water absorption, control of satiety, and secretion of selective gut hormones (incretins) that act on pancreatic β cells to stimulate insulin secretion. The breadth of these biological effects implies participation of several cell types in the intestinal tract, including the epithelial cells, enteroendocrine cells, various types of immune cells, and enteric neurons. One of the molecular mechanisms by which SCFAs, the predominant metabolites of bacterial fermentation in the colonic lumen, elicit at least some of these effects is through inhibition of HDACs. Butyrate (and also propionate) inhibit HDAC1 and HDAC3. This represents the intracellular actions of these bacterial metabolites in target cells. As such, this mode of action depends on the entry of these metabolites into target cells. In colonic epithelial cells, which are in contact with luminal contents, carrier-mediated processes as well as diffusion contribute to the entry of SCFAs across the apical membrane (Figure 1). Once inside the cells, butyrate is used as an energy source through metabolism via β-oxidation. The findings that butyrate is present in portal blood only at micromolar concentrations in spite of its occurrence in the colonic lumen at millimolar levels and the presence of effective transporters and diffusional processes in colonic epithelial cells highlights the fact that most of the butyrate that enters the cells is metabolized to provide cellular energy. In addition, inhibition of HDACs by butyrate (and propionate) also impact on the epigenetic profile (histone acetylation as well as DNA methylation) and the transcriptome landscape in these cells. Even though butyrate is present in the lamina propria only at micromolar concentrations, the high-affinity transporter SLC5A8, with its energetic coupling to transmembrane Na^+ gradient and membrane potential, has the ability to mediate the uphill transport of butyrate in immune cells to cause HDAC inhibition and modulate cellular function. For example, it has been shown that butyrate suppresses the differentiation of bone marrow-derived precursor cells into the antigen-presenting dendritic cells in a SLC5A8-dependent manner [32]. This mechanism of butyrate action agrees with the findings that HDACs are required for the differentiation of dendritic cells [53]. Since inhibition of HDACs also induces the immunosuppressive enzyme indoleamine 2,3-dioxygenase in dendritic cells [54], butyrate as an inhibitor of HDACs may also impact on the dendritic cell function in a SLC5A8-dependent manner. Recent studies have shown that butyrate also regulates the function of enteric neurons through a mechanism involving HDAC inhibition, but the H^+-coupled monocarboxylate transporter MCT2 is implicated in the process [16]. Since the Na^+-coupled high-affinity transporter SLC5A8 is expressed in neurons in the central nervous system [33], it remains a possibility that enteric neurons also express this transporter, which might promote butyrate entry into cells for its subsequent function as an HDAC inhibitor.

SLC5A8 and Colon Cancer

Li et al. [55] identified SLC5A8 as a putative tumor suppressor in colon. The transporter is silenced in colon cancer and in colon cancer cell lines; when the colon cancer cells are forced to express SLC5A8, the cells undergo apoptosis. Subsequent studies have shown that the ability of the transporter to mediate cellular entry of butyrate underlies its tumor-suppressive function in colon [56-58]. However, despite the overwhelming in vitro evidence for SLC5A8 as a tumor suppressor, in vivo studies by Frank et al. [59] with *Slc5a8*$^{-/-}$ mice under conditions of optimal dietary fiber intake failed to support such a function. Recently we used the same *Slc5a8*$^{-/-}$ mice generated by Frank et al. to investigate the potential tumor-suppressive role of Slc5a8 in mammary gland. Quite contrary to the findings in the colon, the absence of *Slc5a8* accelerated breast cancer growth [60], which constituted the first in vivo evidence for the tumor-suppressive role of Slc5a8 in any tissue. The marked differences in the in vivo findings between the two tissues are puzzling. We speculate that the vastly varying levels of butyrate in the colonic lumen (~15 mM) versus the blood (<10 μM) might provide a logical explanation for these differences. Since SLC5A8 is a high-affinity transporter for butyrate, SLC5A8-mediated entry of butyrate into colon cells might represent only a small fraction of the total entry process, rendering the transporter dispensable for the biological functions of butyrate when the dietary fiber intake is optimal. The transporter might become essential only when the luminal butyrate levels are low (e.g., low-fiber diet). This is not the case in mammary gland; circulating levels of butyrate are always low irrespective of the dietary fiber content. Based on this logic, we hypothesize that SLC5A8 is a conditional tumor suppressor in colon with its ability to suppress cancer becoming evident only under conditions of low dietary fiber intake; this hypothesis however remains to be tested.

Role of MCTs in Colon Cancer and Colitis

There are conflicting reports in the literature on the relative expression of the H^+-coupled monocarboxylate transporters (MCTs) in colon cancer versus normal colon [61, 62]. Initial reports showed downregulation of MCT1 in colon cancer [63], but later studies have refuted these earlier observations and showed upregulation of MCT1 and MCT4 in colon cancer [64, 65]. Considering the fact that MCT1 is upregulated in cancers of various non-colonic tissues [62, 66], it is likely that a similar phenomenon occurs in colon cancer. Since butyrate is well known for its ability to block carcinogenesis in colon, it might seem paradoxical that MCT1 is upregulated in colon cancer, but this can be explained [66]. First, colonic epithelial cells lose their polarity and the monolayer phenotype when transformed; as such, MCT1 does not function solely to facilitate butyrate entry from the lumen into cancer cells. Second, even more important and more compelling than the first, MCT1 transports lactate with much higher affinity than it does butyrate. Cancer cells generate lactate as the glycolytic end product, and unless effluxed out of the cell, this metabolite would decrease the intracellular pH and kill the tumor cells. Therefore, cancer cells have a reason to upregulate MCT1 because of its functional features being ideal to prevent intracellular acidification caused by overproduction of lactic acid. Since lactate transport via MCT1 occurs via symport with H^+, upregulation of this transporter in cancer cells is necessary to enhance the export lactate and H^+. Stated differently, MCT1 in colon cancer cells does not mediate the cellular entry of the bacterial metabolite butyrate from the lumen but rather the efflux of cellular lactic acid generated in tumor cell-specific metabolic pathways. A similar function could also be attributed to MCT4 in colon cancer. The molecular pathways known to increase the expression of MCT1 and MCT4 have direct relevance to cancer and cancer-associated upregulation of these transporters. MCT1 is a target gene for the oncogene c-MYC and the tumor suppressor p53; c-MYC induces MCT1 expression whereas p53 suppresses its expression [67, 68]. In the case of MCT4, the hypoxia-inducible factor 1α is likely to have a role in cancer-associated upregulation of the transporter [69].

In contrast to cancer, the expression of MCT1 in colon is decreased during inflammation [70, 71]. Since butyrate serves as the primary source of metabolic energy to colonic epithelial cells, decreased expression of MCT1 might result in energy deficit, thus contributing to the colonic pathology seen in colitis.

BIOLOGICAL FUNCTIONS OF BUTYRATE: ROLE OF BUTYRATE RECEPTORS

GPR41 and GPR43

The enteroendocrine cells located in the intestinal tract play a key role in the control of appetite, intestinal motility, and pancreatic insulin secretion. This control occurs through secretion of the hormones peptide YY (PYY) and glucagon-like peptide 1 (GLP-1). GPR41 as well as GPR43 are expressed in specific enteroendocrine cells that secrete PYY and GLP-1, and luminal SCFAs, including butyrate, stimulate secretion of both hormones into blood by serving as agonists for the receptors [72-74]. PYY is a satietogenic peptide that controls appetite whereas GLP-1 stimulates insulin secretion by pancreas and thus improves glucose tolerance. In addition, GPR43 is also expressed in serotonin-positive intestinal mast cells [75] and in adipocytes [36] where SCFAs stimulate the secretion of serotonin and leptin, respectively. Serotonin is an important regulator of electrolyte and water absorption/secretion in the intestinal tract, and leptin is known for its actions as a promoter of energy expenditure and a suppressor of food intake. There is also evidence indicating that GPR41 is expressed in the neuronal cells of the submucosal and myenteric ganglia where SCFAs could potentially regulate intestinal and colonic motility through the receptor [76]. As such, GPR41 and GPR43 elicit a plethora of biological effects on the intestinal tract and these effects are dependent on the activation of these receptors by SCFAs present in the gut lumen.

GPR41 and GPR43 are expressed also in intestinal and colonic epithelial cells as well as in several subtypes of immune cells, implying a potential role for these receptors in mucosal inflammation. However, the findings reported in the literature do not project a clear and uniform picture, with some studies indicating a protective role against inflammation [77, 78] while others indicating the opposite [79, 80]. In the case of the former, deletion of *Gpr43* in mice leads to exacerbated or unresolving inflammation in an experimental model of colitis (treatment of dextran sulfate sodium in drinking water) [77]. In the same colitis model, *Gpr43*$^{-/-}$ mice showed increased disease activity index along with increased immune cell recruitment and increased production of tumor necrosis factor α and interleukin 17 [78]. In contrast, another study yielded totally opposite results, surprisingly using the same experimental colitis model in which *Gpr43*$^{-/-}$ mice showed decreased immune cell recruitment but increased mortality if the colitis was acute and decreased immune cell recruitment but protection against inflammatory tissue damage if the colitis was chronic [79]. A similar proinflammatory function of Gpr41 and Gpr43 was demonstrated in another study using three distinct experimental models of colitis: administration of ethanol, administration of trinitrobenzene sulfonic acid, or infection with *Citrobacter rodentium* [80]. Deletion of either *Gpr41* or *Gpr43* in mice showed reduced inflammatory response in all three models. The expression of Gpr41 and Gpr43 in epithelial cells and different types of immune cells suggest a complex role for these receptors in gut inflammation; further studies are certainly needed in this area.

There is some evidence suggesting a tumor-suppressive role for Gpr43 in colon. Tang et al. [81] have shown recently that GPR43 is silenced in colon cancer tissues and in colon cancer cell lines and that forced expression of the receptor in cancer cell lines leads to cell cycle arrest and increased apoptotic cell death in the presence of SCFAs. These findings have not yet been confirmed or corroborated by others.

GPR109A

The intestinal and colonic expression of GPR109A, which is activated solely by butyrate among the SCFAs produced by bacterial fermentation in the intestinal lumen, is under the control of commensal bacteria; the expression is decreased markedly in germ-free mice [31] as well as in antibiotic-treated mice [82]. Bacteria per se or specific bacterial metabolites are most likely responsible for the maintenance of optimal expression of the receptor in the intestinal tract, but details of the regulatory mechanism remain unknown. Butyrate induces the expression of its transporter MCT1 in colonic epithelial cells, and this effect is mediated via GPR109A signaling [83]. Since germ-free mice also show markedly decreased expression of the other butyrate transporter SMCT1 [31], it is possible that GPR109A signaling is necessary for optimal expression of not only MCT1 but also that of SMCT1, but this remains to be investigated. There is strong evidence in vitro as well as in vivo showing that GPR109A signaling in the intestinal tract is anti-inflammatory [39, 84]. With the experimental model of colitis induced by dextran sulfate sodium, it has been shown recently that *Gpr109a*$^{-/-}$ mice experience increased signs of inflammation compared to wild type mice [84]. In wild type mice, Gpr109a signaling induces anti-inflammatory properties in colonic immune cells and promotes the differentiation of Treg cells and interleukin-10-producing cells and suppresses Th17 cells. The receptor is also necessary for the ability of butyrate to generate interleukin-18 in the colon. Since Tregs, IL-10, and IL-18 are immunosuppressive whereas IL-17 is pro-inflammatory, it is clear that activation of Gpr109a with butyrate shifts the balance of the cytokine profile in the colon in favor of immunosuppression.

GPR109A also functions as a tumor suppressor in colon [39, 84]. The expression of this receptor is silenced in primary colon cancer tissues and in colon cancer cell lines. Ectopic expression of GPR109A in cancer cells induces apoptosis but only in the presence of its agonists, including butyrate. In vivo studies comparing the incidence and progression of colon cancer between wild type and *Gpr109a*$^{-/-}$ mice have shown that absence of the receptor enhances intestinal and colon carcinogenesis in two different experimental models: inflammation-driven colon cancer and *Apc*^{Min}-driven intestinal and colon cancer.

BUTYRATE AND THE IMMUNOSUPPRESSIVE PHENOTYPE OF THE MUCOSAL IMMUNE SYSTEM

The gut-associated immune system by nature has to perform a paradoxical role in dealing with microorganisms. On one hand, it has to be tolerant towards the commensal bacteria but on the other hand it has to mount an attack against pathogenic bacteria. Even with the commensal bacteria, the mucosal immune system is tolerogenic only as long as the mucosal barrier function is intact. When the barrier is compromised, an immune attack ensues even against the commensal bacteria. What makes the mucosal immune system "friendly" to the commensal bacteria? Recent studies have begun to shed some light on this important question. The bacterial fermentation products seem at least partly responsible for the immunosuppressive phenotype of the gut-associated immune system. Butyrate and propionate, two of the SCFAs generated by the bacteria, induce the tryptophan-degrading enzyme indoleamine 2,3-dioxygenase in colonic epithelial cells and in mucosal immune cells through their ability to inhibit HDACs. Increased expression of this enzyme depletes the essential amino acid tryptophan and suppresses the proliferation of cytotoxic T cells. Another immune cell type that is relevant to immunosuppressive phenotype of the mucosal immune system is the regulatory T cells (Tregs); these cells are essential to maintain host-commensal homeostasis in colon [85]. Recently three different groups of investigators have shown that butyrate and propionate, but not acetate, induce Tregs [86-88]. Even though there is agreement among these studies on the involvement of HDAC inhibition in the induction of Tregs, the role of cell-surface receptors in this process remains controversial. The studies by Smith et al. [86] concluded that signaling through Gpr43 is necessary for butyrate-induced HDAC inhibition and consequent Treg induction whereas those by Furusawa et al. [87] and Arpaia et al. [88] supported direct inhibition of HDACs by butyrate, thus discounting a role for Gpr43. In both of the latter studies, the induction of Tregs does not occur in the presence of acetate, an agonist for Gpr43 but with no inhibitory activity against HDACs. A more recent study by Singh et al. [84] has implicated Gpr109a in the process. Irrespective of the controversy as to the specific mechanism involved, there is no disagreement with regard to a key role for butyrate in the maintenance of the immunosuppressive phenotype of the mucosal immune system.

BUTYRATE AS A POTENTIAL ANTI-DIARRHEAL AGENT

Absorption as well as secretion of electrolytes and fluid constitutes one of the primary physiologic functions of the small intestine and large intestine. The normal fluid load to the intestinal tract is approximately 8.5 liters, of which 6.5 liters are absorbed in the small intestine. The remaining 2 liters are presented to the large intestine, which absorbs approximately 1.9 liters, leaving about 100-200 ml to be lost in the feces. Water movement across intestinal and colonic epithelial cells is coupled to ion and/or solute movement. A functional coupling between Na^+/H^+ exchanger (NHE2 and NHE3) and Cl^-/HCO_3^- exchanger (also known as DRA, an acronym for Down-Regulated in Adenoma) in the ileum and colon brings about a net absorption of Na^+ and Cl^-, and a net secretion of HCO_3^-. Secretion of Cl^- occurs primarily in the crypt cells of the small intestine and large intestine via an electrogenic process mediated by a Cl^- channel which is identical at the molecular level to cystic fibrosis transmembrane conductance regulator (CFTR), the protein affected in cystic fibrosis. Numerous chemical mediators regulate the function of these three transporters, and cAMP is the most important among them. Increase in cellular levels of cAMP in the intestinal tract blocks the absorption of NaCl by inhibiting the two exchangers (Na^+/H^+ exchanger and Cl^-

$/HCO_3^-$ exchanger) and promotes Cl^- secretion by stimulating CFTR. Diarrheal diseases such as cholera and Traveller's diarrhea are caused by the actions of bacterial toxins (cholera toxin and *E. coli* heat-labile enterotoxin) on intestinal and colonic epithelial cells; these toxins elevate cAMP levels within the cells. As such, agents that possess the ability to antagonize the cAMP-elevating effects of these bacterial toxins would be clinically valuable in the treatment of diarrhea. Activation of GPR43 and GPR109A by SCFAs does exactly that. We speculate that the bacterial fermentation products such as butyrate function to promote water and electrolyte absorption in the intestinal tract under physiological conditions and that these bacterial metabolites might also protect against diarrhea under pathological conditions such as cholera and Traveller's diarrhea. Based on this logic, pharmacological agonists of these receptors have potential as effective anti-diarrheal agents.

CONCLUSION

Butyrate elicits a broad spectrum of beneficial effects on the intestinal tract, and thus serves as a chemical messenger between commensal bacteria and the host. The SCFA transporters and the recently identified SCFA receptors provide a molecular link between butyrate and the host. Optimal generation of SCFAs in the colon is critical for maintenance of normal colonic health and the host-microbe homeostasis. This is supported by the recent observations that butyrate-producing bacteria are decreased in the colon of patients with inflammatory bowel disease [89-92]. The progression and severity of colonic inflammation can be controlled either by therapeutic administration of butyrate and other SCFAs into colon or by promotion of butyrate production in colon through increased intake of dietary fiber. Nutritional supplementation with prebiotics (t.e., chemically defined complex carbohydrates that can serve as the substrates for bacterial fermentation in the colon to generate SCFAs) and/or probiotics (i.e., live cultures of specific strains of bacteria that can be used to colonize the intestinal tract to promote generation of SCFAs) also has potential to prevent colonic inflammation. Similar strategies would also be beneficial in the prevention of colon cancer.

REFERENCES

[1] Dankert J, Zijlstra JB, Wolthers BG. Volatile fatty acids in human peripheral and portal blood: quantitative determination vacuum distillation and gas chromatography. *Clin Chim Acta* 1981;110:301-307.

[2] Cummings JH, Pomare EW, Branch WJ, Naylor CP, Macfarlane GT. Short-chain fatty acids in human large intestine, portal, hepatic and venous blood. *Gut* 1987;28:1221-1227.

[3] Wolever TM, Chiasson JL. Acarbose raises serum butyrate in human subjects with impaired glucose tolerance. *Br J Nutr* 2000;84:57-61.

[4] Weaver GA, Tangel CT, Krause JA, Parfitt MM, Jenkins PL, Rader JM, Lewis BA, Miller TL, Wolin MJ. Acarbose enhances human colonic butyrate production. *J Nutr* 1997;127:717-723.

[5] Topping DL, Clifton PM. Short-chain fatty acids and human colonic function: roles of resistant starch and non-starch carbohydrates. *Physiol Rev* 2001;81:1031-1064.

[6] Louis P, Flint HJ. Diversity, metabolism and microbial ecology of butyrate-producing bacteria from the human large intestine. *FEMS Microbiol Lett* 2009;294:1-8.

[7] Louis P, Duncan SH, McCrae SI, Millar J, Jackson MS, Flint HJ. Restricted distribution of the butyrate kinase pathway among butyrate-producing bacteria from the human colon. *J Bacteriol* 2004;186:2099-2106.

[8] Louis P, McCrae SI, Charrier C, Flint HJ. Organization of butyrate synthetic genes in human colonic bacteria: phylogenetic conservation and horizontal gene transfer. *FEMS Microbiol Lett* 2007;269:240-247.

[9] Fung KY, Cosgrove L, Lockett T, Head R, Topping DL. A review of the potential mechanisms for the lowering of colorectal oncogenesis by butyrate. *Br J Nutr* 2012;108:820-831.

[10] Denslow SA, Wade PA. The Mi-2/NuRD complex and gene regulation. *Oncogene* 2007;26:5433-5438.

[11] Thangaraju M, Carswell KN, Prasad PD, Ganapathy V. Colon cancer cells maintain low levels of pyruvate to avoid cell death caused by inhibition of HDAC1/HDAC3. *Biochem J* 2009;417:379-389.

[12] Thangaraju M, Gopal E, Martin PM, Ananth S, Smith SB, Prasad PD, Sterneck E, Ganapathy V. SLC5A8 triggers tumor cell apoptosis through pyruvate-dependent inhibition of histone deacetylases. *Cancer Res* 2006;66:11560-11564.

[13] Halestrap AP. The SLC16 gene family – structure, role and regulation in health and disease. *Mol Aspects Med* 2013;34:337-349.

[14] Gill RK, Saksena S, Alrefai WA, Sarwar Z, Goldstein JL, Carroll RE, Ramaswamy K, Dudeja PK. Expression and membrane localization of MCT isoforms along the length of the human intestine. *Am J Physiol Cell Physiol* 2005;289:C846-C852.

[15] Englund G, Rorsman F, Ronnblom A, Karlbom U, Lazorova L, Grasjo J, Kindmark A, Artursson P. Regional levels of drug transporters along the human intestinal tract: co-expression of ABC and SLC transporters and comparison with Caco-2 cells. *Eur J Pharm Sci* 2006;29:269-277.

[16] Soret R, Chevalier J, De Coppet P, Poupeau G, Derkinderen P, Segain JP, Neunlist M. Short-chain fatty acids regulate the enteric neurons and control gastrointestinal motility in rats. *Gastroenterology* 2010;138:1772-1782.

[17] Garcia CK, Goldstein JL, Pathak RK, Anderson RG, Brown MS. Molecular characterization of a membrane transporter for lactate, pyruvate, and other monocarboxylates: implications for the Cori cycle. *Cell* 1994;76:865-873.

[18] Iwanaga T, Takebe K, Kato I, Karaki S, Kuwahara A. Cellular expression of monocarboxylate transporters (MCT) in the digestive tract of the mouse, rat, and humans, with special reference to slc5a8. *Biomed Res* 2006;27:243-254.

[19] Shimoyama Y, Kirat D, Akihara Y, Kawasako K, Komine M, Hirayama K, Matsuda K, Okamoto M, Iwano H, Kato S, Taniyama H. Expression of monocarboxylate transporter 1 (MCT1) in the dog intestine. *J Vet Med Sci* 2007;69:599-604.

[20] Kirat D, Kondo K, Shimada R, Kato S. Dietary pectin up-regulates monocarboxylate transporter 1 in the rat gastrointestinal tract. *Exp Physiol* 2009;94:422-433.

[21] Kirat D, Matsuda Y, Yamashiki N, Hayashi H, Kato S. Expression, cellular localization, and functional role of monocarboxylate transporter 4 (MCT4) in the gastrointestinal tract of ruminants. *Gene* 2007;391:140-149.

[22] Hadjiagapiou C, Schmidt L, Dudeja PK, Layden TJ, Ramaswamy K. Mechanism(s) of butyrate transport in Caco-2 cells: role of monocarboxylate transporter 1. *Am J Physiol Gastroenterol Liver Physiol* 2000;279:G775-G780.

[23] Goncalves P, Araujo JR, Martel F. Characterization of butyrate uptake by nontransformed intestinal epithelial cell lines. *J Membr Biol* 2011;240:35-46.

[24] Cuff MA, Lambert DW, Shirazi-Beechey SP. Substrate-induced regulation of the human colonic monocarboxylate transporter MCT1. *J Physiol* 2002;539:361-371.

[25] Wright EM. Glucose transport families SLC5 and SLC50. *Mol Aspects Med* 2013;34:83-96.

[26] Miyauchi S, Gopal E, Fei YJ, Ganapathy V. Functional identification of SLC5A8, a tumor suppressor down-regulated in colon cancer, as a Na^+-coupled transporter for short-chain fatty acids. *J Biol Chem* 2004;279:13293-13296.

[27] Coady MJ, Chang MH, Charron FM, Plata C, Wallendorff B, Sah JF, Markowitz SD, Romero MF, Lapointe JY. The human tumour suppressor gene *SLC5A8* expresses a Na^+-monocarboxylate transporter. *J Physiol* 2004;557:719-731.

[28] Srinivas SR, Gopal E, Zhuang L, Itagaki S, Martin PM, Fei YJ, Ganapathy V, Prasad PD. Cloning and functional identification of slc5a12 as a sodium-coupled low-affinity transporter for monocarboxylates (SMCT2). *Biochem J* 2005;392:655-664.

[29] Gopal E, Fei YJ, Sugawara M, Miyauchi S, Zhuang L, Martin PM, Smith SB, Prasad PD, Ganapathy V. Expression of slc5a8 in kidney and its role in Na^+-coupled transport of lactate. *J Biol Chem* 2004;279:44522-44532.

[30] Gopal E, Miyauchi S, Martin PM, Ananth S, Roon P, Smith SB, Ganapathy V. Transport of nicotinate and structurally related compounds by human SMCT1 (SLC5A8) and its relevance to drug transport in the mammalian intestinal tract. *Pharm Res* 2007;24:575-584.

[31] Cresci GA, Thangaraju M, Mellinger JD, Liu K, Ganapathy V. Colonic gene expression in conventional and germ-free mice with a focus on the butyrate receptor GPR109A and the butyrate transporter SLC5A8. *J Gastrointest Surg* 2010;14:449-461.

[32] Singh N, Thangaraju M, Prasad PD, Martin PM, Lambert NA, Boettger T, Offermanns S, Ganapathy V. Blockade of dendritic cell development by bacterial fermentation products butyrate and propionate through a transporter (Slc5a8)-dependent inhibition of histone deacetylases. *J Biol Chem* 2010;285:27601-27608.

[33] Martin PM, Gopal E, Ananth S, Zhuang L, Itagaki S, Prasad BM, Smith SB, Prasad PD, Ganapathy V. Identity of SMCT1 (SLC5A8) as a neuron-specific Na^+-coupled transporter for active uptake of L-lactate and ketone bodies in the brain. *J Neurochem* 2006;98:279-288.

[34] Brown AJ, Goldsworthy SM, Barnes AA, Eilert MM, Tcheang L, Daniels D, Muir AI, Wigglesworth MJ, Kinghorn I, Fraser NJ, Pike NB, Strum JC, Steplewski KM, Murdock PR, Holder JC, Marshall FH, Szekeres PG, Wilson S, Ignar DM, Foord SM, Wise A, Dowell SJ. The orphan G protein-coupled receptors GPR41 and GPR43 are activated by propionate and other short chain carboxylic acids. *J Biol Chem* 2003;278:11312-11319.

[35] Le Poul E, Loison C, Struyf S, Springael JY, Lannoy V, Decobecq ME, Brezillon S, Dupriez V, Vassart G, Van Damme J, Parmentier M, Detheux M. Functional characterization of human receptors for short chain fatty acids and their role in polymorphornuclear cell activation. *J Biol Chem* 2003;278:25481-25489.

[36] Xiong Y, Miyamoto N, Shibata K, Valasek MA, Motoike T, Kedzierski RM, Yanagisawa M. Short-chain fatty acids stimulate leptin production in adipocytes through the G protein-coupled receptor GPR41. *Proc Natl Acad Sci* USA 2004;101:1045-1050.

[37] Regard JB, Sato IT, Coughlin SR. Anatomical profiling of G protein-coupled receptor expression. *Cell* 2008;135:561-571.

[38] Karaki S, Tazoe H, Hayashi H, Kashiwabara H, Tooyama K, Suzuki Y, Kuwahara A. Expression of the short-chain fatty acid receptor GPR43 in the human colon. *J Mol Histol* 2008;39:135-142.

[39] Thangaraju M, Cresci GA, Liu K, Ananth S, Gnana-Prakasam JP, Browning DD, Mellinger JD, Smith SB, Digby GJ, Lambert NA, Prasad PD, Ganapathy V. GPR109A is a G protein-coupled receptor for the bacterial fermentation product butyrate and functions as a tumor suppressor in colon. *Cancer Res* 2009;69:2826-2832.

[40] Tunaru S, Kero J, Schaub A, Wufka C, Blaukat A, Pfeffer K, Offermanns S. PUMA-G and HM74 are receptors for nicotinic acid and mediate its anti-lipolytic effect. *Nat Med* 2003;9:352-355.

[41] Wise A, Foord SM, Fraser NJ, Barnes AA, Elshourbagy N, Eilert M, Ignar DM, Murdock PR, Steplewski K, Green A, Brown AJ, Dowell SJ, Szekeres PG, Hassall DG, Marshall FH, Wilson S, Pike NB. Molecular identification of high and low affinity receptors for nicotinic acid. *J Biol Chem* 2003;278:9869-9874.

[42] Taggart AKP, Kero J, Gan X, Cai TQ, Cheng K, Ippolito M, Ren N, Kaplan R, Wu K, Wu TJ, Jin L, Liaw C, Chen R, Richman J, Connolly D, Offermanns S, Wright SD, Waters MG. (D)-β-Hydroxybutyrate inhibits adipocyte lipolysis via the nicotinic acid receptor PUMA-G. *J Biol Chem* 2005;280:26649-26652.

[43] Ganapathy V, Thangaraju M, Prasad PD, Martin PM, Singh N. Transporters and receptors for short-chain fatty acids as the molecular link between colonic bacteria and the host. *Curr Opin Pharmacol* 2013;13:869-874.

[44] Offermanns S, Colletti SL, Lovenberg TW, Semple G, Wise A, Ijzerman AP. International Union of Basic and Clinical Pharmacology. LXXXII: Nomenclature and classification of hydroxyl-carboxylic acid receptors (GPR81, GPR109A, and GPR109B). *Pharmacol Rev* 2011;63:269-290.

[45] Benyo Z, Gille A, Kero J, Csiky M, Suchankova MC, Nusing RM, Moers A, Pfeffer K, Offermanns S. GPR109A (PUMA-G/HM74A) mediates nicotinic acid-induced flushing. *J Clin Invest* 2005;115:3634-3640.

[46] Tang H, Lu JY, Zheng X, Yang Y, Reagan JD. The psoriasis drug monomethylfumarate is a potent nicotinic acid receptor agonist. *Biochem Biophys Res Commun* 2008;375:562-565.

[47] Yajima T, Inoue R, Yajima M, Tsuruta T, Karaki S, Hira T, Kuwahara A. The G-protein on cholesterol-rich membrane microdomains mediates mucosal sensing of short-chain fatty acid and secretory response in rat colon. *Acta Physiol* 2011;203:381-389.

[48] Tolhurst G, Heffron H, Lam YS, Parker HE, Habib AM, Diakogiannaki E, Cameron J, Grosse J, Reimann F, Gribble FM. Short-chain fatty acids stimulate glucagon-like peptide-1 secretion via the G-protein-coupled receptor FFAR2. *Diabetes* 2012;61:364-371.

[49] Richman JG, Kanemitsu-Parks M, Gaidarov I, Cameron JS, Griffin P, Zheng H, Guerra NC, Cham L, Maciejewski-Lenoir D, Behan DP, Boatman D, Chen R, Skinner P, Ornelas P, Waters MG, Wright SD, Semple G, Connolly DT. Nicotinic acid receptor agonists differentially activate downstream effectors. *J Biol Chem* 2007;282:18028-18036.

[50] Walters RW, Shukla AK, Kovacs JJ, Violin JD, DeWire SM, Lam CM, Chen JR, Muehlbauer MJ, Whalen EJ, Lefkowitz RJ. β-Arrestin 1 mediates nicotinic acid-induced flushing, but not its antilipolytic effect, in mice. *J Clin Invest* 2009;119:1312-1321.

[51] Lee SU, In HJ, Kwon MS, Park BO, Jo M, Kim MO, Cho S, Lee S, Lee HJ, Kwak YS, Kim S. β-Arrestin 2 mediates G protein-coupled receptor 43 signals to nuclear factor-κB. *Biol Pharm Bull* 2013;36:1754-1759.

[52] Li Y, Kokrashvili Z, Mosinger B, Margolskee RF. Gustducin couples fatty acid receptors to GLP-1 release in colon. *Am J Physiol Endocrinol Metab* 2013;304:E651-E660.

[53] Sebastian C, Serra M, Yeramian A, Serrat N, Lloberas J, Celada A. Deacetylase activity is required for STAT5-dependent GM-CSF functional activity in macrophages and differentiation to dendritic cells. *J Immunol* 2008;180:5898-5906.

[54] Sun Y, Chin YE, Weisiger E, Malter C, Tawara I, Toubai T, Gatza E, Mascagni P, Dinarello CA, Reddy P. Cutting edge: Negative regulation of dendritic cells through acetylation of the nonhistone protein STAT-3. *J Immunol* 2009;182:5899-5903.

[55] Li H, Myeroff L, Smiraglia D, Romero MF, Pretlow TP, Kasturi L, Lutterbaugh J, Rerko RM, Casey G, Issa JP, Willis J, Willson JK, Plass C, Markowitz SD. SLC5A8, a sodium transporter, is a tumor suppressor gene silenced by methylation in human colon aberrant crypt foci and cancers. *Proc Natl Acad Sci* USA 2003;100:8412-8417.

[56] Thangaraju M, Cresci G, Itagaki S, Mellinger J, Browning DD, Berger FG, Prasad PD, Ganapathy V. Sodium-coupled transport of the short-chain fatty acid butyrate by SLC5A8 and its relevance to colon cancer. *J Gastrointest Surg* 2008;12:1773-1782.

[57] Ganapathy V, Gopal E, Miyauchi S, Prasad PD. Biological functions of SLC5A8, a candidate tumour suppressor. *Biochem Soc Trans* 2005;33:237-240.

[58] Gupta N, Martin PM, Prasad PD, Ganapathy V. SLC5A8 (SMCT1)-mediated transport of butyrate forms the basis for the tumor suppressive function of the transporter. *Life Sci* 2006;78:2419-2425.

[59] Frank H, Groger N, Diener M, Becker C, Braun T, Boettger T. Lactaturia and loss of sodium-dependent lactate uptake in the colon of SLC5A8-deficient mice. *J Biol Chem* 2008;283:24729-24737.

[60] Elangovan S, Pathania R, Ramachandran S, Ananth S, Padia R, Srinivas SR, Babu E, Howthorn L, Schoenlein PV, Boettger T, Smith SB, Prasad PD, Ganapathy V, Thangaraju M. Molecular mechanism of SLC5A8 inactivation in breast cancer. *Mol Cell Biol* 2013;33:3920-3935.

[61] Goncalves P, Martel F. Butyrate and colorectal cancer: the role of butyrate transport. *Curr Drug Metab* 2013;14:994-1008.

[62] Pinheiro C, Longatto-Filho A, Azevedo-Silva J, Casal M, Schmitt FC, Baltazar F. Role of monocarboxylate transporters in human cancers: state of the art. *J Bioenerg Biomembr* 2012;44:127-139.

[63] Lambert DW, Wood IS, Ellis A, Shirazi-Beechey SP. Molecular changes in the expression of human colonic nutrient transporters during the transition from normality to malignancy. *Br J Cancer* 2002;86:1262-1269.

[64] Koukourakis MI, Giatromanolaki A, Harris AL, Sivridis E. Comparison of metabolic pathways between cancer cells and stromal cells in colorectal carcinomas: a metabolic survival role for tumor-associated stroma. *Cancer Res* 2006;66:632-637.

[65] Pinheiro C, Longatto-Filho A, Scapulatempo C, Ferreira L, Martins S, Pellerin L, Rodrigues M, Alves VA, Schmitt F, Baltazar F. Increased expression of monocarboxylate transporters 1, 2, and 4 in colorectal carcinomas. *Virchows Arch* 2008;452:139-146.

[66] Ganapathy V, Thangaraju M, Prasad PD. Nutrient transporters in cancer: relevance to Warburg hypothesis and beyond. *Pharmacol Ther* 2009;121:29-40.

[67] Doherty JR, Yang C, Scott KE, Cameron MD, Fallahi M, Li W, Hall MA, Amelio AL, Mishra JK, Li F, Tortosa M, Genau HM, Rounbehler RJ, Lu Y, Dang CV, Kumar KG, Butler AA, Bannister TD, Hooper AT, Unsal-Kacmaz K, Roush WR, Cleveland JL. Blocking lactate export by inhibiting the Myc target MCT1 disables glycolysis and glutathione synthesis. *Cancer Res* 2013; in press.

[68] Boidot R, Vegran F, Meulle A, Le Breton A, Dessy C, Sonveaux P, Lizard-Nacol S, Feron O. Regulation of monocarboxylate transporter MCT1 expression by p53 mediates inward and outward lactate fluxes in tumors. *Cancer Res* 2012;72:939-948.

[69] Ullah MS, Davies AJ, Halestrap AP. The plasma membrane lactate transporter MCT4, but not MCT1, is up-regulated by hypoxia through a HIF-1α-dependent mechanism. *J Biol Chem* 2006;281:9030-9037.

[70] Thibault R, De Coppet P, Daly K, Bourreille A, Cuff M, Bonnet C, Mosnier JF, Galmiche JP, Shirazi-Beechey S, Segain JP. Down-regulation of the monocarboxylate transporter 1 is involved in butyrate deficiency during intestinal inflammation. *Gastroenterology* 2007;133:1916-1927.

[71] Thibault R, Blachier F, Darcy-Vrillon B, de Coppet P, Bourreille A, Segan JP. Butyrate utilization by the colonic mucosa in inflammatory bowel diseases: a transport deficiency. *Inflamm Bowel Dis* 2010;16:684-695.

[72] Tazoe H, Otomo Y, Kaji I, Tanaka R, Karaki SI, Kuwahara A. Roles of short-chain fatty acid receptors, GPR41 and GPR43, on colonic functions. *J Physiol Pharmacol* 2008;59 (Suppl. 2):251-262.

[73] Kim S, Kim YM, Kwak YS. A novel therapeutic target, GPR43: Where it stands in drug discovery. *Arch Pharm Res* 2012;35:1505-1509.

[74] Bindels LB, Dewulf EM, Delzenne NM. GPR43/FFAR2: physiopathological relevance and therapeutic prospects. *Trends Pharmacol Sci* 2013;34:226-232.

[75] Karaki SI, Mitsui R, Hayashi H, Kato I, Sugiya H, Iwanaga T, Furness JB, Kuwahara A. Short-chain fatty acid receptor GPR43 is expressed by enteroendocrine cells and mucosal mast cells in rat intestine. *Cell Tissue Res* 2006;324:353-360.

[76] Nohr MK, Pedersen MH, Gille A, Egerod KL, Engelstoft MS, Husted AS, Sichlau RM, Grunddal KV, Poulsen SS, Han S, Jones RM, Offermanns S, Schwartz TW. GPR41/FFAR3 and GPR43/FFAR2 as cosensors for short-chain fatty acids in enteroendocrine cells vs FFAR3 in enteric neurons and FFAR2 in enteric leukocytes. *Endocrinology* 2013;154:3552-3564.

[77] Maslowski KM, Vieira AT, Ng A, Kranich J, Sierro F, Yu D, Schilter HC, Rolph MS, Mackay F, Artis D, Xavier RJ, Teixeira MM, Mackay CR. Regulation of inflammatory responses by gut microbiota and chemoattractant receptor GPR43. *Nature* 2009;461:1282-1286.

[78] Masui R, Sasaki M, Funaki Y, Ogasawara N, Mizuno M, Iida A, Izawa S, Kondo Y, Ito Y, Tamura Y, Yanamoto K, Noda H, Tanabe A, Okaniwa N, Yamaguchi Y, Iwamoto T, Kasugai K. G protein-coupled receptor 43 moderates gut inflammation through cytokine regulation from mononuclear cells. *Inflamm Bowel Dis* 2013;19:2848-2856.

[79] Sina C, Gavrilova O, Forster M, Till A, Derer S, Hildebrand F, Raabe B, Chalaris A, Scheller J, Rehmann A, Franke A, Ott S, Hasler R, Nikolaus S, Folsch UR, Rose-John S, Jiang HP, Li J, Schreiber S, Rosenstiel P. G protein-coupled receptor 43 is essential for neutrophil recruitment during intestinal inflammation. *J Immunol* 2009;183:7514-7522.

[80] Kim MH, Kang SG, Park JH, Yanagisawa M, Kim CH. Short-chain fatty acids activate GPR41 and GPR43 on intestinal epithelial cells to promote inflammatory responses in mice. *Gastroenterology* 2013;145:396-406.

[81] Tang Y, Chen Y, Jiang H, Robbins GT, Nie D. G-protein-coupled receptor for short-chain fatty acids suppresses colon cancer. Int J Cancer 2011;128:847-856.

[82] Cresci G, Nagy LE, Ganapathy V. *Lactobacillus GG* and tributyrin supplementation reduce antibiotic-induced intestinal injury. J Parenter Enteral Nutr 2013;37:763-774.

[83] Borthakur A, Priyamvada S, Kumar A, Natarajan AA, Gill RK, Alrefai WA, Dudeja PK. A novel nutrient sensing mechanism underlies substrate-induced regulation of monocarboxylate transporter-1. *Am J Physiol Gastrointest Liver Physiol* 2012;303:G1126-G1133.

[84] Singh N, Gurav A, Sivaprakasam S, Brady E, Padia R, Shi H, Thangaraju M, Prasad PD, Manicassamy S, Munn DH, Lee JR, Offermanns S, Ganapathy V. Activation of Gpr109a, receptor for niacin and the commensal metabolite butyrate, suppresses colonic inflammation and carcinogenesis. *Immunity* 2014;40:1-12.

[85] Tanoue T, Honda K. Induction of Treg cells in the mouse colonic mucosa: A central mechanism to maintain host-microbiota homeostasis. *Sem Immunol* 2012;24:50-57.

[86] Smith PM, Howitt MR, Panikov N, Michaud M, Gallini CA, Bohlooly M, Glickman JN, Garrett WS. The microbial metabolites, short-chain fatty acids, regulate colonic Treg cell homeostasis. *Science* 2013;341:569-573.

[87] Furusawa Y, Obata Y, Fukuda S, Endo TA, Nakato G, Takahashi D, Nakanishi Y, Uetake C, Kato K, Kato T, Takahashi M, Fukuda NN, Murakami S, Miyauchi E, Hino S, Atarashi K, Onawa S, Fujimura Y, Lockett T, Clarke JM, Topping DL, Tomita M, Hori S, Ohara O, Morita T, Koseki H, Kikuchi J, Honda K, Hase K, Ohno H. Commensal microbe-derived butyrate induces the differentiation of colonic regulatory T cells. *Nature* 2013;504:446-450.

[88] Arpaia N, Campbell C, Fan X, Dikiy S, van der Veeken J, deRoos P, Liu H, Cross JR, Pfeffer K, Coffer PJ, Rudensky AY. Metabolites produced by commensal bacteria promote peripheral regulatory T-cell generation. *Nature* 2013;504:451-455.

[89] Frank DN, St Amand AL, Feidman RA, Boedeker EC, Harpaz N, Pace NR. Molecular-phylogenetic characterization of microbial community imbalances in human inflammatory bowel diseases. *Proc Natl Acad Sci* USA 2007;104:13780-13785.

[90] Frank DN, Robertson CE, Hamm CM, Kpadeh Z, Zhang T, Chen H, Zhu W, Sartor RB, Boedeker EC, Harpaz N, Pace NR, Li E. Diease phenotype and genotype are associated with shifts in intestinal-associated microbiota in inflammatory bowel diseases. *Inflamm Bowel Dis* 2011;17:179-184.

[91] Wang W, Chen L, Zhou R, Wang X, Song L, Huang S, Wang G, Xia B. Increased proportion of *Bifidobacterium* and the *Lactobacillus* group and loss of butyrate-producing bacteria in inflammatory bowel disease. *J Clin Microbiol* 2013; in press.

[92] Machiels K, Joossens M, Sabino J, De Preter V, Arijs I, Eeckhaut V, Ballet V, Claes K, Van Immerseel F, Verbeke K, Ferrante M, Verhaegen J, Rutgeerts P, Vermeire S. A decrease of the butyrate-producing species Roseburia hominis and Faecalibacterium prausnitzii defines dysbiosis in patients with ulcerative colits. *Gut* 2013; in press.

In: Butyrate: Food Sources, Functions and Health Benefits ISBN: 978-1-63117-657-9
Editor: Cong-Jun Li © 2014 Nova Science Publishers, Inc.

Chapter 10

EPIGENETIC INFLUENCE OF BUTYRATE PRODUCING BACTERIA IN METABOLIC SYNDROME

Marlene Remely, Ines Tesar and Alexander G. Haslberger
Department of Nutritional Sciences, University Vienna, Vienna, Austria

ABSTRACT

Bacteria or bacteria-derived metabolites may reverse or change epigenetic regulation patterns such as DNA methylation and histone modifications, thus altering the expression of critical genes associated in pathologic processes, for example in metabolic syndrome. Fermentation end products, especially butyrate, have been suggested as bioactive metabolites influencing epigenetic modifications, either by directly influencing enzymes catalyzing epigenetic modifications, by altering the availability of substrates, or by interactions with receptors. The most important butyrate producers appear to be *Faecalibacterium prausnitzii*, belonging to *Clostridium cluster IV*, and *Eubacterium rectale/Roseburia spp*., belonging to *Clostridium cluster XIVa* of *Firmicutes*. Both are also detectable via analysis of the *butyryl-CoA: acetate CoA-transferase* gene.

Butyrate is well known for its epigenetic activity as a histone deacetylase inhibitor in apoptosis and cell arrest, and it may contribute to obesity through anti-inflammatory effects. Activities of histone deacetylases and methyl CpG binding proteins may also then influence DNA methylation. Our recent study of the methylation status of the FFAR3 promoter region in connection with butyrate producers revealed a significant lower methylation status in obese and type 2 diabetics compared to lean participants. These results revealed a significant correlation between a higher body mass index and lower methylation% of FFAR3. Biological functions of FFAR3 include the modulation of lipid metabolism, impact on leptin production, and control of host energy metabolism influenced by microbial dysbiosis. An overexpression of FFAR3 receptor was reported to induce the expression of satiety hormones. However, in obese individuals leptin is no longer able to contribute to satiety, as a cause of the insensitivity of the cells. The diversity of the microbiota as well as abundance of *Faecalibacterium prausnitzii* were significantly lower in obese and type 2 diabetic patients. *Clostridium cluster IV* and *Clostridium cluster XIVa* showed a decreasing trend in type 2 diabetics in comparison to analysis with the *butyryl-CoA: acetate CoA-transferase* gene.

The GI microbiota composition may contribute to body health by influencing epigenetic regulation of the host. Research provides evidence for butyrate in the prevention/treatment of the chronic low grade inflammation seen in obesity and type 2 diabetes. However, current knowledge of nutritional epigenetics is limited, and further studies are needed to better understand the use of bioactive food components for maintaining health and disease prevention through modifiable epigenetic mechanisms.

Keywords: *Butyryl-CoA:acetate CoA-transferase* gene – *Faecalibacterium prausnitzii* – FFAR3 – DNA Methylation – Histon modifications

INTRODUCTION

At least 2.8 million people worldwide die each year as a result of being overweight (BMI 25-30 kg/m2) or obese (BMI >30 kg/m2). In addition, high blood glucose kills about 3.4 million people annually. Overweight and obesity have been estimated to account for about 65–80% of new cases of type 2 diabetes. A high body weight impairs blood pressure, cholesterol, triglycerides, and insulin resistance. The consequences are an increased risk for coronary heart disease, ischemic stroke, and type 2 diabetes mellitus, as well as increased risk for cancer [1]. The invested costs are escalating; thus prevention is imperative. One target may be the gut microbiota as an option to influence the host metabolism.

The human gut microbiota plays an important role in digestion and metabolism: it is essential for a normal gut physiology [2]. A wide range of inflammatory and metabolic diseases are associated with microbial imbalance [3, 4]. These differences affect the host metabolism: energy extraction, immune system modulation, the modification of the lipid metabolism, and epigenetic regulation. Body weight for example is influenced by the gut microbial composition, food ingredients [5], and the energy harvest from the diet [6]. Thus obesity is associated with a higher abundance of *Firmicutes* and a decreased abundance of *Bacteroidetes* in animal studies [7], and also a relation between an aberrant *Firmicutes/ Bacteroidetes* ratio and obesity is mentioned in human studies [3, 8]. Schwiertz et al. (2011) reported a lower ratio of *Firmicutes/Bacteroidetes* in overweight human adults compared to lean controls [8], while Duncan et al. (2008) showed no correlation between the ratio composition and human obesity [9]. A higher *Firmicutes/ Bacteroidetes* ratio is hypothesized to increase the fermentation end-products butyrate and acetate, as many *Firmicutes* are butyrate producers [10]. After a hypocaloric diet the number of *Bacteroidetes* depends on weight loss whereas the *Firmicutes* group remains unchanged, and no correlation with total caloric intake is detectable [11]. *Roseburia* and *Faecalibacterium prausnitzii* are well-known for butyrate synthesis and are associated with improved insulin sensitivity [12]. *Faecalibacterium prausnitzii* provides anti-inflammatory activity by decreasing the rates of NF-κB (nuclear factor-κB) activation and IL-8 (interleukin) secretion, increasing IL-12, IL-10, and IFN-γ (interferon-γ) [13]. Type 2 diabetes has often been associated with lower abundance of *Firmicutes*, while *Bacteroidetes,* and *Proteobacteria* tended to be more abundant [3]. However, a lower abundance of *Bacteroidetes vulgatus* and *Bifidobacterium* spp. and a higher one of *Clostridium leptum cluster* in diabetics compared to healthy volunteers are also mentioned [14]. The relative abundance of *Bacilli* is increased in diabetic mouse models [3] and humans, with a positive correlation of *Lactobacillus gasseri* and HbA_{1c}

values [12, 15]. *Lactobacilli* together with *Enterobacteria* are named as contributors to low-grade inflammation of obesity and type 2 diabetes. Both species are suggested to influence inflammation via their immune-modulating properties and to provoke the macrophage-mediated adipose tissue inflammation [15] and also gut permeability [16].

In particular, butyrate-producing bacteria are of increasing interest because of their potential role in colonic health [17]. Gut bacteria partially convert proteins, peptides, and especially sugars [17] to short-chain fatty acids (SCFAs), which are used by the host as an energy source [18]. The major SCFAs in the intestinal lumen are butyrate (C4), propionate (C3), and acetate (C2). They interact with the intestinal mucosa through an increase in intracellular pH, modulation of sodium absorption and chloride secretion, stimulation of mucin-release, and enhancing blood flow in the mucosa [19]. Acetate for example is important for muscles, heart, and brain cells, and propionate is used in hepatic neoglucogenic processes [20]. In comparison butyrate is of key importance for gut health as it is not only the preferred energy source of the colonic epithelial cells, but also has important effects on gene expression and the development of intestinal cells. It is generally thought to play a protective role against colorectal cancer and colitis [21] as it provides anti-carcinogenic and anti-inflammatory potential. Effects on the intestinal barrier, satiety, adipose tissue expansion, and epigenetic regulation are also described [20, 22].

Epigenetic factors are somatically heritable states of gene expression resulting from changes in chromatin structure without alterations in the DNA sequence, including DNA methylation, histone modifications, and chromatin remodeling [23]. They have been implicated in orchestrating a seemingly infinite variety of molecular and cellular processes essential for higher nervous system functions and evolutionary innovations [24-27]. These modifications are altered by external or internal environmental factors resulting in permanent maintenance of the acquired phenotype. Internal factors, nutrients, and bioactive food components can modify epigenetic regulation and alter the gene-expression at the transcriptional level [23]. Hence it has become clear that epigenetic modifications play important roles in diseases, including cancer, inflammatory bowel disease, obesity, and type 2 diabetes [17].

BUTYRYL-COA: ACETATE COA-TRANSFERASE GENE

Most of the butyrate in the gut is taken up by the intestinal mucosa and metabolized. Thu,s fecal butyrate concentrations give only little information about the butyrate-producing capacity of the gut microbiota and are biased by nutritional intake. A function-based approach has been suggested for the enumeration of butyrate-producing bacteria [17]. Two pathways of butyrate production are described. The more important pathway, used by more than 90% of the carriers of the gene in culture-based assays, is via butyryl-CoA: acetate CoA-transferase, using acetate as co-substrate [28, 29]. A minority of bacteria are able to use butyrate kinase and phosphotransbutyrylase as an alternative final step [28]. In addition, butyrate producers do not form a monophyletic group, as butyrate producers and non-butyrate producers are in the same phylogenetic clusters [17]. Recent findings from the 16S rRNA study conducted by Louis et al. (2010) suggest the numerical importance of butyrate production in two groups of *Lachnospiraceae*: *Roseburia/ Eubacterium rectale* within *Clostridium cluster XIVa* and

Faecalibacterium prausnitzi within *cluster IV* (figure 1). The most abundant species within the *Roseburia/E. rectale* group is *Eubacterium rectale* with 54%, with the four *Roseburia* species (*R. faecis, R. hominis, R. inulinivorans, R. intestinalis*) accounting for 45%. These findings suggest an abundance of a third group of as yet unnamed bacteria, SS2/1. All butyrate producers represent about 25% of total bacteria [30].

Dietary components and prebiotics affect the growth of butyrate producers. For example the consumption of inulin stimulates the growth of *F. prausnitzii*, strain SS2/1, and *E. rectale* [31]. A reduction in these species was observed during low-carb diets, but no changes were shown during moderate carbohydrate intake [9]. Hippe et al. (2011) also showed the important influence of diet on butyrate production in the GI tract. The microbiota of elder study participants is characterized by decreased butyrate production capacity in response to a lower fiber intake. In contrast a vegetarian diet leads to an increase of butyryl-CoA:acetate CoA-transferase gene copy number [28]. Recently research investigates the role of these bacteria on the host epigenetic regulation.

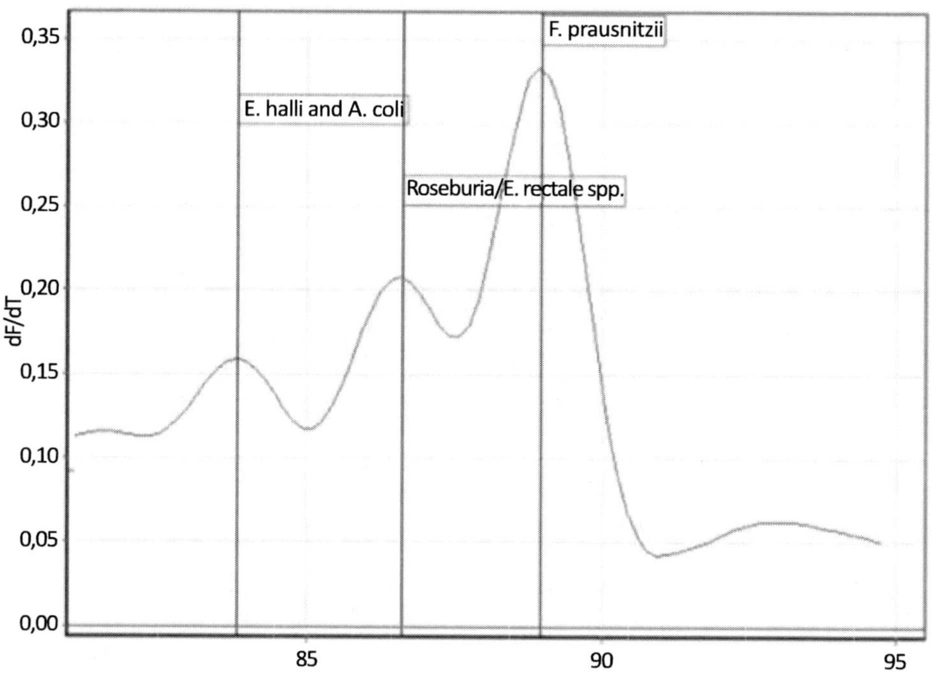

Figure 1. Melt curves of butyryl-CoA: acetate CoA-transferase gene representing the peaks related to *E. hallii* and *A. coli* (82.5–85.0), *Roseburia/E. rectale spp.* (85.5–89.0) and *F. prausnitzii* (89.5–92.5).

Table 1. Primers for quantification of butyryl CoA:acetate CoA-transferase gene (BCoAT gene)

Target	Primer/Probe	Sequence (5' - 3')	Conc. [pmol/μL]	Reference
BCoAT gene	Fwd primer	GCI GAI CAT TTC ACI TGG AAY WSI TGG CAY ATG	27	[17]
	Rev primer	CCT GCC TTT GCA ATR TCI ACR AAN GC	27	

DNA METHYLATION

DNA methylation means the modification of the 5'-position of a cytosine base at the CpG dinucleotide with methyl groups catalyzed by DNA-methyltransferases (Dnmts). Five different Dnmts are known: Dnmt1, Dnmt2, Dnmt3a, Dnmt3b, and DnmtL. Changes in global DNA methylation affect chromosomal integrity, and gene specific promoter DNA methylation is associated with impaired gene expression [23]. A high methylation rate in the promoter region is proposed to decrease transcriptional activity of the downstream gene [32].

Folate is one of the best-known methyl group donors; however, other substances such as methionine, choline, and butyrate are also able to influence the DNA methylation status [32]. Theoretically every nutrient affecting S-adenosylmethionine (SAM), a methyl donor for methylation reactions, or S-adenosylhomocystein (AdoHcy), an inhibitor of methyltransferases, can alter the DNA methylation and histone methylation. In addition Dnmts work in a complex network with other enzymes catalyzing other epigenetic modifications. DNA methylation is involved in the suppression of the expression of endogenous retroviral genes and other harmful stretches as well as in X-chromosome inactivation [33]. Demethylation of CpGs also plays an important role, but it is not well understood yet. It is known to result in the activation of specific genes with an influence on cellular regulatory mechanisms [34]. For example 5-hyrdoxymethylcytosine (5-hmC) is suggested to be involved in DNA demethylation, as it is significantly represented in mammalian DNA. Further studies are needed to determine the role of 5-hmC for example in aging or cancer, as both are characterized by DNA hypomethylation [23].

EFFECTS OF BUTYRATE ON DNA METHYLATION

Although most of the butyrate is metabolized by the colonic epithelium and extracted by the liver, the remaining concentrations (0.5-3.3 μmol) in the venous system [21] act as a signalling molecule [35] mediated by the G-protein coupled receptors (GPRs). The affinity of SCFAs to GPR41 (FFAR3; free fatty acid receptor) and GPR43 (FFAR2) depends on the length of the fatty acids. FFAR3 has a higher affinity for the ligands butyrate and propionate, whereas FFAR2 is activated by acetate and propionate [36, 37]. Additionally, GPR40 binds LCFAs (long chain fatty acid) but not SCFAs and is located upstream close to the GPR41 gene. Halpern et al. (2012) indicated that GPR41 may have no promoter region and thus is transcribed by the promoter of GPR40 [38]. Biological functions of FFARs include the modulation of lipid metabolism [39], influences on leptin production [39, 40] and other satiety hormones [41], and the control of host energy metabolism [40].

Investigations of a potential interaction of the gut microbiota with the epigenetic regulation of FFAR3 in obese and type 2 diabetes patients compared to a lean control group showed a significant lower abundance of *Faecalibacterium prausnitzii* and lower microbial diversity in type 2 diabetics and obese patients. Results from *Clostridium cluster IV* and *Clostridium cluster XIVa* showed a decreasing trend in type 2 diabetics in comparison to the butyryl-CoA:acetate CoA-transferase gene and according to melt curve analysis. Therefore missing differences in butyryl-CoA:acetate CoA-transferase gene might only be a result of difficulties in detection; as already mentioned above not all butyrate producers are included

[42]. The analysis of five CpGs in the promoter region of FFAR3 showed different methylation levels in the three analysed groups, type 2 diabetics, obese patients, and lean controls. Thus, lean controls showed significantly higher methylation than obese and type 2 diabetics. These results disclosed a significant correlation between a higher body mass index and lower methylation of FFAR3 [42]. Accordingly Canani et al. (2011) has observed lower expression of FFAR3 receptor in the lean control group [32]. The lower methylation in FFAR3 promoter region of type 2 diabetics was supposed to cause an overexpression of FFAR3 receptors, confirmed by the high expression of the named receptor in adipose tissue with an influence on the leptin resistant state, as a positive correlation of leptin plasma levels and body fat mass was already indicated [43].

Leptin is produced exclusively in adipose tissue and influences the hunger-satiety cycle by suppression of the appetite and contribution to the fat metabolism. In mice, increased leptin production caused by an overexpression of FFAR3 was observed after oral doses of propionate [44], and a knockdown of FFAR3 inhibits the ability of propionate to induce leptin expression, mainly in adipocytes [45]. In addition Ichimura et al. (2009) showed a dose dependent SCFA activation of FFAR3 and regulation of leptin production in adipocytes. A higher FFAR3 expression might induce a higher leptin production [44]. Therefore, supplementation with SCFAs may help to improve the sensitivity or the production of leptin. However, few obese patients suffer from leptin deficiency, and therapies with leptin or even SCFAs might be affected. Studies on increased consumption of dietary fibres resulted in reduced inflammation and increased butyrate production with an increased FFAR3 activation [32].

Besides hypophagic effects of leptin, studies from Samuel et al. (2008) show that deficiency in FFAR3 results in decreased PYY (Peptide YY) expression [41]. The main functions of PYY are the ability to control appetite and caloric intake, inhibition of gut motility, and enhancement of nutrient absorption. Further it inhibits stomach emptying and increases the water and electrolyte absorption in the gastrointestinal tract. In general obese patients show lower fasting PYY-levels compared to lean patients, and the postprandial release of the peptide is decreased leading to diminished satiety [43]. These results are underlined by a study with FFAR3-deficient mice and conventionally raised mice, in which a deficiency of the receptor was associated with a lower expression of PYY and as a consequence with a higher energy harvest from diet. An inhibition of FFAR3 may cause a decreased energy extraction and leaner individuals [41]. However, current researches indicate a FFAR3-independent influence of butyrate and propionate on body weight and food intake.

Wu et al. (2012) suggest a possible involvement of FFAR3 in histone acetylation, proliferation, apoptosis, and cell cycle regulation. Their results showed a dose dependent increase of pro-apoptotic Bax proteins and decreased anti-apoptotic Bcl-2 proteins after butyrate induction. In FFAR3 cells the expression of anti-apoptotic Bcl-2 proteins was increased. Consequently it is supposed that FFAR3 prevents butyrate induced pro-apoptotic impacts. Finally, an inclusion of FFAR3 in cell cycle alteration could also be shown. Therefore, flow cytometry analysis of relative DNA content was used to establish the inclusion of butyrate in cell cycle alterations. It was shown that FFAR3 is able to transfer more cells from G1- (post mitotic) phase to S- (DNA synthesis) phase checkpoint. Almost no effects could be observed in cells without FFAR3. These results may explain the lowered anti-proliferative effect of FFAR3 induced by butyrate. Interestingly, FFAR3 is able to inhibit an increase of p21, a cyclin-dependent kinase (Cdk) inhibitor, which is able to inhibit Cdk 2 and Cdk 4, after butyrate induction [45].

Recent studies emphasize a cooperation of DNA methylation, miRNA expression, and histone modifications to silence genes and to repress the transcription. It is supposed that histone deacetylation and H3K9 (histone H3 lysine 9) methylation clear the way for CpG methylation. An interaction of these two mechanisms is also discussed and supposed to result in long-term transcriptional silencing [46].

HISTONE MODIFICATIONS

Histones are alkaline proteins in eukaryotic cell nuclei, are surrounded by DNA molecules and can undergo posttranslational modification at their N-terminal tails of 15–38 amino acids. Possible modifications include acetylation, methylation, phosphorylation, sumoylation, ubiquitination, biotinylation, and ADP ribosylation. These modifications can alter DNA-histone interactions and further chromatin structure [23]. Histone acetylation and phosphorylation can activate gene expression, whereas histone deacetylation, sumoylation, and biotinylation silence gene expression [47, 48]. Methylation and ubiquitination of histones are more complex and can act as silencers or activators depending on the affected histone residue [49]. In addition, different combinations of histone modifications act together and modify the overall conformation of the chromatin [50, 51]. The histone code hypothesis terms this effect of specific histone modifications in specific region of the genome on specific biological functions, resulting in locus-specific gene regulation [52]. The enzymatic regulation of histone methylation, for example, is conducted by histone methyltransferases (HMTs) and histone demethylases, although SAM is necessary for the activation of HMTs [52].

Histone acetylation is regulated by histone acetyl-transferase (HAT) and three classes of histone deacetylase (HDAC). Classes I and II can be inhibited by short-chain carboxylic acids and polyphenols. Class III needs nicotinamide adenine dinucleotide (NAD+) as cofactor [52]. An acetylation of the N-terminal lysine residues (position 9, 14, 18 of H3; position 5, 8, 1 2, 16 of H4) affects histone and DNA interactions and facilitates the access and binding of transcription factors. Bioactive food components directly influence the enzymes involved, for example resveratrol, butyrate, and sulforaphane inhibit HDAC, and curcumin inhibits HAT. HDAC inhibitors are named as potential therapeutics in cancer, as they induce cell cycle arrest and apoptosis by enhancing the expression of proapoptotic or cell mediating genes [23].

EFFECTS OF BUTYRATE ON HISTONE MODIFICATIONS

The ability of butyrate to induce inhibition of histone deacetylase helps to reduce inflammatory symptoms [32] by reduction of macrophages, B-lymphocytes, and T-lymphocytes [53]. Butyrate restrains the LPS- and cytokine-stimulated production of TNF-α, IL-6, and NO (nitric oxide) and also suppresses the major Th1-skewing factors IL-12 and IFN-γ, which might seriously influence the development of a subsequent T-cell response. In addition, butyrate increases the secretion of anti-inflammatory cytokine IL-10, but this effect is not confirmed in all studies [54-56]. Park et al. (2007) investigated the anti-inflammatory effects of sodium butyrate (NaB), sodium phenylbutyrate (NaPB) and sodium phenylacetate (NaPA) in IFN-γ-stimulated macrophage cells. The results showed that SCFAs significantly repressed IFN-γ-mediated NO generation. NaB inhibited the production of TNF-α, iNOS (Nitric oxide synthases), and IL-6 and enhanced the IFN-γ-induced production of IL-10. Moreover, SCFAs inhibited the IFN-γ-induced NF-κB activity. They had no effect on the IFN-γ-induced JAK/STAT activation, but they repressed IFN-γ-induced ERK (extracellular regulated kinase) phosphorylation. In summary, the study demonstrates that the major anti-inflammatory mechanisms of SCFAs in macrophage cells seem to be the inhibition of NF-κB and ERK, but not the JAK/STAT pathway. The order of effectiveness was NaB>NaPB>NaPA [55]. Bailón et al. (2010) also reported a significant inhibition of the proliferation of bone marrow-derived macrophages by butyrate in a concentration-dependent manner. They suggested that butyrate is able to inhibit both lymphocyte and macrophage proliferation while only suppressing T-cell activation [57]. In addition, Usami, Kishimoto et al. (2008) reported a reduced LPS-induced TNF-α secretion by 0.5 mM butyrate, indicating a therapeutic potential of butyrate by intravenous or oral administration [58].

The main mechanisms described for the anti-inflammatory effects are the reduction of HDAC activity [54-56], and the suppression of NF-κB, the inhibition of IFN-γ production, and the up-regulation of peroxisome proliferator-activated receptor γ (PPARγ) [32]. PPARγ occurs mostly in adipose tissue and is able to regulate genes involved in fatty acid uptake, inflammation, and glucose homeostasis [59].

In inflammatory bowel disease (IBD) butyrate induced the inhibition of histone deacetylase and therefore reduced abdominal symptoms and inflammation after increased consumption of dietary fibers [32]. The inflammatory profile of patients with ulcerative colitis could be improved by reduction of macrophages, B-lymphocytes, and T-lymphocytes. Processes responsible for the improvement in IBD may be the suppression of NF-κB, inhibition of IFN-γ production, and the up-regulation of peroxisome PPARγ [32].

CONCLUSION

A different composition of the gut microbiota and therefore SCFA-production influences the epigenetic modifications of host genes and thus helps to maintain intestinal symbiosis. These interactions between microbiota and epigenetic regulation of genes influence not only regulatory mechanisms, for example hunger-satiety cycle, but also disease patterns. There is increasing evidence that gut microbiota composition maintains host health. Butyrate in particular is a candidate to take a role in regenerative medicine by promoting epigenetic remodelling. Although to delineate the precise effect of nutrients is very hard as the effects, depend on their structure, physiologic and pathologic processes in our body, nutrient interaction, but also interaction with other lifestyle factors. Therefore, more gene-specific studies and expression analysis are necessary for a better understanding of the involvement of gut microbiota and SCFA in epigenetic regulation and expression. A consistent and improved detection of SCFA and butyrate-producing bacteria would be desirable.

REFERENCES

[1] WHO. http://www.euro.who.int/en/health-topics/noncommunicable-diseases/ 2013 [cited 2013 18/10/2013].

[2] Aziz, Q., et al., Gut microbiota and gastrointestinal health: current concepts and future directions. *Neurogastroenterol Motil,* 2013. 25(1): p. 4-15.

[3] Larsen, N., et al., Gut microbiota in human adults with type 2 diabetes differs from non-diabetic adults. *PLoS One,* 2010. 5(2): p. e9085.

[4] Vrieze, A., et al., The environment within: how gut microbiota may influence metabolism and body composition. *Diabetologia,* 2010. 53(4): p. 606-13.

[5] Harris, K., et al., Is the gut microbiota a new factor contributing to obesity and its metabolic disorders? *J Obes, 2012.* 2012: p. 879151.

[6] Musso, G., R. Gambino, and M. Cassader, Obesity, diabetes, and gut microbiota: the hygiene hypothesis expanded? *Diabetes Care,* 2010. 33(10): p. 2277-84.

[7] Turnbaugh, P.J., et al., An obesity-associated gut microbiome with increased capacity for energy harvest. *Nature,* 2006. 444(7122): p. 1027-31.

[8] Schwiertz, A., et al., Microbiota and SCFA in lean and overweight healthy subjects. *Obesity* (Silver Spring), 2010. 18(1): p. 190-5.

[9] Duncan, S.H., et al., Human colonic microbiota associated with diet, obesity and weight loss. *Int J Obes* (Lond), 2008. 32(11): p. 1720-4.

[10] Turnbaugh, P.J. and J.I. Gordon, The core gut microbiome, energy balance and obesity. *J Physiol,* 2009. 587(Pt 17): p. 4153-8.

[11] Cani, P.D., et al., Changes in gut microbiota control metabolic endotoxemia-induced inflammation in high-fat diet-induced obesity and diabetes in mice. *Diabetes,* 2008. 57(6): p. 1470-81.

[12] Karlsson, F.H., et al., Gut metagenome in European women with normal, impaired and diabetic glucose control. *Nature,* 2013. 498(7452): p. 99-103.

[13] Furet, J.P., et al., Differential adaptation of human gut microbiota to bariatric surgery-induced weight loss: links with metabolic and low-grade inflammation markers. *Diabetes,* 2010. 59(12): p. 3049-57.

[14] Wu, X., et al., Molecular characterisation of the faecal microbiota in patients with type II diabetes. *Curr Microbiol,* 2010. 61(1): p. 69-78.

[15] Remely, M., et al., Abundance and diversity of microbiota in type 2 diabetes and obesity. *Diabetes Metab Res Rev,* 2013. 4(4).

[16] de Kort, S., D. Keszthelyi, and A.A. Masclee, Leaky gut and diabetes mellitus: what is the link? *Obes Rev,* 2010. 12(6): p. 449-58.

[17] Louis, P. and H.J. Flint, Development of a semiquantitative degenerate real-time pcr-based assay for estimation of numbers of butyryl-coenzyme A (CoA) CoA transferase genes in complex bacterial samples. *Appl Environ Microbiol,* 2007. 73(6): p. 2009-12.

[18] Macfarlane, S. and G.T. Macfarlane, Regulation of short-chain fatty acid production. *Proc Nutr Soc,* 2003. 62(1): p. 67-72.

[19] Piekarska, J., et al., Trichinella spiralis: the influence of short chain fatty acids on the proliferation of lymphocytes, the goblet cell count and apoptosis in the mouse intestine. *Exp Parasitol,* 2011. 128(4): p. 419-26.

[20] Qin, J., et al., A human gut microbial gene catalogue established by metagenomic sequencing. *Nature,* 2010. 464(7285): p. 59-65.

[21] Hamer, H.M., et al., Review article: the role of butyrate on colonic function. *Aliment Pharmacol Ther,* 2008. 27(2): p. 104-19.

[22] Delzenne, N.M. and P.D. Cani, Interaction between obesity and the gut microbiota: relevance in nutrition. *Annu Rev Nutr,* 2011. 31: p. 15-31.

[23] Choi, S.W. and S. Friso, Epigenetics: A New Bridge between Nutrition and Health. *Adv Nutr,* 2010. 1(1): p. 8-16.

[24] Klose, R.J. and A.P. Bird, Genomic DNA methylation: the mark and its mediators. *Trends Biochem Sci,* 2006. 31(2): p. 89-97.

[25] Kondo, T., Epigenetic alchemy for cell fate conversion. *Curr Opin Genet Dev,* 2006. 16(5): p. 502-7.

[26] Mehler, M.F. and J.S. Mattick, Noncoding RNAs and RNA editing in brain development, functional diversification, and neurological disease. *Physiol Rev,* 2007. 87(3): p. 799-823.

[27] Tsankova, N., et al., Epigenetic regulation in psychiatric disorders. *Nat Rev Neurosci,* 2007. 8(5): p. 355-67.

[28] Hippe, B., et al., Quantification of butyryl CoA:acetate CoA-transferase genes reveals different butyrate production capacity in individuals according to diet and age. *FEMS Microbiol Lett,* 2011. 316(2): p. 130-5.

[29] Louis, P., et al., Restricted distribution of the butyrate kinase pathway among butyrate-producing bacteria from the human colon. *J Bacteriol,* 2004. 186(7): p. 2099-106.

[30] Louis, P., et al., Diversity of human colonic butyrate-producing bacteria revealed by analysis of the butyryl-CoA:acetate CoA-transferase gene. *Environ Microbiol,* 2010. 12(2): p. 304-14.

[31] Louis, P. and H.J. Flint, Diversity, metabolism and microbial ecology of butyrate-producing bacteria from the human large intestine. *FEMS Microbiol Lett,* 2009. 294(1): p. 1-8.

[32] Canani, R.B., et al., Epigenetic mechanisms elicited by nutrition in early life. *Nutr Res Rev,* 2011. 24(2): p. 198-205.

[33] McKay, J.A. and J.C. Mathers, Diet induced epigenetic changes and their implications for health. *Acta Physiol (Oxf),* 2011. 202(2): p. 103-18.

[34] Franchini, D.M., K.M. Schmitz, and S.K. Petersen-Mahrt, 5-Methylcytosine DNA demethylation: more than losing a methyl group. *Annu Rev Genet,* 2012. 46: p. 419-41.

[35] Brown, A.J., et al., The Orphan G protein-coupled receptors GPR41 and GPR43 are activated by propionate and other short chain carboxylic acids. *J Biol Chem,* 2003. 278(13): p. 11312-9.

[36] Layden, B.T., et al., Short chain fatty acids and their receptors: new metabolic targets. *Transl Res,* 2012.

[37] Lin, H.V., et al., Butyrate and propionate protect against diet-induced obesity and regulate gut hormones via free fatty acid receptor 3-independent mechanisms. *PLoS One,* 2012. 7(4): p. e35240.

[38] Halpern, K.B., et al., PR41 Gene Expression Is Mediated by Internal Ribosome Entry Site (IRES)-dependent Translation of Bicistronic mRNA Encoding GPR40 and GPR41 Proteins. *Journal of Biological Chemistry* 2012. 287 (24): p. 20154-20174.

[39] Kebede, M.A., et al., Lipid receptors and islet function: therapeutic implications? *Diabetes Obes Metab,* 2009. 11 Suppl 4: p. 10-20.
[40] Talukdar, S., J.M. Olefsky, and O. Osborn, Targeting GPR120 and other fatty acid-sensing GPCRs ameliorates insulin resistance and inflammatory diseases. *Trends Pharmacol Sci,* 2011. 32(9): p. 543-50.
[41] Samuel, B.S., et al., Effects of the gut microbiota on host adiposity are modulated by the short-chain fatty-acid binding G protein-coupled receptor, Gpr41. *Proc Natl Acad Sci U S A,* 2008. 105(43): p. 16767-72.
[42] Remely, M., et al., Effects of short chain fatty acid producing bacteria on epigenetic regulation of FFAR3 in type 2 diabetes and obesity. 2013.
[43] 43. Schloegl, H., et al., Peptide hormones regulating appetite--focus on neuroimaging studies in humans. *Diabetes Metab Res Rev,* 2010. 27(2): p. 104-12.
[44] Ichimura, A., et al., Free fatty acid receptors act as nutrient sensors to regulate energy homeostasis. *Prostaglandins Other Lipid Mediat,* 2009. 89(3-4): p. 82-8.
[45] Wu, J., et al., Butyrate-induced GPR41 activation inhibits histone acetylation and cell growth. *J Genet Genomics,* 2012. 39(8): p. 375-84.
[46] Fuks, F., DNA methylation and histone modifications: teaming up to silence genes. *Curr Opin Genet Dev,* 2005. 15(5): p. 490-5.
[47] Brosch, G., P. Loidl, and S. Graessle, Histone modifications and chromatin dynamics: a focus on filamentous fungi. *FEMS Microbiol Rev,* 2008. 32(3): p. 409-39.
[48] Oliver, S.S. and J.M. Denu, Dynamic interplay between histone H3 modifications and protein interpreters: emerging evidence for a "histone language". *Chembiochem,* 2011. 12(2): p. 299-307.
[49] Sawicka, A. and C. Seiser, Histone H3 phosphorylation - a versatile chromatin modification for different occasions. *Biochimie,* 2012. 94(11): p. 2193-201.
[50] Brandl, A., T. Heinzel, and O.H. Kramer, Histone deacetylases: salesmen and customers in the post-translational modification market. *Biol Cell,* 2009. 101(4): p. 193-205.
[51] Haberland, M., R.L. Montgomery, and E.N. Olson, The many roles of histone deacetylases in development and physiology: implications for disease and therapy. *Nat Rev Genet,* 2009. 10(1): p. 32-42.
[52] Jimenez-Chillaron, J.C., et al., The role of nutrition on epigenetic modifications and their implications on health. *Biochimie,* 2012. 94(11): p. 2242-63.
[53] Vieira, E.L., et al., Oral administration of sodium butyrate attenuates inflammation and mucosal lesion in experimental acute ulcerative colitis. *J Nutr Biochem,* 2012. 23(5): p. 430-6.
[54] Vinolo, M.A., et al., Suppressive effect of short-chain fatty acids on production of proinflammatory mediators by neutrophils. *J Nutr Biochem,* 2011. 22(9): p. 849-55.
[55] Park, J.S., et al., Anti-inflammatory effects of short chain fatty acids in IFN-gamma-stimulated RAW 264.7 murine macrophage cells: involvement of NF-kappaB and ERK signaling pathways. *Int Immunopharmacol,* 2007. 7(1): p. 70-7.
[56] Liu, L., et al., Butyrate interferes with the differentiation and function of human monocyte-derived dendritic cells. *Cell Immunol.* 277(1-2): p. 66-73.
[57] Bailon, E., et al., Butyrate in vitro immune-modulatory effects might be mediated through a proliferation-related induction of apoptosis. *Immunobiology,* 2010. 215(11): p. 863-73.

[58] Usami, M., et al., Butyrate and trichostatin A attenuate nuclear factor kappaB activation and tumor necrosis factor alpha secretion and increase prostaglandin E2 secretion in human peripheral blood mononuclear cells. *Nutr Res,* 2008. 28(5): p. 321-8.
[59] Staels, B. and J.C. Fruchart, Therapeutic roles of peroxisome proliferator-activated receptor agonists. *Diabetes,* 2005. 54(8): p. 2460-70.

In: Butyrate: Food Sources, Functions and Health Benefits ISBN: 978-1-63117-657-9
Editor: Cong-Jun Li © 2014 Nova Science Publishers, Inc.

Chapter 11

Butyrate Facilitates Epigenetic Reprogramming

Justin E. Brier-Jones, Jason B. Kiroyan and Xiao-Bing Zhang*
Loma Linda University School of Medicine, CA, US

Abstract

Reprogramming of somatic cells into pluripotency by reshaping the epigenetic landscape of differentiated cells has transformed the field of stem cell research and regenerative medicine. Sodium butyrate, a histone deacetelase inhibitor, has made a substantial impact on reprogramming technology. It significantly improves reprogramming efficiency and allows for the development of potentially "safer" reprogramming strategies. This chapter briefly discusses contemporary reprogramming techniques and the possible mechanisms of sodium butyrate in facilitating cellular reprogramming.

Keywords: Cellular Reprogramming, Sodium Butyrate, HDAC Inhibitor, Induced Pluripotent Stem Cell (iPSC), miR-302/367, NuRD, MBD2

Introduction to Reprogramming

The Impact of Cellular Reprogramming Technology

Over the past decade, it has become possible to readily change the fate of adult somatic cells using the Nobel Prize-winning reprogramming technology [1]. This breakthrough was achieved through forced expression of crucial transcription factors associated with pluripotency, and builds upon the notion that the nucleus of a mature differentiated cell still contains all the necessary genetic information to create all cell types of the adult organism [2].

* Corresponding Author: Xiao-Bing Zhang, Division of Regenerative Medicine MC1528B, Department of Medicine, Loma Linda University. 11234 Anderson Street, Loma Linda, California 92350, USA;.E-mail: xzhang@llu.edu.

This discovery may be one of the most profound scientific breakthroughs of this century, and will undoubtedly contribute to the treatment of countless diseases once reprogramming technology becomes safe and efficient enough to introduce into clinical practice. In this chapter, we focus on the reprogramming of adult somatic cells into induced pluripotent stem cells (iPSCs), and how sodium butyrate, a histone deacetylation inhibitor, has made a significant impact on advancing reprogramming technology.

The Basic Principles of Cellular Reprogramming

The cell is the smallest functional unit of a biological organism, and within each cell itself contains a relatively intact and comprehensive library of instructions that it uses to replicate itself known as the genome. However, a cell's structure and function is largely restricted by its current epigenomic status and chromatin availability, which dictates the delicate balance of proteins expressed at a given time [3]. Epigenetic reprogramming is to convert specified somatic cells into what is called a stem cell by manipulating the epigenome [3]. Reprogramming of somatic cells to pluripotency leads to the generation of iPSCs, which are capable of generating tissues from all 3 germ layers (endoderm, mesoderm and ectoderm), similar to what is seen in a developing embryo. Stem cells are known for their ability to 1) self-renew, or proliferate without losing their ability to differentiate into phenotypically mature cells, and 2) differentiate into cell types of one or more lineages [4-5]. Stem cells are more practically known for their ability to regenerate functional cells and replace damaged tissues. This regeneration process competes with injury repair, which often re-establishes tissue continuity and basic structural integrity through fibroblastic invasion that does not always preserve the tissues original functionality [6]. Furthermore, the potential for regeneration wanes as our species grows older due to a dwindling number of stem cells and/or a diminished capacity for their recruitment and differentiation at the site of injury [7]. Tissues may ultimately become fibrotic to the point of disability. It is here that the marvel of reprogramming technology can be realized: We can now remodel cellular expression profiles to better resemble natural pluripotent stem cells well enough to convert adult mouse cells into iPSCs capable of developing into a healthy animal [8]. The sheer number of potential clinical applications of reprogramming technology is staggering.

Cellular Reprogramming Technique, and How Butyrate Fits in

Somatic cell nuclear transfer technology pioneered by John Gurdon [2] in the 1960's brought forth decades of hope in someday eradicating disease by simply replacing our age-feebled selves with new cells, tissues and organs. Cloning large animals soon became possible after triumphs in life science research with the famous birth of Dolly the Sheep in 1996; the first mammal successfully cloned by transferring a somatic cell nucleus from healthy mammary tissue into an unfertilized oocyte [9]. The fetus matured in a surrogate mother until birth and proved to the world that a nucleus from a determined cell still had the ability to function as a totipotent cell that can proliferate and differentiate into all three germ layers of the developing embryo, as well as into the placenta that will cradle it to life. This feat reminds us of an earlier Nobel Prize-winning discovery as well: the oocyte cytoplasm is packed with maternal RNA and translational regulatory proteins that restrict transcriptional control of the developing zygote until several divisions are made, known as maternal effect [10]. Harnessing transcriptional control in a similar fashion was necessary to change the fate of committed cells in the future.

The first successful reprogramming experiments in the 2000's made it possible to generate a viable stem cell line without compromising ethical principles by harvesting the embryonic stem cells formed shortly after fertilization [1]. It was first accomplished by overexpressing four key pluripotency-related transcription factors OCT4, SOX2, KLF4, and MYC (OSKM), coined "Yamanaka Factors" in honor of Shinya Yamanaka's seminal contribution [1]. Shortly after, Thomson et al. [11] discovered a slightly different cocktail of factors that were found to induce pluripotency in human cells (OCT4, SOX2, NANOG, and LIN28). Many labs have ever since extensively explored the mechanism of reprogramming and translation of iPSCs technology.

Table 1. Summary of human cellular reprogramming studies

Author / Year	Cell Source	Butyrate Concentration	Factor	Mode of Introduction	Reprogramming Efficiency	Date Colonies Picked
Takahashi et al. 2007	Fibroblasts	None	OSKM	pMX Retrovirus	0.02%	Day 30
Aasent et al. 2008	Keritinocytes	None	OSKM	pMSCV Retrovirus	0.80%	NR
Zhou et al. 2011	Urine Cells	None	OSKM	pMX Retrovirus	0.01-4%	Day 16
Staerk et al. 2010	Peripheral Blood MNCs	None	OSKM	LentiVirus	0.001-0.002%	Day 25-40
Li et al. 2009	Amniotic Cells	None	OSKM	pMX Retrovirus	NR	Day 20
Sugii et al. 2010	Adipose	None	OSK	pMX Retrovirus	0.0002%-0.02%	Day 29-42
Giorgetti et al. 2009	Cord Blood CD133+	None	OS	pMX Retrovirus	0.006%	Day 12-15
Kim et al. 2009	Neural Stem Cells	None	O	pMX Retrovirus	0.004%-0.006%	Week 10-11
Anokye-Danso et al. 2011	Fibroblasts	None	miR-302/367 cluster	Lenti Virus	10.40%	Day 18
Mali et al. 2010	Fibroblasts	0.25 mM (Day 7-12)	OSKM	pMX Retrovirus	0.003%	Day 12-24
Shimada et al. 2011	Adipose	0.25 mM	OSKM	pMX Retrovirus	NR	Day 10
Meng et al. 2011	Cord Blood CD34+	0.25 mM (Day 2-12)	OS	Episomal Vector	2%	Week 2
Zhu et al.	Keritinocytes	0.25 mM	O	Lenti Virus	0.004%	Week 4
Zhu et al.	Amniotic Cells	0.25 mM	O	Lenti Virus	0.004%	Week 5-6
Su et al. 2013	Peripheral Blood MNCs	0.25 mM (Day 2-12)	OSMK+BCL-XL	Episomal Vector	0.001%	Week 3

There are three techniques capable of generating stem cells that demonstrate pluripotent properties: somatic cell nuclear transfer (SCNT), cell-fusion mediated reprogramming, and transcription factor mediated reprogramming [2, 12-14]. All three techniques show different strengths and limitations, and we will primarily focus on transcription factor mediated reprogramming. However, a common theme emerges amongst these techniques that reinforce the notion that reprogramming requires substantial epigenetic change, and that current reprogramming techniques often lead to incomplete epigenetic reprogramming [2, 13-14]. For example, Dr. Gurdon and his associates have reported that nuclei retain "epigenetic memory" of their cell of origin for many cell divisions after nuclear transfer, even after activation of the embryonic gene expression program [15].

Low reprogramming efficiency has been a major roadblock in the reprogramming process. Evidence suggests that histone acetylation plays a positive role in the acquisition and maintenance of pluripotency [16-17]. Histone deacetylase (HDAC) inhibitors were soon found to promote reprogramming at different times along the reprogramming process [4, 18-19]. It became apparent that the role of sodium butyrate was complicated and its contribution to reprogramming seemed to depend on the cell type, culture conditions and reprogramming factor cocktail used [18]. Table 1 summarizes relevant information of human cell sources, reprogramming efficiency and cocktail of factors used as reported from several groups. A schematic representation of the reprogramming process is shown in Figure 1.

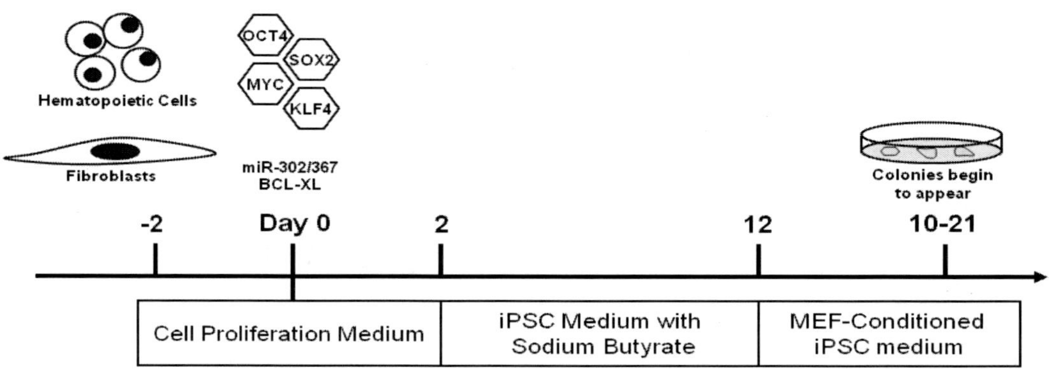

Figure 1. Schematics of ectopic factor expression-induced reprogramming. Addition of sodium bytyrate at the early stage of reprogramming generally increases efficiency by 3- to 10-fold.

Mechanistic Insight: Reprogramming with Sodium Butyrate

Sodium Butyrate Improves Reprogramming Efficiency and Safety

Despite so much promise, current reprogramming technology suffers several pitfalls that prevent its clinical application [4]. The most notable limitation we will discuss is a low reprogramming efficiency, which prevents large numbers of high quality iPSCs from being generated using adult cells [4]. Many small molecule compounds have been used to increase efficiency, among which sodium butyrate shows a very impressive ability to increase reprogramming efficiency when in combination with members of the OSKM factor cocktail [4, 18-23]. Small molecule inhibitors of HDACs, and most notably butyrate, worked so well to improve efficiency that it allowed experimentation with low efficiency non-integrating

OSKM expression systems and novel reprogramming strategies to better explore the mechanism of inducing pluripotency [24].

It is also important to recognize that sodium butyrate acts as a major regulator of the fatty acid β-oxidation pathway in which it is metabolized [25-26]. Butyrate acts in an intriguing fashion described as the "butyrate paradox", where this fatty acid demonstrates toxicity to cancer cell lines while simultaneously promoting proliferation of healthy cells [25]. While not the focus of this chapter, it is advisable to recognize that butyrate serves as a fuel source as well as an epigenetic modulator. The individual metabolism of each cell source used in reprogramming likely dictates the availability of intracellular sodium butyrate, and undoubtedly relates to its discriminative toxicity as can be seen in glycolytic cancer populations [27].

Sodium butyrate has gained the attention of the cellular reprogramming field due to its potency in inhibiting HDAC [18-20, 22-23, 28], and thus promoting gene transcription by increasing histone acetylation and increasing accessibility of chromatin [29]. Reprogramming efficiencies nearing 100% were achieved last year (2013) by depleting Mbd3, a member of the NuRD (nucleosome remodeling and deacetylation) repressor complex, together with OSKM transduction [30]. Later in this chapter we will discuss evidence that butyrate may facilitate reprogramming in a similar way, through its activity as an HDAC inhibitor and a modulator of miRNA that further inhibits NuRD activity [23, 31-32]. Butyrate as a reprogramming supplement has improved efficiency and made it possible to explore new strategies for increasing reprogramming safety. Proto-oncogenes MYC, Kruppel-like factor 4 (KLF4), and even SOX2 can be omitted in specific instances with combined butyrate supplementation, such as when reprogramming human keratinocytes with OCT4 alone [18, 20, 33-34]. Safer, non-integrating approaches for factor delivery are now viable strategies in iPSC reprogramming because efficiency can be raised to acceptable levels to pick iPSC colonies [20-21, 35]. We showed that human cord blood hematopoietic progenitors or $CD34^+$ cells can be efficiently reprogrammed to pluripotency with EBNA1-based episomal vectors expressing only OCT4 and SOX2 with 0.25 mM butyrate added days 2-12 post-transduction [21]. We also found that in the absence of sodium butyrate, OCT4 and SOX2 alone failed to generate integration-free iPSCs [21].

The potency of butyrate in reprogramming may be due to its role in converting partially reprogrammed cells into full pluripotency [19, 23-24, 36-37]. It has been suggested that butyrate also facilitates reprogramming of cells that are typically more difficult to induce pluripotency *in vitro,* such as human skeletal myoblasts or cells from older patients [20, 22]. Additional studies suggest that butyrate also promotes pluripotency through upregulated expression of pluripotency-related miRNAs [23, 36, 38]. Unfortunately, the precise mechanisms of most of the apparent benefits of butyrate have yet to be reported. The bulk of the remaining chapter will focus on a concise review of reported evidence that sheds light on how this small molecule played such a significant role in facilitating reprogramming: **1)** Butyrate acts as a potent histone deacetylase inhibitor that facilitates OSKM access to nuclear chromatin [19-20, 24], and **2)** butyrate induces miR-302/367 cluster expression in an OCT4/SOX2 dependent manner to serve as a key regulator of stemness and promote self-renewal [23, 32].

Sodium Butyrate As a Histone Deacetylase Inhibitor

Early reprogramming reports by Mali et al. [19], and Liang et al. [20] demonstrate that butyrate significantly improves reprogramming efficiency of cells from different species. Mali et al. [20] reprogrammed human adult and fetal fibroblasts using retrovirus or the non-viral *piggyback* transposon vectors expressing OSKM and demonstrated a 15- to 50-fold increase in reprogramming efficiency when 0.5 mM NaB was added at 2 to 11 days post transduction. Mali et al. had reported several findings that butyrate promotes demethylation at 1,174 loci during the reprogramming process, as well further promoting acetylation of H3K9, a major epigenetic barrier to iPSC reprogramming when it remains methylated [20]. This study also reported that the addition of butyrate increased expression of endogenous pluripotency genes DPPA2, NANOG, and OCT4, while downregulating genes specific to fibroblasts. Increasing endogenous expression of pluripotency genes may in part explain butyrate facilitated reprogramming, but detailed investigation is required to be certain. Conversely, Liang et al. [19] reported that mouse embryonic fibroblast (MEF) specific genes were not downregulated after butyrate treatment, nor was endogenous pluripotency gene expression seen to increase. Butyrate was also found to require exogenous MYC in order to show a modest improvement in MEF reprogramming efficiency [19]. Butyrate treatment was found to be most beneficial in the early stages of reprogramming in MEFs (2-4 days after factor transduction). They performed microarray analysis of gene expression during MEF reprogramming 48 hours after adding 1 mM butyrate and found that 19 of the upregulated genes are also expressed in embryonic stem cells. These studies demonstrate the ability of butyrate to improve reprogramming through inhibiting HDAC function.

Sodium Butyrate Induces Expression of miR-302/367 Cluster

It has been suspected that modulating HDAC activity is not the only mechanism involved in butyrate-mediated reprogramming efficiency increases. Recently, Zhang et al. [23] found that 0.5 mM butyrate induced miR-302/367 gene cluster expression in primary human foreskin fibroblasts (HFFs) when OSKM were used in reprogramming. OSKM were found necessary to upregulate miRNAs expressed from this cluster, and can in part be explained by OCT4 and SOX2 binding regions in its promoter [23]. The miR-302/367 cluster expresses miR-302 a/b/c/d and miR-367, and is associated with mesenchymal-to-epithelial transition, a critical process in development and the initiation of somatic cell reprogramming [39]. MiR-302 has also been found to target NR2F2, which directly inhibits the activity of the OCT4 promoter, thus promoting positive feedback regulation between miR-302 and OCT4 [38]. Butyrate treatment also increases stability of miRNA from the expression of miR-302/367 transduced HFFs (an experiment performed without OSKM) [23]. In this case, RNA stability was determined by comparing miRNA expression by RT-qPCR at several time points after transcriptional inhibition [23]. A later study by the same team showed that knocking out the miR-302/367 cluster completely prevented reprogramming and was rescued after its replacement through retroviral transduction [32]. Furthermore, HFFs and human dermal fibroblasts can be induced to pluripotency through overexpression of miR-302/367 alone via lentiviral transduction [40]. The iPSCs derived from this technique showed a remarkable reprogramming efficiency of approximately 10%, reinforcing a powerful and complex connection of intracellular miRNAs in orchestrating reprogramming in certain cell types [32, 36].

Finally, butyrate has also been reported to decrease the portion of partially reprogrammed colonies [19, 23-24, 36-37]. Insight as to why sodium butyrate pushes reprogramming to completion can also be related to its ability to induce the miR-302/367 cluster [40]. MicroRNA expressed from this cluster have been found to inhibit methyl-CpG binding domain protein 2 (MBD2), one of the several components that are associated with the NuRD complex and acts as a reprogramming roadblock by silencing endogenous pluripotency gene expression [30-31, 36, 41-44]. MBD2 also downregulates *NANOG* expression, a critical pluripotency factor that acts downstream of SOX2 and is used to facilitate iPSC reprogramming in several laboratories [32, 36, 45]. Although the miR-302/367 cluster appears critical to the reprogramming process, it should be stated that the exact downstream targets of its miRNAs are not fully known and further investigation is required [23].

CONCLUSION

Reprogramming technology has advanced miraculously in recent decades. We have reached the point where induced pluripotent stem cells can now be derived from many different types of human cells at remarkable efficiency. Sodium butyrate has played a substantial role in the recent evolution of the reprogramming technology by facilitating the development of novel reprogramming protocols. Butyrate has shown to improve reprogramming efficiency through its activity as an HDAC inhibitor [19-20] and modulator of pluripotency-related miRNAs [23, 32, 36], while also converting partially reprogrammed cells into full pluripotency [19, 23-24, 36-37]. Hopefully the insights highlighted in this chapter will serve to enlighten readers as to how butyrate touched the brief history of reprogramming technology, while also reminding that butyrate is a small molecule worthy of attention and further research.

REFERENCES

[1] Takahashi, K.; Yamanaka, S., Induction of pluripotent stem cells from mouse embryonic and adult fibroblast cultures by defined factors. *Cell* 2006, *126* (4), 663-76.

[2] Gurdon, J. B., The developmental capacity of nuclei taken from intestinal epithelium cells of feeding tadpoles. *J Embryol Exp Morphol* 1962, *10*, 622-40.

[3] Ramalho-Santos, M.; Yoon, S.; Matsuzaki, Y.; Mulligan, R. C.; Melton, D. A., "Stemness": transcriptional profiling of embryonic and adult stem cells. *Science* 2002, *298* (5593), 597-600.

[4] Stadtfeld, M.; Hochedlinger, K., Induced pluripotency: history, mechanisms, and applications. *Genes Dev* 2010, *24* (20), 2239-63.

[5] Jankowski, R. J.; Deasy, B. M.; Huard, J., Muscle-derived stem cells. *Gene Ther* 2002, *9* (10), 642-7.

[6] Krafts, K. P., Tissue repair: The hidden drama. *Organogenesis* 2010, *6* (4), 225-33.

[7] Piccin, D.; Morshead, C. M., Potential and pitfalls of stem cell therapy in old age. *Dis Model Mech* 2010, *3* (7-8), 421-5.

[8] Quinlan, A. R.; Boland, M. J.; Leibowitz, M. L.; Shumilina, S.; Pehrson, S. M.; Baldwin, K. K.; Hall, I. M., Genome sequencing of mouse induced pluripotent stem cells reveals retroelement stability and infrequent DNA rearrangement during reprogramming. *Cell Stem Cell* 2011, *9* (4), 366-73.

[9] McLaren, A., Cloning: pathways to a pluripotent future. *Science* 2000, *288* (5472), 1775-80.

[10] Cohen, B., Nobel committee rewards pioneers of development studies in fruitflies. *Nature* 1995, *377* (6549), 465.

[11] Yu, J.; Vodyanik, M. A.; Smuga-Otto, K.; Antosiewicz-Bourget, J.; Frane, J. L.; Tian, S.; Nie, J.; Jonsdottir, G. A.; Ruotti, V.; Stewart, R.; Slukvin, II; Thomson, J. A., Induced pluripotent stem cell lines derived from human somatic cells. *Science* 2007, *318* (5858), 1917-20.

[12] Pereira, C. F.; Lemischka, I. R.; Moore, K., Reprogramming cell fates: insights from combinatorial approaches. *Ann N Y Acad Sci* 2012, *1266*, 7-17.

[13] Serov, O. L.; Matveeva, N. M.; Khabarova, A. A., Reprogramming mediated by cell fusion technology. *Int Rev Cell Mol Biol* 2011, *291*, 155-90.

[14] Watanabe, A.; Yamada, Y.; Yamanaka, S., Epigenetic regulation in pluripotent stem cells: a key to breaking the epigenetic barrier. *Philos Trans R Soc Lond B Biol Sci* 2013, *368* (1609), 20120292.

[15] Ng, R. K.; Gurdon, J. B., Epigenetic memory of active gene transcription is inherited through somatic cell nuclear transfer. *Proc Natl Acad Sci U S A* 2005, *102* (6), 1957-62.

[16] Jafarpour, F.; Hosseini, S. M.; Hajian, M.; Forouzanfar, M.; Ostadhosseini, S.; Abedi, P.; Gholami, S.; Ghaedi, K.; Gourabi, H.; Shahverdi, A. H.; Vosough, A. D.; Nasr-Esfahani, M. H., Somatic cell-induced hyperacetylation, but not hypomethylation, positively and reversibly affects the efficiency of in vitro cloned blastocyst production in cattle. *Cell Reprogram* 2011, *13* (6), 483-93.

[17] Isaji, Y.; Murata, M.; Takaguchi, N.; Mukai, T.; Tajima, Y.; Imai, H.; Yamada, M., Valproic acid treatment from the 4-cell stage improves Oct4 expression and nuclear distribution of histone H3K27me3 in mouse cloned blastocysts. *J Reprod Dev* 2013, *59* (2), 196-204.

[18] Huangfu, D.; Maehr, R.; Guo, W.; Eijkelenboom, A.; Snitow, M.; Chen, A. E.; Melton, D. A., Induction of pluripotent stem cells by defined factors is greatly improved by small-molecule compounds. *Nat Biotechnol* 2008, *26* (7), 795-7.

[19] Liang, G.; Taranova, O.; Xia, K.; Zhang, Y., Butyrate promotes induced pluripotent stem cell generation. *J Biol Chem* 2010, *285* (33), 25516-21.

[20] Mali, P.; Chou, B. K.; Yen, J.; Ye, Z.; Zou, J.; Dowey, S.; Brodsky, R. A.; Ohm, J. E.; Yu, W.; Baylin, S. B.; Yusa, K.; Bradley, A.; Meyers, D. J.; Mukherjee, C.; Cole, P. A.; Cheng, L., Butyrate greatly enhances derivation of human induced pluripotent stem cells by promoting epigenetic remodeling and the expression of pluripotency-associated genes. *Stem Cells* 2010, *28* (4), 713-20.

[21] Meng, X.; Neises, A.; Su, R. J.; Payne, K. J.; Ritter, L.; Gridley, D. S.; Wang, J.; Sheng, M.; Lau, K. H.; Baylink, D. J.; Zhang, X. B., Efficient reprogramming of human cord blood CD34+ cells into induced pluripotent stem cells with OCT4 and SOX2 alone. *Mol Ther* 2012, *20* (2), 408-16.

[22] Trokovic, R.; Weltner, J.; Manninen, T.; Mikkola, M.; Lundin, K.; Hamalainen, R.; Suomalainen, A.; Otonkoski, T., Small molecule inhibitors promote efficient generation of induced pluripotent stem cells from human skeletal myoblasts. *Stem Cells Dev* 2013, *22* (1), 114-23.

[23] Zhang, Z.; Wu, W. S., Sodium butyrate promotes generation of human induced pluripotent stem cells through induction of the miR302/367 cluster. *Stem Cells Dev* 2013, *22* (16), 2268-77.

[24] Zhang, Z.; Gao, Y.; Gordon, A.; Wang, Z. Z.; Qian, Z.; Wu, W. S., Efficient generation of fully reprogrammed human iPS cells via polycistronic retroviral vector and a new cocktail of chemical compounds. *PLoS One* 2011, *6* (10), e26592.

[25] Vanhoutvin, S. A.; Troost, F. J.; Hamer, H. M.; Lindsey, P. J.; Koek, G. H.; Jonkers, D. M.; Kodde, A.; Venema, K.; Brummer, R. J., Butyrate-induced transcriptional changes in human colonic mucosa. *PLoS One* 2009, *4* (8), e6759.

[26] Davie, J. R., Inhibition of histone deacetylase activity by butyrate. *J Nutr* 2003, *133* (7 Suppl), 2485S-2493S.

[27] Donohoe, D. R.; Collins, L. B.; Wali, A.; Bigler, R.; Sun, W.; Bultman, S. J., The Warburg effect dictates the mechanism of butyrate-mediated histone acetylation and cell proliferation. *Mol Cell* 2012, *48* (4), 612-26.

[28] Apostolou, E.; Hochedlinger, K., Chromatin dynamics during cellular reprogramming. *Nature* 2013, *502* (7472), 462-71.

[29] Plath, K.; Lowry, W. E., Progress in understanding reprogramming to the induced pluripotent state. *Nat Rev Genet* 2011, *12* (4), 253-65.

[30] Rais, Y.; Zviran, A.; Geula, S.; Gafni, O.; Chomsky, E.; Viukov, S.; Mansour, A. A.; Caspi, I.; Krupalnik, V.; Zerbib, M.; Maza, I.; Mor, N.; Baran, D.; Weinberger, L.; Jaitin, D. A.; Lara-Astiaso, D.; Blecher-Gonen, R.; Shipony, Z.; Mukamel, Z.; Hagai, T.; Gilad, S.; Amann-Zalcenstein, D.; Tanay, A.; Amit, I.; Novershtern, N.; Hanna, J. H., Deterministic direct reprogramming of somatic cells to pluripotency. *Nature* 2013, *502* (7469), 65-70.

[31] Fujita, N.; Watanabe, S.; Ichimura, T.; Ohkuma, Y.; Chiba, T.; Saya, H.; Nakao, M., MCAF mediates MBD1-dependent transcriptional repression. *Mol Cell Biol* 2003, *23* (8), 2834-43.

[32] Zhang, Z.; Xiang, D.; Heriyanto, F.; Gao, Y.; Qian, Z.; Wu, W. S., Dissecting the Roles of miR-302/367 Cluster in Cellular Reprogramming Using TALE-based Repressor and TALEN. *Stem Cell Reports* 2013, *1* (3), 218-25.

[33] Zhu, S.; Li, W.; Zhou, H.; Wei, W.; Ambasudhan, R.; Lin, T.; Kim, J.; Zhang, K.; Ding, S., Reprogramming of human primary somatic cells by OCT4 and chemical compounds. *Cell Stem Cell* 2010, *7* (6), 651-5.

[34] Palma, C. S.; Tannous, M. A.; Malta, T. M.; Russo, E. M.; Covas, D. T.; Picanco-Castro, V., Forced expression of OCT4 influences the expression of pluripotent genes in human mesenchymal stem cells and fibroblasts. *Genet Mol Res* 2013, *12* (2), 1054-60.

[35] Chou, B. K.; Mali, P.; Huang, X.; Ye, Z.; Dowey, S. N.; Resar, L. M.; Zou, C.; Zhang, Y. A.; Tong, J.; Cheng, L., Efficient human iPS cell derivation by a non-integrating plasmid from blood cells with unique epigenetic and gene expression signatures. *Cell Res* 2011, *21* (3), 518-29.

[36] Lee, M. R.; Prasain, N.; Chae, H. D.; Kim, Y. J.; Mantel, C.; Yoder, M. C.; Broxmeyer, H. E., Epigenetic regulation of NANOG by miR-302 cluster-MBD2 completes induced pluripotent stem cell reprogramming. *Stem Cells* 2013, *31* (4), 666-81.

[37] Chan, E. M.; Ratanasirintrawoot, S.; Park, I. H.; Manos, P. D.; Loh, Y. H.; Huo, H.; Miller, J. D.; Hartung, O.; Rho, J.; Ince, T. A.; Daley, G. Q.; Schlaeger, T. M., Live cell imaging distinguishes bona fide human iPS cells from partially reprogrammed cells. *Nat Biotechnol* 2009, *27* (11), 1033-7.

[38] Hu, S.; Wilson, K. D.; Ghosh, Z.; Han, L.; Wang, Y.; Lan, F.; Ransohoff, K. J.; Burridge, P.; Wu, J. C., MicroRNA-302 increases reprogramming efficiency via repression of NR2F2. *Stem Cells* 2013, *31* (2), 259-68.

[39] Esteban, M. A.; Bao, X.; Zhuang, Q.; Zhou, T.; Qin, B.; Pei, D., The mesenchymal-to-epithelial transition in somatic cell reprogramming. *Curr Opin Genet Dev* 2012, *22* (5), 423-8.

[40] Anokye-Danso, F.; Trivedi, C. M.; Juhr, D.; Gupta, M.; Cui, Z.; Tian, Y.; Zhang, Y.; Yang, W.; Gruber, P. J.; Epstein, J. A.; Morrisey, E. E., Highly efficient miRNA-mediated reprogramming of mouse and human somatic cells to pluripotency. *Cell Stem Cell* 2011, *8* (4), 376-88.

[41] Noh, E. J.; Jang, E. R.; Jeong, G.; Lee, Y. M.; Min, C. K.; Lee, J. S., Methyl CpG-binding domain protein 3 mediates cancer-selective cytotoxicity by histone deacetylase inhibitors via differential transcriptional reprogramming in lung cancer cells. *Cancer Res* 2005, *65* (24), 11400-10.

[42] Gu, P.; Xu, X.; Le Menuet, D.; Chung, A. C.; Cooney, A. J., Differential recruitment of methyl CpG-binding domain factors and DNA methyltransferases by the orphan receptor germ cell nuclear factor initiates the repression and silencing of Oct4. *Stem Cells* 2011, *29* (7), 1041-51.

[43] Liao, H. F.; Tai, K. Y.; Chen, W. S.; Cheng, L. C.; Ho, H. N.; Lin, S. P., Functions of DNA methyltransferase 3-like in germ cells and beyond. *Biol Cell* 2012, *104* (10), 571-87.

[44] Elabd, C.; Cousin, W.; Chen, R. Y.; Chooljian, M. S.; Pham, J. T.; Conboy, I. M.; Conboy, M. J., DNA methyltransferase-3-dependent nonrandom template segregation in differentiating embryonic stem cells. *J Cell Biol* 2013, *203* (1), 73-85.

[45] Ichida, J. K.; Blanchard, J.; Lam, K.; Son, E. Y.; Chung, J. E.; Egli, D.; Loh, K. M.; Carter, A. C.; Di Giorgio, F. P.; Koszka, K.; Huangfu, D.; Akutsu, H.; Liu, D. R.; Rubin, L. L.; Eggan, K., A small-molecule inhibitor of tgf-Beta signaling replaces sox2 in reprogramming by inducing nanog. *Cell Stem Cell* 2009, *5* (5), 491-503.

In: Butyrate: Food Sources, Functions and Health Benefits ISBN: 978-1-63117-657-9
Editor: Cong-Jun Li © 2014 Nova Science Publishers, Inc.

Chapter 12

Role and Function of Short Chain Fatty Acids in Rumen Epithelial Metabolism, Development and Importance of the Rumen Epithelium in Understanding Control of Transcriptome

***Ransom L. Baldwin, VI*[1,*] *and Kyle R. McLeod*[2]**
[1]Bovine Functional Genomics Laboratory, Agricultural Research Service, US Department of Agriculture, Beltsville Agricultural Research Center, Maryland, US
[2]Department of Animal Sciences, University of Kentucky, Lexington, KY, US

Abstract

Short chain fatty acids play a critical role in the development and energy metabolism of productive ruminant. The epithelial lining of the rumen has several distinctive characteristics which make it an important model for the study of nutrient-gene interactions relating to animal production. Understanding the metabolism of this organ in relationship to the whole animal is fundamental to interpreting findings using this organ in vivo and in vitro for analysis of SCFA actions on the tissue. Research into the processes of development and differentiation of the rumen epithelium has received interest in the past due to the obvious importance to production systems. In light of new abilities to assess the molecular control of mammalian function, the interaction between microbial populations and host, and the epigenetic level changes occurring in the cells, more use of this model system is likely. This chapter seeks to facilitate greater use of this model system by reviewing the formative findings relevant to the interpretation of future results. The unique occurrence of high SCFA concentrations found under normal physiological circumstances in the rumen provides for a powerful model system to enhance our understanding of complex control systems.

* Corresponding author: Ransom L. Baldwin. Bovine Functional Genomics Laboratory, Agricultural Research Service, US Department of Agriculture 10300 Baltimore Ave. Beltsville Agricultural Research Center, Maryland, 20705. E-mail: ransom.baldwin@ars.usda.gov, Tel: (301) 504-8964.

Introduction

The epithelial lining of the rumen is uniquely placed to have impact on the nutrient metabolism of the animal. The symbiotic relationship with the microbial populations that inhabit the rumen, serves to provide a constant supply of nutrients from roughage that would otherwise be unusable. Metabolically the tissue serves as a protective yet permeable barrier to diffusion of end products of fermented feedstuffs, but cannot simply be considered as a sieve. The tissue structure, metabolism and the development are all functions of the symbiosis with the rumen environment. The interplay between the use of short chain fatty acids (SCFA) and their concomitant effect on this organ are characteristics make the rumen epithelium a tissue of great interest to not only the animal science community but also those studying colonic health.

Moreover, epigenetic and transcriptomic control exerted by SCFA need to be understood in order to develop better feeding paradigms for our production animals and aid in our understanding of gastrointestinal tissue health. Physically, metabolically and developmentally this tissue has served to provide great insight into the metabolic and transcriptomic control of mammalian genes expression.

The continued study of this unique tissue will also provide insight into the epigenetic responses dictating long term changes in function of this dynamic tissue. To use this model system, it is important to understand its unique character as an organ.

Structure and Function of the Ruminal Epithelium

The rumen epithelium is responsible for several physiologically important functions, including absorption, transport, volatile fatty acid metabolism and protection [1, 2]. The ruminal epithelium is a stratified squamous epithelium consisting of four strata: *stratum basale*, *stratum spinosum*, *stratum granulosum*, and *stratum corneum* [3]. The number of cell layers present in each strata is highly variable and is dependent upon diet, stage of ruminal development and feeding pattern. The *stratum basale* is the layer of cells immediately adjacent to the basal lamina. These cells contain fully functional mitochondria and other organelles, and are the cells of the rumen which contribute most significantly to the metabolic properties of the tissue, i.e., ketogenesis which occurs in the mitochondria of the ruminal epithelium.

Consequently, these cells would be the most important cells of the rumen with regard to whole animal energy metabolism. The *stratum spinosum* and *stratum granulosum* are the intermediate cell layers and are not separated by a distinct division [2]. As the cells migrate through these intermediate layers they contain progressively fewer numbers of mitochondria, and take on a less uniform appearance. In the *stratum granulosum* the cells have established tight gap junctions (desmosomes) which maintain the integrity of metabolite concentration gradients across the rumen wall [3]. Cells in the *stratum corneum*, the most external cell strata, are highly cornified, and presumably function as a defensive barrier against the physical environment of the rumen. The desmosomal integrity of the *stratum corneum* has degenerated and large gaps exist between individual cells [3]. The number of cell layers present in the *stratum corneum* is highly related to the dietary composition [4].

High concentrate rations, decreased ruminal pH, increased propionate:acetate ratios, and increased molar proportions of butyrate all result in a *stratum corneum* of up to 15 cell layers in thickness [4]. Conversely, in an animal maintained on a high roughage diet the *stratum corneum* may consist of as few as four cell layers [4]. Although feeding regime (i.e., how and when the feed is presented) has been implicated as affecting the *stratum corneum* [5, 6], these adaptations are more likely attributable to the subsequent alterations in the ruminal environment [1].

METABOLISM OF MATURE RUMINAL EPITHELIUM

The rumen and reticulum account for more than 70% of the total digestive tract volume by weight [7]. Vast numbers of papillae protrude from the ruminal surface into the lumen, greatly increasing the surface area available for absorption of volatile fatty acids or short chain fatty acids (SCFA; [8]). A large majority (>75%; [9]) of the SCFA are absorbed through the epithelial lining of the rumen and reticulum, with less than 10% of the ruminally produced SCFA passing into the small intestine [8]. Rate and capacity for SCFA removal from the ruminal lumen is influenced by the pH of the rumen contents. When ruminal pH is near neutrality (7.2), all of the SCFA are absorbed at similar rates. When ruminal pH falls below 6.0 the rate of SCFA absorption declines concomitantly [2]. Acetate and propionate absorption are more sensitive to decreases in pH. Thus, at low ruminal pH butyrate absorption increases as a proportion of total SCFA absorbed, although rates of butyrate absorption are still below those observed at near neutral pH [2]. However, the ruminal epithelium is not simply a barrier to nutrient diffusion, but through the metabolism of SCFA, primarily butyrate, acts to maintain the integrity of metabolite concentration gradients. In addition, ruminal SCFA metabolism protects against potentially detrimental decreases in blood pH [1, 2]. Acetate, propionate and butyrate are metabolized to different extents by the ruminal epithelium.

VOLATILE FATTY ACID METABOLISM

Acetate

Acetate is present in the rumen in the highest concentrations of all of the SCFA produced by the rumen microbes. Acetate is utilized for fat synthesis by the adipose tissue and as an energy substrate by all extrahepatic tissues of the animal. Appearance of acetate in portal blood is highly correlated with acetate concentration within the ruminal lumen [10]. The absorption of acetate increases with ruminal development and decreases in response to high concentrate diets [11] presumably due to decreases in ruminal pH and acetate to propionate ratio. *In vitro* experiments indicate that acetate is absorbed readily by the ruminal epithelia [12]. However, acetate addition fails to induce an increase in oxygen uptake by rumen tissue slices [12], indicating that the tissue does not metabolize acetate to a great extent. However, Baldwin reported [13] using isolated rumen epithelial cells enriched for the metabolically active cells of the tissue, that acetate addition decreased butyrate conversion to ß-hydroxybutyrate (ßHBA) produced. They attributed that Acetyl-CoA formation may result an inhibition of butyryl-CoA synthesis and thus, decreased butyrate metabolism. Regardless, the extent to which acetate was oxidized to CO_2 was minimal in those same experiments.

Propionate

Propionate is the primary gluconeogenic substrate utilized by ruminant liver, and can account for 60% of the glucose utilized by the animal [8]. Propionate seems to undergo limited metabolism to lactate and pyruvate by the ruminal epithelium [14, 15]. However, some question remains as to how much propionate carbon is metabolized by ruminal epithelium. Estimates range from 3% to 15% of absorbed propionate undergoing metabolism, primarily to lactate and pyruvate [11, 15, 16].

Addition of propionate *in vitro* to rumen slices resulted in no change in oxygen uptake by the rumen pieces [12]. Despite the apparently low utilization of propionate by the ruminal epithelium, disappearance of propionate carbon from the rumen cannot be completely accounted for by the lactate, pyruvate and propionate appearing in the portal blood. Using an isolated cell preparation Baldwin and Jesse [17] addressed the role of propionate metabolism, and found significant interactions with butyrate metabolism and hypothesized that these changes were largely due to redox status in the cells dictating net outputs of ketone bodies in the form of acetoacetate vs. ßHBA.

Propionate activation to propionyl-CoA by propionyl-CoA synthetase is the limiting step in propionate metabolism [14]. Propionyl-CoA synthetase activity is sensitive to developmental state of the rumen and to the molar proportion of propionate in the ruminal fluid [11, 14]. Following activation to propionyl-CoA the propionate carbon is converted to methylmalonyl-CoA and subsequently enters the TCA cycle as succinyl-CoA.

Propionate metabolism to lactate and pyruvate may serve to maintain the balance of cytosolic NAD/NADH in the ruminal epithelium of concentrate fed animals [16]. In ruminant liver, propionate has been shown to have an inhibitory effect upon ketogenesis [18], while in the ruminal epithelium contradictory findings have been reported (inhibitory, [14]; stimulitory, [16]; no change, [15]). Some of these differences may be explained due to the differences in the incubation conditions utilized and the tissue sources investigated.

Metabolism of propionate to lactate and pyruvate may also result in preservation of propionate-derived carbon for gluconeogenesis, as the liver quantitatively removes pyruvate and lactate from the portal blood [19].

Butyrate

Unlike non-ruminants where ketone bodies (ß-hydroxybutyrate, ßHBA) and acetoacetate (AcAc)) are utilized as a last resort during hypoglycemia, usually fasting, conditions, ketone bodies are continuously utilized as an energy source by the extra hepatic tissues of the ruminant animal [20]. In the fed ruminant animal, the rumen and the liver are the primary producers of ketone bodies [20]. Ruminally derived AcAc is quantitatively removed from portal blood by the liver and metabolized to ßHBA. Thus, in the fed state, the ruminal epithelium is the primary source of circulating ketone bodies in the ruminant animal [20].

The majority (85% to 90%) of ruminally absorbed butyrate carbon appearing in portal blood is in the form of ßHBA and AcAc [21]. The balance of the absorbed butyrate carbon can be accounted for as CO_2 produced as a result of oxidation [12].

Ketogenesis in the ruminal epithelium is carried out exclusively in the mitochondria [22] due to the compartmentalization of the ketogenic enzymes. Two pathways of ketogenesis are available to the ruminal epithelium. Ketogenesis can progress through 3-hydroxy-3-methyl-glutaryl-CoA (HMG-CoA) synthase and HMG-CoA lyase, as in the liver, or via deacylation of AcAc-CoA catalyzed by succinyl-CoA transferase. Both of these pathways result in the production of AcAc. The final step in ruminal ketogenesis is the production of ßHBA catalyzed by ßHBA dehydrogenase. In the fed ruminant this pathway is favored due to the NADH: NAD ratio of the mitochondria [20]. All of these ketogenic enzymes are present within the ruminal epithelium at sufficient activities to account for the ketogenic capacity of the rumen [22-24].

Metabolism of Neonatal Ruminal Epithelium

Few reports are available concerning neonatal ruminal epithelial metabolism. In the milk fed animal, due to the reflexive closure of the esophageal groove and the lack of SCFA in the ruminal lumen, the primary source of energetic substrate is blood borne, derived from intestinally absorbed nutrients. Fatty acids and glucose, absorbed in the small intestine, must first pass through the liver. Thus, it has been assumed that glucose is the primary energy substrate of the immature tissue as is the case with other neonatal tissues [25]. Experiments *in vitro* evaluated oxygen uptake by rumen slices from 14 day old calf ruminal epithelium (undeveloped) or mature ruminal papillae in the presence of various oxidizable substrates, such as glucose, butyrate and lactate. Oxygen uptake by neonatal rumen was greatest when glucose was present as the oxidizable substrate. Oxygen consumption by mature rumen papillae increased above basal oxygen uptake when glucose was added, but did not respond as dramatically as neonatal rumen slices [26]. Lactate addition to the media induced a similar pattern of oxygen uptake as observed with glucose [26]. Oxygen uptake by mature rumen papillae was stimulated to a higher degree than that by neonatal rumen with butyrate addition. Ketogenesis from butyrate was also substantially lower in the neonatal rumen as compared to the mature tissue. In further studies with ruminal epithelium from 10 wk old milk fed calves, ketogenic capacity remained depressed when compared to ruminal epithelium isolated from grain fed control calves [26].

Rumen Development

Development of the Ruminal Epithelium

The rumen is incompletely developed both physically and metabolically at birth [27]. In the neonate, the rumen does not exhibit the high degree of keratinization characteristic of the mature organ [28]; metabolically, the rumen is essentially non-functional with respect to ketogenic capacity [27].

Following the initiation of solid feed intake by the neonate and the subsequent establishment of the ruminal fermentation, the rumen undergoes both physical and metabolic development. Physical development of the rumen can be further partitioned into two aspects: increases in rumen mass and growth of the papillae. Early research indicated that physical stimulation by feed in the rumen could account for measurable increases in both rumen weight and musculature development. The presence of physical bulk does not, however, promote papillary development [29]. Thus, for normal development of the ruminal epithelium to progress, a viable ruminal fermentation must be established, suggesting that there is a requirement for the presence of SCFA in the ruminal lumen to promote normal papillary development [30].

When compared to grain and hay fed control animals, neonatal ruminants maintained solely on milk during the first months of life exhibit limited ruminal development with respect to rumen weight [31], capacity [31, 32], papillary growth [27, 31], degree of keratinization [28], pigmentation [31] and musculature development [27, 29, 31, 32].

The lack of development is likely due to the effective shunting of milk directly to the abomasum by the reflexive closure of the esophageal groove [33], thus preventing substrate for the establishment of a ruminal fermentation from entering the rumen. Accordingly, when milk was infused directly into the rumen, resulting in SCFA production, papillary growth is stimulated [31].

Similarly, Lane and Jesse [34] reported that infusing 50% of the lamb's estimated net energy requirement in the form of SCFA at physiological concentrations resulted in increases in papillae length. Conversely, use of ruminally inert materials such as nylon bristles [27], plastic sponges [31], wood shavings [32], and plastic cubes [29] to simulate the physical stimulus of feed in the rumen resulted in no significant papillary development. Infusions of sodium propionate and sodium butyrate, but not sodium acetate, sodium chloride or glucose, resulted in marked development of the ruminal papillae in calves [30, 31].

A mixture of SCFA salts (propionate and butyrate included) fed as 10% (wt./wt.) of a concentrate starter ration resulted in increased incidence of ruminal parakeratosis, and in all treated animals a thickening of the *stratum corneum* was reported in calves [28] and lambs [35]. Increasing amounts of concentrate in the diet resulted in no change in rumen muscularity but did result in increased papillae density and papillae height in calves [7] and lambs [35]. None of these studies were able to definitively distinguish the mechanism responsible for the induction of papillary development.

The possibility that butyrate and propionate metabolism by the ruminal epithelium induces an increase in blood flow through the rumen cannot be disregarded as a factor [30], nor can the possibility of a direct effect of butyrate or propionate on gene expression within the rumen [1, 36].

Wang et al. [37] reported the selection and identification of cDNA clones encoding two small proline-rich proteins which are characteristically associated with the development of the cornified envelope of stratified squamous epithelial tissues (skin, rumen epithelium) and thus, may represent excellent molecular level markers of physical development.

Although these clones exhibited a differential expression pattern throughout development in normally reared lambs, the expression increased gradually, thereby indicating a more ontological control rather than a trigger driven change in expression of these gene products.

Control of Proliferation

Ruminal epithelial cell proliferation has been studied both *in vivo* [38, 39] and *in vitro* [1] by measuring ^{3}H-thymidine incorporation and mitotic indices. Butyric acid infused directly into the rumen of sheep resulted in a stimulation of mitotic indices (number of basal cell nuclei showing mitotic figures/total basal cell nuclei counted; [38, 40].

However, only two animals were observed in this study, and data are confounded by the fact that both animals were fasted throughout the 5 and 7 d and the effect of butyrate did not appear until 3 or 4 d subsequent to the initiation of the fast. Thus, from this experiment it is difficult to determine if butyrate is stimulatory or permissive in promoting mitosis. In a series of similar trials, a single pulse dose of sodium butyrate followed by continuous saline infusion stimulated mitotic indices to a greater extent than a pulse-chase regime with sodium butyrate [38, 39].

Thus, a rapid but transient increase in butyrate in the rumen, which is not observed physiologically, stimulates cell proliferation as indicated by greater mitotic indices. To a lesser extent than with butyrate, both propionate and acetate have been shown to stimulate mitotic indices when administered as a single dose [41].

Contrary to results *in vivo*, ^{3}H-thymidine incorporation into cellular DNA by isolated ruminal epithelial cells was inhibited over a 24 h period in a dose dependent manner by the presence of sodium butyrate (2 mM and 10 mM) in the medium [42]. Further studies with butyrate in cultures of tissue explants indicate that butyrate tends to arrest cell division of cells in the basal lamina, while increasing the keratinization and protein expression of the other cell types. This results in increased size and cornification of the explant [1]. Moreover, Baldwin [43] used isolated rumen epithelial cells in 48-h cultures to demonstrate decreased cell proliferation, as determined by MTT-assay, in the presence of butyrate or propionate alone, with half-maximal inhibition occurring at concentrations of 0.52 mM butyrate and 0.93 mM propionate.

The vastly different responses observed *in vivo* and *in vitro*, and the seemingly contradictory nature of the *in vivo* reports, is suggestive of an indirect pathway of cell stimulation. Ruminal epithelial mitotic indices have been shown to be stimulated by intravenous insulin infusions [44]. Because propionate has been shown to be a stimulator of insulin release *in vivo* [44] it is possible that insulin could be a mediator in the stimulation of mitosis in the ruminal epithelium.

In fact, administration of pentagastrin, insulin and glucagon to isolated ruminal cells all resulted in stimulation of cell proliferation (as detected by ^{3}H-thymidine incorporation), while responses to cortisol were inconsistent [39, 41]. Of the additions tested, only insulin was able to overcome the inhibitory effect of butyrate on ^{3}H-thymidine incorporation by isolated cells of the *stratum basale* [45].

Similar results were observed by Baldwin [43], where insulin, epidermal growth factor (EGF), and IGF-I stimulated cell proliferation to rates 75%, 97%, and 96% (MTT-assay) of the rates observed in 5% fetal calf serum (FCS) treated controls, respectively. Moreover, the inhibitory action of 1 mM butyrate was completely overcome by the addition of IGF-I and EGF and to a lesser extent by insulin (66% of the 5% FCS stimulated rate of proliferation).

Thus, factors other than direct action by nutrients cannot be eliminated as possible agents controlling ruminal epithelial proliferation, although clear primary candidates have not yet been delineated conclusively.

Neonatal Ruminal Epithelial Metabolism

In the milk-fed ruminant, due to the reflexive closure of the esophageal groove and the lack of SCFA in the ruminal lumen, the primary source of energetic substrates are blood borne, derived from intestinally absorbed nutrients.

Fatty acids and glucose absorbed in the small intestine must first pass through the liver; thus it has been assumed that glucose is a primary energy substrate of the immature tissue, as is the case with other neonatal tissues [25].

Early experiments *in vitro* evaluated rates of oxygen uptake by rumen slices from 14-d old calf ruminal epithelium (undeveloped) or mature ruminal papillae in the presence of various oxidizable substrates such as glucose, butyrate and lactate [26]. Oxygen uptake by neonatal rumen was greatest when glucose was present as the oxidizable substrate; however, oxygen consumption by mature rumen papillae increased above basal oxygen uptake when glucose was added, but did not respond as dramatically as neonatal rumen slices [26]. Lactate addition to the media induced a similar pattern of oxygen uptake as that observed with glucose [26].

In contrast, the addition of butyrate stimulated oxygen uptake to a greater degree in mature rumen papillae than in the neonatal rumen. Ketogenesis from butyrate was also substantially lower in the neonatal rumen as compared to the mature tissue.

Baldwin and Jesse [46] used an isolated rumen epithelial cell system that compared the metabolic capabilities of stratum basale and stratum spinosal cells isolated from lambs at seven ages during normal development. They observed that glucose was oxidized at moderate rates by cells isolated from 1-, 4- and 7-day old lambs and at very high rates from 14- to 49-d old lambs.

However, by weaning at 56 days, glucose oxidation by the ruminal cells had declined to rates below those observed in ruminal cells from newborn lambs. Butyrate oxidation exhibited a similar pattern; initially rates of oxidation were low followed by high rates of oxidation from 7 d through weaning. Both butyrate and glucose oxidation rates decreased in the presence of the other oxidizable substrate. Thus, although the ruminal epithelium can use glucose and butyrate as its energetic substrate, neither appears to be the favored substrate. In the same experiments, ketogenic capacity of the isolated cells was apparent by 4 days of age and did not increase until weaning when an 8-fold increase in β-hydroxybutyrate production was observed [46].

Lane et al. [47] assessed rumen metabolic development of ruminal epithelium in the absence of solid feed intake by maintaining lambs solely on milk replacer and observed the characteristic and marked increase in ketogenic capacity at 42 d regardless of dietary regimen. While other metabolic parameters did not follow this characteristic development, this is again indicative of an ontogenic response rather than a nutrient triggered event.

Moreover, using rumen epithelial RNA isolated from these same experimental animals, Lane et al. [48] were able to demonstrate an increase in gene transcripts for 3-hydroxy-3-methylglutaryyl-CoA synthase (HMG-CoA synthase; E.C. 4.1.3.5), despite the lack of significant SCFA production in the rumen.

Thus, ontological control of some of the critical development changes occurring in the developing ruminant cannot be eliminated as a causative factor, despite the large volume of evidence implicating butyrate as the putative trigger for development.

Moreover, these processes need not be mutually exclusive events.

ALIMENTATION, GUT MASS AND TOTAL METABOLIC ACTIVITY

Cost of Service Functions

A large portion of the absorbed nutrients from ruminant gut are modified or used, during microbial fermentation in the foregut and also by absorptive tissues of the calf, prior to their release into circulation. This results in a decrease in supply of energy and amino acid precursors from a given feed source that are available to productive tissues of the calf. However, this energy and amino acid use cannot be considered a total loss to the calf because the absorptive gut tissues perform a vital service to the productive tissues of the animal. Yet, it does represent a decrease in productive efficiency per unit feed energy supplied. By functional necessity, the gut and liver are anatomically placed to have access to absorbed nutrients before peripheral tissues.

Therefore, gut and liver metabolism determine the availability of most carbon based nutrients for the support of productive functions and thus, are crucial to the health and growth of the calf. In fact, the portal drained viscera (PDV; includes the digestive tract, pancreas, spleen, and omental and mesenteric fat) represents only 8 to 10% of body tissues [49], yet accounts for 18 to 25% of the O_2 consumption of the animal with an additional 25% being accounted for by the liver. While a portion of the energy expended by the gut epithelium is directly associated with the cost of actively absorbing and transporting nutrients for subsequent use by the productive tissues, a majority of the energy expended is used for maintenance of tissue integrity and mass. These maintenance functions of the visceral organs primarily include Na^+- K^+-ATPase activity, protein synthesis and degradation, substrate cycling and urea synthesis [50]. In fact, the ruminant gastrointestinal tract as a whole is responsible for 40% of the whole body ATP use [50].

Additionally, a simulation of protein turnover in growing lambs predicts that 19% of total body ATP expenditure is due to protein turnover and that 25 - 27% is due to gastrointestinal tract (GIT) protein turnover [51]. Based on the aforementioned energetic and nutrient costs, the maintenance of the GIT tissues in the growing ruminant has an extensive impact on whole body metabolism. However, defining the actual cost of the gut tissues is further complicated by the fact that the mass of these tissues changes in response to plane of nutrition, dietary chemical composition, and physiological status of the animal.

Gut Growth and Metabolic Activity

While extensive research has focused on the role of milk and colostral growth factors on ruminant neonatal intestinal development [52], a paucity of data are available describing the intestinal response during weaning and development of the rumen. Baldwin [53], using isocaloric diets of either milk replacer or pelleted lamb starter demonstrated that the physical form of the diet does not impact intestinal mass. However, ruminal mass was exceptionally responsive to the change in form of the diet, likely reflecting the successful shunting of the milk replacer diet past the rumen and disruption of the establishment of a ruminal fermentation. This is consistent with observations made in rats, where weaning has been demonstrated to have no casual role in the growth and differentiation of the intestine [54].

Although intestinal mass changes are not apparent, capacity for nutrient assimilation may be affected. Shirazi-Beechey [55] demonstrated that intestinal digestive enzymes are not regulated by solid feed intake. However, Na-glucose co-transporter expression is clearly regulated by the delivery of hexose post-ruminally, indicating the potential for specific nutrient gene interactions controlling metabolic function of the intestine [56]. In the growing post-weaning ruminant model, a number of data sets are available to assess the impact of dietary energy intake and density on gut growth and oxidative metabolism as it affects the nutrients available for production. Gut mass changes dramatically with changes in ME intake and is highly responsive to changes in level of alimentation [57-63]. Research by Ferrell and coworkers has convincingly demonstrated a positive relationship between plane of nutrition (level of energy intake) and increased maintenance energy costs associated with the splanchnic tissues [58-63]. The influence of energy intake and density was further defined by Reynolds et al. [66], who demonstrated in growing heifers a positive relationship between PDV O_2 use and both ME intake (1 X vs. 2 X maintenance energy intake) and fiber content of the diet (75% forage diet vs. 75% concentrate diet). The increase in PDV O_2 use associated with decreased dietary energy density of the diet resulted in a reduction in the partial efficiency of ME for tissue gain. A series of experiments [64, 65] using a similar feeding protocol to that of Reynolds et al. [66] in growing lambs to determine whether the increase in PDV heat production associated with dietary forage level is due to increased mass or mass specific metabolism. In these experiments, they demonstrated that increasing ME intake and dietary forage resulted in increased ruminal and intestinal growth via cellular hyperplasia [64]. Moreover, the increase in intestinal mass response associated with both ME intake and dietary forage level was largely (> 90%) a result of proliferation within the mucosa. In an effort to delineate mass specific metabolic activity changes associated with ME intake and dietary forage content, isolated rumen epithelial cells and intestinal enterocytes were subjected to *in vitro* analysis of oxidative metabolism. Oxygen consumption and Na^+- K^+-ATPase activity were unaffected by dietary regime [64], which is consistent with earlier work demonstrating that *in vitro* rates of O_2 consumption by sheep rumen, duodenal, and jejunal epithelium were unaffected by level of alimentation [67-70]. Similarly, V_{max} (maximal rate of substrate oxidation) and K_{ox} (concentration of substrate at which half V_{max} oxidation rate is achieved) estimates for the metabolism of specific oxidative substrates by rumen epithelial cells [65] and intestinal enterocytes were unaffected by ME intake and dietary forage content. This demonstration that cellular oxidative capacity remains constant despite differences in gut cellularity indicates that changes in PDV O_2 consumption are due to changes in mass rather than mass specific activity.

The regulation of gut growth is complex because it is affected by metabolic and trophic hormones as well as chemical and physical dietary factors. Moreover, the cause and effect relationship between ME intake and gut growth is largely speculative due to confounding factors such as dietary chemical composition and DM intake. In an attempt to define the role of dietary bulk on gut growth, Rompala et al. [68] demonstrated that inert bulk, in the form of polyethylene, stimulated increases in ruminal and colonic tissue mass but failed to elicit a growth response in the small intestine. Similarly, Hamada et al. [29] found that plastic cubes placed in the rumen of milk-fed steers increased musculature development of the rumen, but did not elicit normal epithelial development. Conversely, McLeod et al. [71] reported that ruminal infusion of starch hydrolyzed at 20% of ME intake increased ruminal mass in growing steers but, abomasal starch infusion failed to elicit an intestinal growth response.

This suggests that ruminal growth is responsive to the energy substrate supply, but intestinal tissue growth is not responsive to energy delivery per se. The latter is consistent with the data of Orskov et al. [72] and Gross et al. [73], which demonstrated that intestinal atrophy occurs in animals maintained on total intragastric infusion. Furthermore, the results of Gross et al. [73] tend to suggest O_2 consumption by the PDV tissues is lower in animals maintained on total intragastric infusion than those fed alfalfa. In fact, when this data is plotted against ME intake, total intragastrically infused animals fall well below the expected PDV heat energy expenditure predicted using a regression equation developed from several published PDV heat energy data sets using animals fed a wide range of diets differing in ME intake [49]. Taken together, these data show that gut growth is not simply a function of energy substrate supply or dietary chemical composition, but rather a plexus of nutritional and physiological inputs.

A comprehensive discussion of all the growth factors associated with the regulation of gastrointestinal tissues is beyond the scope of this review; however, a brief description of a number of factors that may be of interest is included. Epidermal growth factor and transforming growth factor-α interact with the epidermal growth factor receptor to elicit proliferative responses in epithelial cell types including, intestinal mucosa [74-77] and keratinocytes [43, 78]. Epidermal growth factor has also been shown to stimulate ornithine decarboxylase activity [79], which is the rate limiting step in the conversion of ornithine to polyamines. Polyamines have been linked to increased RNA synthesis [80] and interestingly, are high in rumen microbial protein fractions. Locally released hormones such as gastrin, cholecystokinin, enteroglucagon, secretin and bombesin have also been shown to have proliferative effects in intestinal tissue of nonruminants; however, it remains equivocal as to whether they are centrally involved in gut growth and development [80]. In contrast to the aforementioned proliferative factors, somatostatin has been shown to exhibit anti-proliferative and anti-secretory actions on the gut and pancreatic tissues in nonruminants [81]. Although substantially less documented in ruminants, Fachney and Barry [82] demonstrated that continuous somatostatin infusion (72 hours) in sheep decreased gut tissue mass. Furthermore, McLeod et al. [83] reported that somatostatin infusion decreased net PDV glucose and alpha-amino nitrogen absorption and reduced splanchnic O_2 consumption in sheep. McLeod et al. [83] further demonstrated that depletion of endogenous somatostatin had opposite effects to those observed for somatostatin infusion, suggesting that somatostatin has a physiological role in the regulation of splanchnic metabolism. Baldwin and McLeod [84] subsequently asserted that somatostatin exerts its effects via direct action at the cellular level from a series of experiments which demonstrated that increasing somatostatin resulted in a linear decline in glucose oxidation to CO_2. However, it is uncertain if the reduction in glucose oxidation is transporter related or represents a change in cellular oxidation.

Impact of Butyrate and Weaning on the Transcriptome

Using the rumen epithelial tissue responses to short-chain fatty acids (SCFAs), such as butyrate, have clearly defined butyrate as a signaling molecule which exerts its impact on multiple signaling pathways. Baldwin et al. [85] demonstrated the temporal effects of elevated butyrate concentrations on the transcriptome of the rumen epithelium using serial biopsy sampling from cows ruminally infused with butyrate for 7 d combined with high-throughput RNA-sequencing technology and bioinformatic tools. The initial reaction of the rumen epithelium to elevated exogenous butyrate may represent a stress response as Gene Ontology (GO) terms identified as enriched were predominantly related to biological processes such as response to bacteria and biotic stimuli. In addition butyrate induced, at least 16 other tight junction related genes in *in vitro* studies. A strong up-regulation of the major macromolecular components, such as claudins (CLDN1, CLDN3, CLDN4, CLDN7, CLDN 12, and CLDN23), tight junction protein 3 (TJP3), and junctional adhesion molecules 2 and 3 (JAM2 and JAM3), by butyrate supports the contention that these genes may play an important role in maintaining and/or restoring intestinal barrier function. Several regulatory networks putatively controlled by transcription factors, such as CREBBBP and TTF2, which were regulated by butyrate, were involved in distinct functions including solute transport and enzymes affecting SCFA and intermediary metabolites [85]. Another putative activated transcription factor important to the control of gene expression in the weaning animal was reported by Connor et al. [86], as PPAR-alpha. Downstream gene targets (32 identified) of PPAR-alpha were responsive to the transition from milk replacer to solid feed in developing calf rumen epithelium. The majority of the genes identified participate in beta-oxidation of lipids; however other functions include apoptosis, organ development, nutrient metabolism, and the immune response. Bünger et al. [87] attributed PPAR-alpha expression pattern in mice intestine to its critical role in the absorption of long-chain fatty acids by the intestinal villus and suggested that PPAR-alpha serves as a mechanism by which fatty acids can influence their own uptake and processing by enterocytes. Thus a role in the rumen epithelium is possible, however the distribution of PPAR-alpha protein or mRNA expression has not yet been investigated in the rumen papillae. It does not appear that expression of PPAR-alpha mRNA itself is affected by SCFA concentration in bovine rumen [88], although it appears that SCFA such as butyrate can serve as a PPAR ligand in the colon [89].

Moreover, the expression of 2 gene targets of PPAR-alpha, mitochondrial acetyl-CoA acetyltransferase (*ACAT1*) and mitochondrial hydroxymethylglutaryl-CoA synthase (*HMGC S2*) that function in metabolic organ development were upregulated during weaning.

The products of these genes play a crucial role in ketogenesis by the rumen epithelium of sheep during development [48]. Furthermore, *ACAT* expression has been shown previously to be increased in mature rumen epithelium in heifers fed high- versus low-concentrate diets [90]. Combined, these observations support the hypothesis that increased production of SCFA in response to introducion of solid feed during weaning may promote ketogenesis in rumen epithelium. Thus, while dramatic changes in mature tissue gene expression are often not observed, the changes seen in the developmental model may serve to aid in elucidating the mechanisms involved in the control of metabolism in the mature differentiated tissue, during critical changes in metabolic demand such as lactation.

A final area of obvious importance to the role of the ruminal epithelium as a service function tissue in the ruminant is nutrient transport. Changes in specific transporter activity have been recognized specifically those functioning in SCFA and ion transport of ruminants fed high-concentrate [90] or high-protein [91] diets. Connor also identified a large number of transport-related genes including the water channel protein *aquaporin 5*, *copper transport protein*, the intestinal proton-dependent peptide transporter *adherin 17*, *chloride channel 2*, *sodium channel (non-voltage-gated 1, gamma subunit)*, *transient receptor potential cation channel (subfamily M, member 6)*, and 20 different solute carrier (*SLC*) family members changed in response to weaning from milk to either forage or concentrate based rations.

However, these changes were not always consistent in direction with upregulation of some (*SLC14A1*, *SLC16A1*, and *SLC26A3*) and decreases in others (*SLC4A4*). Expression of these same genes and other transporters were affected by age rather than calf diet in reports from Naeem et al. [91]. This is an exciting area where clearly additional study of specific transporters needs further focus but will undoubtedly lead to elucidation of the impact of dietary changes and rumen developmental changes relating to control of rumen epitheial metabolism of the ruminant.

CONCLUSION

The rumen epithelial metabolism of SCFA and the role of SCFA in the stimulation and control of development have a clear and major impact on the digestive capabilities and supply of substrates to the growing and mature ruminant. Although a number studies have been conducted to elucidate the process of rumen development, and differential expression of key regulatory gene products have been identified, the mechanisms controlling ruminal differentiation are not sufficiently understood. Moreover it is still equivocal as to whether ontological control and/or nutrient and endocrine factors are the primary mechanism regulating these important processes. While intestinal development occurs during the fetal and the perinatal period, nutrient transport capacity changes as the preruminant animal becomes a ruminant as a result of specific nutrients supplied. In the growing ruminant, dietary effects, i.e., energy intake and dietary energy density, on ruminal and intestinal mass clearly alter protein and energy maintenance requirements. However, it is unclear whether these changes in gut mass affect digestive and absorptive capacities. Given the more recent studies focused on transcriptomic changes, and epigenetic modifications, it is becoming clear that whole families of genes are affected by the nutrient delivery system present in the functioning ruminant. Because SCFA concentrations are rarely found at the high levels observed in the rumen, it has served, and will continue to serve as a unique model to enhance our understanding of complex control systems.

REFERENCES

[1] Galfi, P., S. Neogrady and T. Sakata. 1991. Effects of volatile fatty acids on the epithelial cell proliferation of the digestive tract and its hormonal mediation. Tsuda, T., Y. Sasaki and R. Kawashima (eds.) *Physiological Aspects of Digestion and Metabolism in Ruminants: Proceedings of the Seventh International Symposium on Ruminant Physiology*. pp. 49-59. Academic Press, Inc., San Diego.

[2] Stevens, C. E. 1969. Fatty acid transport through the rumen epithelium. Phillipson, A. T. (ed.) *Physiology of Digestion and Metabolism in the Ruminant*. pp. 101-112. Oriel Press, Ltd., Newcastle upon Tyne, England.

[3] Steven, D. H. and A. B. Marshall. 1969. Organization of the rumen epithelium. Phillipson, A. T. (ed.) *Physiology of Digestion and Metabolism in the Ruminant*. pp. 80-100. Oriel Press, Ltd., Newcastle upon Tyne, England.

[4] Gaebel, G., H. Martens, M. Suendermann and P. Galfi. 1987. The effect of diet, intraruminal pH and osmolarity on sodium, chloride and magnesium absorption from the temporarily isolated and washed reticulo-rumen of sheep. *Quart. J. Exp. Physiol.* 72:501.

[5] Sakata, T. and H. Tamate. 1974. Effect of intermittent feeding on the mitotic index and the ultrastructure of basal cells of the ruminal epithelium in the sheep. *Tohoku J. Agr. Res.* 25:156.

[6] Tamate, H., T. Kikuchi and T. Sakata. 1974. Ultrastructural changes in the ruminal epithelium after fasting and subsequent refeeding in the sheep. *Tohoku J. Agr. Res.* 25:142.

[7] Stobo, I. J. F., J. H. B. Roy and H. J. Gaston. 1966. Rumen development in the calf. *Br. J. Nutr.* 20:171-188.

[8] Harfoot, C. G. 1978. Anatomy, physiology and microbiology of the ruminant digestive tract. *Prog. Lipid Res.* 17:1-19.

[9] Church, D. C. 1975. *Digestive Physiology and Nutrition of Ruminants.* Vol. 1. D. C. Church Publishing, Corvallis, OR.

[10] Annison, E. F., K. J. Hill and D. Lewis. 1957. Studies on the portal blood of sheep. 2. Absorption of volatile fatty acids from the rumen of the sheep. *Biochem. J.* 66:592.

[11] Nocek, J. E., J. H. Herbein and C. E. Polan. 1980. Influence of ration physical form, ruminal degradable nitrogen and age on rumen epithelial propionate and acetate transport and some enzymatic activities. *J. Nutr.* 110:2355.

[12] Goosen, P. C. M. 1976. Metabolism in rumen epithelium. Oxidation of substrates and formation of ketone bodies by pieces of rumen epithelium. *Zeit. Tierphysiol. Tierernah. Futtermit.* 37:14.

[13] Baldwin, R. L. and B. W. Jesse. 1991. A technical note concerning the isolation and characterization of sheep rumen epithelial cells. *J. Animal Sci.* 69:3603-3609.

[14] Weekes, T. E. C. 1974. The in vitro metabolism of propionate and glucose by the rumen epithelium. *Comp. Biochem. Physiol.* 49B:393.

[15] Weigand, E., J. W. Young and A. D. McGilliard. 1975. Volatile fatty acid metabolism by rumen mucosa from cattle fed hay or grain. *J. Dairy Sci.* 58: 1294.

[16] Emmanuel, B. 1981. Further metabolic studies in the rumen epithelium of camel (camelus dromedarius) and sheep (ovis aries). *Comp. Biochem. Physiol.* 68b: 155.

[17] Baldwin, R. L., VI and B. W. Jesse. 1996. Propionate modulation of ruminal ketogenesis. *J. Anim. Sci.* 74:1694-1700.

[18] Bush, R. S. and L. P. Milligan. 1971. Study of the mechanism of inhibition of ketogenesis by propionate in bovine liver. *Can. J. Animal Sci.* 51:121.

[19] Young, J. W., S. L. Thorp and H. E. De Lumen. 1969. Activity of selected gluconeogenic and lipogenic enzymes in bovine rumen mucosa, liver, and adipose tissue. *Biochem. J.* 114:83.

[20] Heitmann, R. N., D. J. Dawes and S. C. Sensenig. 1987. Hepatic ketogenesis and peripheral ketone body utilization in the ruminant. *J. Nutr.* 117:1174-1180.

[21] Beck, U., B. Emmanuel and D. Giesecke. 1984. The ketogenic effect of glucose in rumen epithelium of ovine (Ovis aries) and bovine (Bos taurus) origin. Comp. *Biochem. Physiol.* 77B:517.

[22] Leighton, B., A. R. Nicholas and C. I. Pogson. 1983. The pathway of ketogenesis in rumen epithelium of the sheep. *Biochem. J.* 216:769.

[23] Baird et al., 1970.
[24] Bush, R. S. and L. P. Milligan. 1971a. Enzymes of ketogenesis in bovine rumen epithelium. *Can. J. Animal Sci.* 51:129.
[25] White, R. G. and R. A. Leng. 1980. Glucose metabolism in feeding and postabsorptive lambs and mature sheep. *Comp. Biochem. Physiol.* 67A:223.
[26] Giesecke, D., U. Beck, S. Wiesmayer and M. Stangassinger. 1979. The effect of rumen epithelial development on metabolic activities and ketogenesis by the tissue *in vitro*. *Comp. Biochem. Physiol.* 62B:459-463.
[27] Warner, R. G., W. P. Flatt and J. K. Loosli. 1956. Dietary factors influencing the development of the ruminant stomach. *Agric. Food Chem.* 4:788-801.
[28] Gilliland, R. L., L. J. Bush and J. D. Friend. 1962. Relation of ration composition to rumen development in early-weaned dairy calves with observations on ruminal parakeratosis. *J. Dairy Sci.* 45:1211-1217.
[29] Hamada, T., S. Maeda and K. Kameoka. 1976. Factors influencing growth of rumen, liver, and other organs in kids weaned from milk replacers to solid foods. *J. Dairy Sci.* 59:1110-1118.
[30] Sander, E. G., H. N. Warner, H. N. Harrison and J. K. Loosli. 1959. The stimulatory effect of sodium butyrate and sodium propionate on the development of rumen mucosa in the young calf. *J. Dairy Sci.* 42:1600-1605.
[31] Tamate, H., A. D. McGilliard, N. L. Jacobson and R. Getty. 1962. Effect of various dietaries on the anatomical development of the stomach in the calf. *J. Dairy Sci.* 45: 408-420.
[32] Smith, R. H. 1961. The development and function of the rumen in milk-fed calves. II. Effect of wood shavings in the diet. *J. Agric. Sci.* 56:105-113.
[33] Orskov, E. R., D. Benzie and R. N. B. Kay. 1970. The effects of feeding procedure on closure of the oesophageal groove in young sheep. *Br. J. Nutr.* 24:785-794.
[34] Lane, M. A. and B. W. Jesse. 1997. Effect of volatile fatty acid infusion on development of the rumen epithelium in neonatal sheep. *J. Dairy Sci.* 80:740-746.
[35] Rickard, M. D. and J. H. Ternouth. 1965. The effect of the increased dietary volatile fatty acids on the morphological and physiological development of lambs with particular reference to the rumen. *J. Agric. Sci.* 65:371-382.
[36] Glauber, J. G., N. J. Wandersee, J. A. Little and G. D. Ginder. 1991. 5'-Flanking sequences mediate butyrate stimulation of embryonic globin gene expressioin in adult erythroid cells. *Molec. Cell. Biol.* 11:4690-4697.
[37] Wang, L.-Q., R. L. Baldwin VI and B. W. Jesse. 1996. Identification of two cDNA clones encoding small proline-rich proteins expressed in sheep ruminal epithelium. *Biochem. J.* 317, 225-233.
[38] Sakata, T. and H. Tamate. 1976b. Effect of n-butyrate administration rate on the epithelial cell proliferation in adult sheep rumen: A preliminary report. *Tohoku J. Agr. Res.* 27:136-138.
[39] Sakata, T. and H. Tamate. 1978. Rumen epithelial cell proliferation accelerated by rapid increase in intraruminal butyrate. *J. Dairy Sci.* 61:1109-1113.
[40] Sakata, T. and H. Tamate. 1976a. Effect of intraruminal injection of n-sodium butyrate on the mitotic indices in sheep ruminal epithelium. *Tohoku J. Agr. Res.* 27:133-135.
[41] Sakata, T. and H. Tamate. 1979. Rumen epithelium cell proliferation accelerated by propionate and acetate. *J. Dairy Sci.* 62:49-52.

[42] Gálfi, P., T. Veresegyházy, S. Neogrády and F. Kutas. 1981. Effect of sodium n- butyrate on primary ruminal epithelial cell culture. *Zender. Veter. Med.* 28:259-261.

[43] Baldwin, R. L., VI. 1999. The proliferative actions of insulin, insulin-like growth factor-I, epidermal growth factor, butyrate and propionate on ruminal epithelial cells in vitro. *Small Ruminant Research*. 32:261-268.

[44] Sakata, T., K. Hikosaka, Y. Shiomura and H. Tamate. 1980. Stimulatory effect of insulin on ruminal epithelium cell mitosis in adult sheep. *Br. J. Nutr.* 44:325-331.

[45] Galfi, P. and S. Neogrady. 1989. Epithelial and non-epithelial cell- and tissue culture from the rumen mucosa. *Asian-Austral. J. Animal Sci.* 2:143-149.

[46] Baldwin, R. L. and B. W. Jesse. 1992. Developmental changes in glucose and butyrate metabolism by isolated sheep ruminal cells. *J. Nutr.* 122: 1149-1153.

[47] Lane, M. A., R. L. Baldwin, VI and B. W. Jesse. 2000. Sheep rumen metabolic development in response to different dietary treatments. *J. Anim. Sci.* 78:1990-1996.

[48] Lane, M. A., R. L. Baldwin and B. W. Jesse. 2002. Developmental Changes in Ketogenic Enzyme Gene Expression During Sheep Rumen Development. *J. Anim. Sci.* 80: 1538-1544.

[49] Seal, C. J. and C. K. Reynolds. 1993. Nutritional implications of gastrointestinal and liver metabolism in ruminants. *Nutrition Research Reviews* 6:185-202.

[50] McBride, B. W. and J. M. Kelly. 1990. Energy cost of absorption and metabolism in the ruminant gastrointestinal tract and liver: a review. *J. Anim. Sci.* 68:2997-3010.

[51] Gill, M., J. France, M. Summers, B. W. McBride and L. P. Milligan. 1989. Simulation of the energy costs associated with protein turnover and Na+,K+-transport in growing lambs. *J. Nutr.* 119:1287-1299.

[52] Blum, J. W. and C. R. Baumrucker. 2002. Colostral and milk insulin-like growth factors and related substances: Mammary gland and neonatal (intestinal and systemic) targets. *Domest. Anim. Endocrinol.* 23:101-110.

[53] Baldwin, R. L., VI. 2000. Sheep gastrointestinal development in response to different dietary treatments. *Small Ruminant Research* 35:39-47.

[54] Morisset, J. 1993. SYMPOSIUM: Physiology of the gastrointestinal tract: Regulation of function and metabolism. Regulation and growth and development of the gastrointestinal tract. *J. Dairy. Sci.* 76:2080-2093.

[55] Shirazi-Beechey, S. P., M. W. Smith, Y. Wang, and P. S. James. 1991b. Postnatal development of lamb intestinal digestive enzymes is not regulated by diet. *J. Physiol.* 437:691-698.

[56] Shirazi-Beechey, S. P., B. A. Hirayama, Y. Wang, D. Scott, M. W. Smith, and E. M. Wright. 1991a. Ontogenic development of lamb intestinal sodium-glucose co-transporter is regulated by diet. *J. Physiol.* 437:699-708.

[57] Johnson, D. E., K. A. Johnson and R. L. Baldwin. 1990. Changes in liver and gastrointestinal tract energy demands in response to physiological workload in ruminants. *J. Nutr.* 120:649-655.

[58] Freetly, H. C., C. L. Ferrell, T. G. Jenkins and A. L. Goetsch. 1995. Visceral oxygen consumption during chronic feed restriction and realimentation in sheep. *J. Anim. Sci.* 73:843-852.

[59] Ferrell, C. L., L. J. Koong and J. A. Nienaber. 1986. Effect of previous nutrition on body composition and maintenance energy costs of growing lambs. *Br. J. Nutr.* 56:595-605.

[60] Ferrell, C. L. 1988. Contribution of visceral organs to animal energy expenditures. *J. Anim. Sci.* 66, supplement 3:23-33.

[61] Burrin, D. G., C. L. Ferrell, J. H. Eisemann, R. A. Britton, and J. A. Nienaber. 1989. Effect of level of nutrition on splanchnic blood flow and oxygen consumption in sheep. *Brit. J. Nutr.* 62:23-34.

[62] Burrin, D. G., C. L. Ferrell, J. H. Eisemann and R. A. Britton. 1991. Level of nutrition and splanchnic metabolite flux in young lambs. *J. Anim. Sci.* 69:1082-1091.

[63] Burrin, D. G., R. A. Britton, C. L. Ferrell and M. L. Bauer. 1992. Level of nutrition and visceral organ protein synthetic capacity and nucleic acid content in sheep. *J. Anim. Sci.* 70:1137-1145.

[64] McLeod, K. R. and R. L. Baldwin, VI. 2000. Effects of Diet Forage-to-Concentrate Ratio and Metabolizable Energy Intake on Visceral Organ Growth and *In vitro* Oxidative Capacity of Gut Tissues in Sheep. *J. Anim. Sci.* 78:760-770.

[65] Baldwin, R. L., VI and K. R. McLeod. 2000. Effects of Diet Forage-to-Concentrate Ratio and Metabolizable Energy Intake on Isolated Rumen Epithelial Cell Substrate Metabolism *In vitro*. *J. Anim. Sci.* 78:771-783.

[66] Reynolds, C. K., H. F. Tyrrell and P. J. Reynolds. 1991. Effects of diet forage-to-concentrate ratio and intake on energy metabolism in growing beef heifers: whole body energy and nitrogen balance and visceral heat production. *J. Nutr.* 121:994-1003.

[67] McBride, B. W. and L. P. Milligan. 1985. Influence of feed intake and starvation on the magnitude of Na+,K+-ATPase(EC3.6.1.3)-dependent respiration in duodenal mucosa of sheep. *Br. J. Nutr.* 53:605-614.

[68] Rompala, R. E., T. A. Hoagland and J. A. Meister. 1988. Effect of dietary bulk on organ mass, fasting heat production and metabolism of the small and large intestines in sheep. *J. Nutr.* 118:1553-1557.

[69] Burrin, D. G., R. A. Britton, C. L. Ferrell, and M. L. Bauer. 1990. Level of nutrition and visceral organ size and metabolic activity in sheep. *Br. J. Nutr.* 64:439-448.

[70] Wester, T. J., R. A. Britton, T. J. Klopfenstein, G. A. Ham, D. T. Hickok and C. R. Krehbiel. 1995. Differential Effects of Plane of Protein or Energy Nutrition on Visceral Organs and Hormones in Lambs. *J. Anim. Sci.* 73:1674.

[71] McLeod, K. R., R. L. Baldwin, VI, D. L. Harmon, C. J. Richards, and W. V. Rumpler. 2002. Influence of Ruminal and Postruminal Starch Infusion on Energy Balance in Growing Steers. In: A. Chwalibog and K. Jakobsen (Eds.), *Energy Metabolism of Farm Animals; Proceedings of the 15th Symposium on Energy Metabolism*. Snekkersten, Denmark. pp. 385-388.

[72] Orskov, E. R., D. A. Grubb, J. S. Smith, A. J. F. Webster and W. Corrigal. 1979. Efficiency of utilisation of volatile fatty acids for maintenance and energy retention in sheep. *British Journal of Nutrition* 41:541-551.

[73] Gross, K. L., D. L. Harmon and T. B. Avery. 1990. Portal-drained visceral flux of nutrients in lambs fed alfalfa or maintained by total intragastric infusion. *J. Anim. Sci.* 68:214-221.

[74] Jaeger, L. A. and C. H. Lamar. 1992. Immunolocalization of epidermal growth factor (EGF) and EGF receptors in the porcine upper gastrointestinal tract. *Am. J. Vet. Res.* 53: 1685-1692.

[75] Kelly, D., M. McFadyen, T. P. King and P. J. Morgan. 1992. Chacterization and autoradiographic localization of the epidermal growth factor receptor in the jejunum of neonatal and weaned pigs. *Reprod. Fertil. Dev.* 4:183-191.

[76] Tarnawski, A., S.-Y. Lu, J. Stachura and I. J. Sarfeh. 1992. Adaptation of gastric mucosa to chronic alcohol administration is associated with increased mucosal expression of growth factors and their receptor. *Scan. J. Gastroenterol.* 27:59-63.

[77] Playford, R. J., A. C. Woodman, P. Clark, P. Watanapa, D. Vesey, P. H. Deprez, R. C. N. Williamson and J. Calam. 1993. Effect of luminal growth factor preservation on intestinal growth. *The Lancet* 341:843-848.

[78] Peter, R. U., A. Beetz, C. Ried, G. Michel, D. van Beuningen and T. Ruzicka. 1993. Increased expression of the epidermal growth factor receptor in human epidermal keratinocytes after exposure to ionizing radiation. *Radiation Research* 136:65-70.

[79] Feldman, E. J., D. Aures and M. I. Grossman. 1978. Epidermal growth factor stimulates ornithine decarboxylase activity in the digestive tract of the mouse. *Proc. Soc. Exp. Boil. Med.* 159:400.

[80] Johnson, L. R. 1987. Regulation of gastrointestinal growth. *Physiology of the Gastro-intestinal Tract* 2:301-319.

[81] Yamada, T. and T. Chiba. 1989. Somatostatin. S. T. Schultz and G. M. Makhlouf (eds.) *Handbook of Physiology: The gastrointestinal system II.* p. 431. Oxford Univ., Press, Oxford.

[82] Faichney, G. J. and T. N. Barry. 1984. Intravenous somatostatin infusion affects gastrointestinal tract in sheep. *Can. J. Anim. Sci.* 64(Suppl.):93.

[83] McLeod, K. M., M. L. Bauer, D. L. Harmon, C. K. Reynolds and G. E. Mitchell. 1997. Effects of somatostatin and cysteamine on net nutrient flux across the portal-drained viscera and liver of sheep during intraduodenal infusion of starch hydrolysate and casein. *J. Anim. Sci.* 75:3026-3037.

[84] Baldwin, R. L., VI and K. R. McLeod. 2002. Glucose Oxidation by Isolated Steer Duodenal Enterocytes *in vitro*. In: A. Chwalibog and K. Jakobsen (Eds.), Energy Metabolism of Farm Animals; *Proceedings of the 15th Symposium on Energy Metabolism.* Snekkersten, Denmark. pp. 217-220.

[85] Baldwin, R. L. VI, S. Wu, W. Li, C. Li, B. J. Bequette and R. W. Li. 2012. Quantification of transcriptome responses of the rumen epithelium to butyrate infusion using RNA-seq technology. *Gene Regulation and Systems Biology.* 6: 67-80.

[86] Connor, E. E., Baldwin, R. L., C. Li, R. W. Li, C. Hoyung. 2013. Characterization of gene expression in bovine rumen epithelium during weaning identifies putative molecular regulators of rumen development and growth. *Functional and Integrative Genomics.* 13:133-142.

[87] Bünger, M., H. M. van den Bosch, J. van der Meijde, S. Kersten, G. J. E. J. Hooiveld, and M. Müller. 2007. Genome-wide analysis of PPARα activation in murine small intestine. *Physiol. Genomics* 30:192-204.

[88] Steele, M. A., G. Vandervoort, O. AlZahal, S. E. Hook, J. C. Matthews, and B. W. McBride. 2011. Rumen epithelial adaptation to high-grain diets involves the coordinated regulation of genes involved in cholesterol homeostasis. *Physiol. Genomics* 43:308–316.

[89] Kinoshita, M., Y. Suzuki and Y. Saito. 2002. Butyrate reduces colonic paracellular permeability by enhancing PPARγ activation. *Biochem. Biophys. Res. Commun*. 293: 827–831.

[90] Penner, G. B., M. A. Steele, J. R. Aschenbach, and B. W. McBride. 2011. Ruminant nutrition symposium: Molecular adaptation of ruminal epithelia to highly fermentable diets. *J. Anim. Sci*. 89:1108-1119.

[91] Naeem, A., J. K. Drackley, J. Stamey, and J. J. Loor. 2012. Role of metabolic and cellular proliferation genes in ruminal development in response to enhanced plane of nutrition in neonatal Holstein calves. *J. Dairy Sci*. 95:1807–1820.

In: Butyrate: Food Sources, Functions and Health Benefits
Editor: Cong-Jun Li
ISBN: 978-1-63117-657-9
© 2014 Nova Science Publishers, Inc.

Chapter 13

REGULATION OF CELLULAR PROCESSES BY EPIGENETIC MECHANISMS OF BUTYRATE

Kasturi Ranganna**, Omana P. Mathew, and Shirlette G. Milton
Department of Pharmaceutical Sciences, College of Pharmacy,
Texas Southern University, Houston, Texas, US

ABSTRACT

Continued prevalence of chronic diseases including cardiovascular diseases, cancer, diabetes, arthritis and neurological disorders which accounts for more than half of the deaths worldwide is becoming a global burden. For years dietary fiber has been linked to the prevention of chronic diseases and one of the mechanisms through which beneficial effects of dietary fiber is mediated is linked to epigenetic mechanisms of butyrate, a colonic fermentation product of dietary fiber. Butyrate exerts a multitude of reversible cellular effects such as inhibition of proliferation, stimulation of cell differentiation, induction of apoptosis, suppression of angiogenesis, activation of antiinflammatory and antioxidant response in a wide variety of cell types, mainly by altering gene expression. Three distinct, but closely interacting epigenetic mechanisms demonstrated to play important roles in the plethora of cellular effects of butyrate. These include DNA methylation, histone modification and non-coding microRNAs (miRNAs), which are responsible for modifying the expression of critical genes required for cellular effects that are associated with normal physiologic or pathologic processes. The chapter presents an overview of the epigenetic mechanisms of butyrate to enhance understanding of epigenetic regulation of cellular processes and to explore its potential in maintaining health and preventing diseases.

Keywords: Butyrate, DNA methylation, histone modification, non-coding microRNAs (miRNAs)

---

* Kasturi Ranganna, PhD, Department of Pharmaceutical Sciences, College of Pharmacy, Texas Southern University, 3100 Cleburne St, Houston, Texas 77004, Ranganna_kx@tsu.edu

Introduction

Epidemiological, animal, and interventional studies suggest an inverse relationship between dietary fiber and colonic health [1-3]. Several new studies suggest a similar relationship for dietary fiber and chronic diseases such as cardiovascular diseases, cancer, diabetes, obesity and hypertension [1-10]. Moreover, dietary fiber has been linked to prevention of chronic diseases and implicated in many pathways of diseases including inflammation, proliferation/cell cycle control, differentiation, apoptosis and angiogenesis [1-10]. However, it is only during the past ten to twenty years intense attention has been focused on exploring the components of fermentation products of dietary fiber that translate to health benefit and disease prevention. Although the specific nutrients and their sites of actions are relatively obscure, fermentation of soluble dietary fiber by colonic microflora generates short-chain fatty acids (SCFAs), which include acetate, butyrate, and propionate along with carbon dioxide, methane, and other gases. Of the SCFAs, butyrate, a four-carbon short chain fatty acid and a histone deacetylase inhibitor (HDACi), is shown to elicit many cytoprotective, chemopreventive and chemotherapeutic activities mainly by modulating expression of genes that contribute to many of the disease pathways via epigenetic mechanisms [1-3]. Interestingly, even though butyrate affects many cellular processes such as proliferation/cell cycle control, differentiation, apoptosis/cell death inflammation and angiogenesis [1-10] by exhibiting antiproliferative, antiinflammatory and antioxidant actions, these same cellular effects influenced by butyrate are deregulated in most of the chronic diseases. However, how these multiple cellular processes are influenced by a small molecule such as butyrate is surprising.

It is recognized that three interrelated epigenetic mechanisms appear to play prominent regulatory roles in cellular effects of butyrate. These include: methylation of DNA at CpG dinucleotides at specific position in the DNA molecule that suppress expression of nearby genes [11]; posttranslational modifications of histones, which alter chromatin structure and changes promoter accessibility, thus modulates gene expression [12]; and small RNA molecules generated from non-coding RNAs (ncRNAs) such as microRNA (miRNA) that inhibit gene expression [13, 14] along with activity of various non-histone proteins that bind to the DNA. Even though role of DNA methylation and chromatin modification in epigenetic regulation of gene expression is relatively well known, we have just begun to understand the contribution of miRNAs in the regulation of gene expression. Available, limited current evidence indicates that cellular effects of butyrate are outcome of these three epigenetic regulations. In this chapter, an overview of involvement of DNA modification, chromatin modification and miRNAs in butyrate regulated cellular processes is provided, which enhances understanding of epigenetic regulation of cellular processes, and health benefit of butyrate in particular and dietary fiber in general.

Epigenetic Code

Epigenetics is an area of biomedical research, which focuses on processes that control how and when certain genes are turned on or off in a cell by promoting or preventing transcription to proceed, thus maintaining cells identity, function and ability to react to internal and external environment by regulating gene expression without changing the nucleotide sequence. In simple terms, epigenetics involves the study of heritable alterations in gene expressions not coded in the DNA sequence of genes. The transcription of genetic information encoded in DNA is regulated by three distinct, but closely interacting mechanisms including epigenetic chemical modifications to N-terminal tails of histones, together with similar chemical modifications to DNA by methylation forming epigenetic code, and non-coding microRNAs. These mechanisms working together modify expression of genes associated with normal physiology and several diseases including chronic diseases such as cardiovascular disease, cancer, diabetes and behavioral pathologies [15, 16]. While the epigenetic codes comprising of specific epigenetic modifications to N-terminal tails of histones, together with chemical modifications to DNA by methylation furnish epigenetic markings on the chromatin that are copied from one cell generation to several generations to establish epigenetic inheritance [17], the non-coding RNAs are processed to short microRNAs that target specific genes for silencing [18]. Because many diseases are associated with changes in the normal program of gene expression that regulate basic cellular processes such as cell proliferation, cell differentiation, cell death/survival, use of epigenetic drugs can reverse anomalous gene expression profiles associated with different diseases, and thus prevent diseases. In this context, butyrate, a dietary-derived histone deacetylase inhibitor (HDACi), with its pleiotropic influence on various cellular processes including cell proliferation, cell differentiation and cell death, exhibits potential therapeutic and chemopreventive effects in the treatment and prevention of various diseases [2,4,8,9,12,19]. Besides its nutritional importance, butyrate has been known for a long time to alter gene expression through its outstanding influence on chromatin structure and dynamics and play a protective role in the prevention of cancer and inflammatory diseases of colon, cancers of other tissues and other diseases [2, 4, 8, 9, 12, 19]. In this chapter, latest update on epigenetic effects of butyrate with potential for clinical implications is presented.

CURRENT STATUS OF EPIGENETIC MODIFICATIONS BY BUTYRATE

DNA Methylation

Genetic code is identical in essentially all cells of an organism, yet each individual cell types have their own gene-expression profile. This specificity is attributed to DNA methylation, one of the epigenetic mechanisms that cells use to detain genes in the “off” position to control gene expression. From the last thirty years of studies, a number of details about DNA methylation has been discovered. It is noticed that DNA methylation occurs at certain regions of the genomes of different organisms and plays an important role in the regulation of gene expression. DNA methylation is recognized to be an important component of various cellular processes that play important role in normal physiological processes and development, chromosome stability, X-chromosome inactivation and genomic imprinting. Furthermore, it is recognized that aberrant DNA methylation profiles are linked to several diseases [20-22]. In mammals, methylation is found sparsely but globally, in definite CpG sequences throughout entire genome. DNA methylation occurs at the cytosine bases of DNA, which are converted to 5-methylcytosine by the action of DNA methyltransferase (DNMT) family of enzymes, DNMT1, DNMT3A and DNMT3B. DNMT1 functions as a maintenance DNMT, copying the methylation profile from parental strands to daughter strands during replication and prefers hemi methylated DNA substrates. DNMT3A and DNMT3B are responsible for de novo methylation by placing the initial pattern of methyl groups in place on DNA sequence. The methylated cytosine is generally flanking to a guanine base resulting in two methylated cytosine bases facing crossway to each other on opposing DNA strands forming what is called as CpG site. Addition of methyl groups changes the appearance and topography of DNA at these sites, which modifies interactions of a gene with its transcriptional machinery needed for its transcription. It is recognized that DNA methylation silences gene expression either by interfering with binding of transcription factors or by attracting methylated DNA-binding proteins (MBDs) that recruit other proteins such as SIN3A and histone modifying enzymes that forms inactive chromatin structure causing silencing of gene expression [23]. Furthermore, there is a tight correlation between DNA methylation patterns and chromatin structure. While active regions of chromatin that enable gene transcription are associated with hypomethylated DNA, particularly at promoter regions, hypermethylated DNA is packaged in inactive chromatin, which are confirmed by analyzing specific genes [23]. Moreover, while methylation status of particular promoter is similar in individual humans, there are considerable differences in overall and specific methylation status between different tissues, and between normal cells and diseased cells from the same tissue.

Importance of DNA methylation for the structure and function of chromatin is clearly established. However, several questions remain open in our understanding of the DNA methylation process, particularly transcriptional silencing of tumor suppressor genes such as retinoblastoma (RB), p53, p15INK4b, p16INK4a, and p21Cip1 [24-26] that regulate cell cycle. Aberrant methylation profiles of these genes is associated with their transcriptional silencing in several different cancers. The genome of cancer cells are generally hypomethylated overall compared to the genome of normal cells, excluding at tumor suppressor genes and genes that are associated with regulation of cell cycle and metastasis where DNA is hypermethylated. Although DNA methylation has been shown to play a vital role in numerous cellular processes, its role is poorly understood in the regulation of cellular processes by butyrate. Antiproliferative effect of butyrate may be linked to DNA methylation status at genes that arrest cell proliferation and promotes cell differentiation such as cyclin-dependent kinases (cdk)-inhibitors [27]. Moreover, one of the universal effect of butyrate is increased expression of p21Cip1, which promotes cell differentiation by inhibiting cell proliferation [12, 19].

Although very limited information is available regarding direct effect of butyrate on DNA methylation, butyrate has been shown to stimulate global DNA methylation in both normal and transformed cells [28, 29], and cause increased expression of fetal hemoglobin in sickle cell patients treated continuously or intermittently with butyrate [30]. This suggests induction of fetal hemoglobin in sickle cell patients is a result of heritable epigenetic modifications. Further studies indicate that butyrate treatment causes a true reversal of normal development switch from gamma-globin to beta-globin expression [31]. This switch is associated with decreased DNA methylation and increased histone acetylation of the gamma-globin gene, and opposite changes on beta-globin gene. Since butyrate is an inhibitor of DNMT3A expression, the enzyme responsible for de novo DNA methylation [32] and an established inhibitor of HDAC activity [2, 12, 14], it is possible that these activities of butyrate contribute to decreased DNA methylation and increased histone acetylation of gamma globin gene. Furthermore, these epigenetic modifications appear to regulate globin gene cluster expression in vivo in a tissue and developmental stage-specific manner [33]. This promoted pharmacological induction of fetal globin genes by agents that target DNA methylation and histone acetylation including butyrate [34]. Interestingly, butyrate with dual effect on chromatin structure through inhibition of DNMT and HDAC activities not only induces reactivation of gene expression by itself [31, 32] but also causes synergistic effect when it is used in combination with DNA methylation inhibitors such as 5-azacytidine and other agents [29,31,32,35,36]. DNA methylation and histone acetylation, the two key epigenetic mechanisms regulate chromatin structure and function. Normally, methylated DNA and deacetylated histones are in "closed" or tightly packed chromatin conformations facilitating suppression of transcription. It is possible that by inhibiting DNMT, butyrate may lower the threshold for DNMT inhibitors to stimulate DNA hypomethylation. This effect combined with stimulation of histone acetylation by butyrate may promote "opened" or relaxed chromatin conformation that contributes to the synergy observed between butyrate and DNMT inhibitors in reactivation of genes that can arrest proliferation and exhibit antitumor activity.

Histone Modification

Chromatin is a nucleoprotein complex consisting of repeating units of nucleosomal core particles that offers a dynamic platform for all DNA-mediated processes within the nucleus. Each nucleosome consisting of 147 base pair of DNA wrapped around an octamer of histone proteins containing two copies of each of the four histone proteins, H3, H4, H2A and H2B, is a building block of chromatin. Each nucleosome is separated by 10-16 base pair linker DNA, which assists compaction of chromatin structure into a higher-order chromatin structure essential for packaging of remarkable lengths of DNA into the cell nucleus. The compact chromatin structure restricts accessibility of DNA to DNA-mediated processes including transcription, DNA replication and repair. However, epigenetic mechanisms including DNA methylation and histone modification change the static chromatin into dynamic chromatin via postsynthetic modifications of DNA and histone proteins. Each of the histones are highly conserved basic proteins with a globular domain and a highly dynamic amino-terminal tail of 20-35 residues rich in basic amino acids. Histone tails are targets of a variety of site-specific modifications such as methylation, acetylation, phosphorylation, biotinylation, ubiquitination, sumoylation and ADP-ribosylation. While DNA methylation is relatively stable and responsible for the stable maintenance of particular gene expression profiles from one generation to the next in somatic cells, profiles of histone modifications are transient, dynamic and reversible, and can change rapidly during the course of the cell cycle. Furthermore, their "on' and "off" modification states are influenced by different physiological, developmental and environmental factors.

Questions about how the process of histone modifications is regulated and how many modifications and at what sites are required for a specific biological effect are still vague. However, histone modifications alters the chromatin structure and gene accessibility resulting in altered expression of genes. Normally, conformationally relaxed and decondensed chromatin structure that is associated with acetylation of histones and hypomethylation of

DNA is the characteristic of transcriptionally active chromatin that is required for gene expression, replication, repair and recombination. On the contrary, compact and condensed chromatin structure that is linked to deacetylation of histones and hypermethylation of DNA is the feature of transcriptionally inactive chromatin, which is essential during cell cycle, mitosis and meiosis. There are more than 100 different discrete posttranslational modifications of histones [11] and various combination of these histone modifications serve as epigenetic marks for the recruitment of different proteins or protein-complexes to regulate disparate functions like gene expression, gene suppression, mitosis, repair, replication and chromosome segregation [37]. Furthermore, there is cross-talk between different histone modifications at independent sites forming a "histone code", which is translated to a specific biological effect through the mediation of various effector proteins [12, 19, 38]. Different families of enzymes, which are referred as histone modification writers, are responsible for the addition of specific functional groups to histones. Most histone modifications are reversible and several families of enzymes catalyze the reactions. Among these, histone acetyltransferases (HATs)/HDACs and histone methyltransferase (HMTs)/histone demethylases (HDMs) exhibit counterbalancing activities that are essential for regulation of gene expression that are fundamental to basic cellular processes such as cell proliferation, differentiation and apoptosis [2, 12].

Mechanisms of Butyrate's Actions and Histone Modification

Hyperacetylation of core histones is the best characterized, and appears to be the main mechanism by which butyrate modulates gene expression, although other posttranslational modification such as histone methylation and phosphorylation also contribute to butyrate action [39-42]. These modifications are pivotal to transcription regulation, DNA replication and repair, gene silencing, and regulation of cellular differentiation and proliferation. Butyrate inhibits HDAC activity and during the inhibition, HAT activity continues, causing changes in the acetylation status of chromatin and other non-histone proteins, resulting in modulation of gene expression leading to various cellular effects including cell cycle arrest, induction of cell differentiation/apoptosis, and inhibition of inflammation and angiogenesis [2, 43, 44]. It is recognized that to enhance histone acetylation and to activate gene transcription, either the activity of HATs has to be increased or the activity of HDACs has to be blocked, which is a part of a transcriptional co-repressor complex that influences various tumor suppressor genes. The later activity is the mode of action of butyrate, which has been exploited in the therapeutic intervention of several diseases [2, 4]. Furthermore, several investigators have investigated gene expression effects of butyrate by array technology to profile anticancer gene expression in cancer cells [45, 46]. A recent study provides an understanding of the changes in transcriptome induced by butyrate in bovine kidney epithelial cells by using deep RNA-sequencing technology [47]. Likewise, the array technology is used to determine antiproliferation/antiatherogenic gene expression profile of butyrate in vascular smooth muscle cells (VSMC) [48]. Taken together, these studies indicate that common cellular processes affected by butyrate include cell proliferation/cell differentiation/apoptosis.

LINK BETWEEN BUTYRATE CELLULAR EFFECTS AND POSTTRANSLATIONAL COVALENT MODIFICATION OF HISTONES

Many of butyrate actions are linked to altered gene expression by modifying chromatin structure and organization via reversible site-specific posttranslational modification of histone amino-terminal tails. It is quite evident that higher order chromatin structure, occurring via modifications of histones plays a crucial role in regulating gene expression and any inappropriate or altered gene expression may lead to disease states. There are five main histones involved in the structure of chromatin in eukaryotic cells, which are posttranslationally modified, but histone H3 is the most extensively modified of the five histones. Histone H3 is important in the emerging field of epigenetics and its variable modification states and sequence variants are believed to play a role in the dynamic and long term regulation of genes. Site-specific modifications of amino-terminal tails of H3 and its sequence variants have been linked to discrete chromatin-based biological activities, such as: acetylation of lysine 9 (H3Lys9) and lysine14 (H3Lys14) to transcriptional activation; methylation of lysine9 (H3Lys9) to transcriptional silencing; methylation of lysine 4 (H3Lys4) to transcriptional activation; and phosphorylation of serine10 (H3Ser10) to cell cycle/mitosis/meiosis and chromosome condensation/segregation [49-53]. Furthermore, certain combinations of acetyl and methyl modifications of lysines in histones tails appear to have antagonistic or cooperative biological effects. However, the reversible posttranslation modification of histone tails by phosphorylation and acetylation has been linked to dynamic condensation and relaxation state of chromatin, respectively [49-51]. While chromatin condensation state is predominantly seen during mitosis, meiosis and cell cycle, relaxed state of chromatin correlates with transcriptional activation. Acting collectively, a combination of different histone modifications cross-talk to each other to form a "histone code" that is translated to a specific biological event such as inhibition of cell proliferation [54]. Histone modifications appear to serve as epigenetic marks and create potential docking sites on histone tails to direct the recruitment of different regulatory proteins or protein complexes to regulate disparate chromatin functions such as gene expression, DNA replication and chromosome segregation.

Concurringly, in VSMC, analysis of histone H3 modifications specific to butyrate arrested proliferation reveals induction of histone H3-Lysine9 acetylation, inhibition of histone H3-Serine10 phosphorylation, reduction of histone H3-Lysine9 dimethylation and stimulation of histone H3-Lysine4 di-methylation, which is linked to transcriptional activation, cell cycle/mitosis, transcriptional suppression and activation, respectively [19]. Conversely, untreated VSMCs exhibit inhibition of H3-Lysine9 acetylation, induction of H3-Serine10 phosphorylation, stimulation of H3- Lysine9 di-methylation and reduction in H3-Lysine4 di-methylation. Butyrate's cooperative effects on H3-Lysine9 acetylation and H3-Serine10 phosphorylation, and contrasting effects on di-methylation of H3-Lysine9 and H3-Lysine4 suggests that the interplay between these site-specific modifications cause distinct chromatin alterations that allow cyclin D1 and D3 induction, G1-specific cdk4, cdk6 and cdk2 downregulation, and upregulation of cdk inhibitors, p15INK4b and p21Cip1 [19]. Regardless of butyrate's effect on D-type cyclins, downregulation of G1-specific cdks and upregulation of cdk inhibitors by butyrate prevents cell cycle progression by failing to inactivate RB protein. Overall, through chromatin remodeling, butyrate appears to differentially alter G1-specific cell cycle proteins to ensure proliferation arrest of VSMC. Unlike in VSMC, butyrate increases both acetylation and di-methylation of histone H3 lysine9 in different non-vascular cells implicating these modifications occurs on independent sets of histone H3 molecules [53]. Butyrate inhibition of HDAC activity enhances derivation of induced pluripotent stem cells by increasing histone H3 acetylation and DNA demethylation providing an effective means for reprogramming various human adult somatic cells [56]. Treatment of rats with tributyrin, a butyrate prodrug is reported to increase hepatic nuclear histone H3Lysine9 acetylation in preneoplastic lesions along with increased p21 Cip1 protein expression, which may be linked to tributyrin-induced HDAC inhibitory activity [57]. Taken together, these studies confirm that butyrate effect on proliferation and differentiation is linked to HDAC inhibition mediated histone modifications.

Epigenetic Regulation of MiRNAs by Butyrate

From the current advances in genome research and RNA biology, now there is evidence indicating that a large section of human and most eukaryotic genome is transcribed as non-coding RNAs (ncRNAs). Only about 2% of the eukaryotic genome sequence codes for protein encoding genes. It is estimated that about 98% of the transcriptional output of their genomes is RNA that does not code for any proteins but mostly contains inept RNA transcripts or ncRNA transcripts that trigger unforeseen functions in eukaryotic biology [14, 58-60]. Recent advancement in new technologies in molecular biology and human genetics has led to the realization that even though ncRNAs do not code for proteins, they play crucial roles in cellular functions via transcriptional and translational regulation of protein coding genes essential for normal development and physiology. Besides, many of the ncRNA are highly conserved and vulnerable to epigenetic and genetic defects that affect normal development and become precursor to disease process [14]. There are different types of ncRNA and among these, the most extensively studied and relatively well understood with reference to their role in normal development and physiology, and to pathogenesis of disease are, small microRNAs (miRNAs). MiRNAs are endogenous, well conserved, 20 to 26 nucleotide small ncRNAs that mediate posttranscriptional gene silencing by complimentary binding to the 3'-untranslated region of their target mRNA, leading to target mRNA degradation or translational repression, a key event for controlling gene expression in a tissue or development-specific manner. These key gene expression regulators control various cellular processes including cell proliferation, differentiation, apoptosis and stem cell derivation particularly in mammalian development [14, 61-64]. Regardless of significant advances in miRNA research, the implications of miRNAs in physiological and pathological processes are just emerging. Furthermore, miRNA deficiencies and excesses have been linked to various diseases including different types of cancers, neurological, metabolic and cardiovascular diseases and other diseases [14].

Recent evidence indicates that epigenetic mechanisms such as promoter methylation and histone acetylation modulate miRNA expression suggesting a connection between epigenetic mechanisms and miRNA expression [65-67]. Both miRNAs and epigenetic mechanisms control gene expression suggesting that they may cross-talk and influence overall gene expression. MiRNAs can play important roles in controlling DNA methylation and histone modification by altering the expression of DNTMs/DNA demethylases and HATs/HDACs. On the other hand, epigenetic mechanisms such as DNA methylation and histone acetylation can also modulate miRNA expression. Consistent with this, a connection between epigenetic mechanisms and miRNAs has been demonstrated in several physiological processes and any disturbance in the balance between them can lead to pathological conditions. The connection between epigenetic mechanisms and miRNA is demonstrated in some of the recent studies by using epigenetic modifiers such as butyrate [14, 66, 67]. In bovine kidney cells, expression of about 35 miRNAs is significantly altered in response to butyrate treatment by using miRNA expression microarrays. Out of these, 11 miRNAs are differentially expressed at very high significance and target some very important gene networks. Furthermore, differentially expressed miRNA may interfere with butyrate-induced modulation of gene expression and cellular functions [67].

In human colon cancer HCT-116 cells, butyrate exhibits chemopreventive and antiproliferative effect, partly, through the mediation of p21Cip1 upregulation. Assessment of miRNA expression profiles of butyrate treated HCT-116 cells by microarray and quantitative PCR, reveals significant alterations in the expression of 44 miRNAs including decreased expression of miR-106b family that targets p21Cip1 expression [68]. Contrary to butyrate treated HCT-116 cells, miRNA microarray analysis of sporadic type human colon cancers reveals increased expression of miR-106b family. Consistent with this, while butyrate-treated cells exhibit upregulation of target p21Cip1 gene expression, which associates with inhibition of HCT-116 cell proliferation, it is decreased in colon cancer tissues. The link between butyrate-induced reduction in miR-106b expression and increased p21Cip1 protein expression is further confirmed by treating the cells with a miR-106b mimic. The addition of miR-106b mimic reversed the increased p21Cip1 expression and decreased cell proliferation stimulaed by butyrate. These results indicate that butyrate by upregulating p21Cip1 expression through the mediation of altered miR-106b restricts cell cycle progression leading to inhibition of colon cancer cell proliferation. Besides miR-106b, several other multiple members of miR-17-92a, miR-18b-106a and miR-25-106b clusters are also significantly decreased in response to butyrate. In another study, examination of role of microRNAs in mediating the cytoprotective effects of butyrate in HT29 and HCT-116 colorectal cancer cells reveals decreased expression of miRNAs of miR-17-92 cluster with a corresponding increase in miR-17-92 target genes, which includes PTEN, BCL2L11 and CDKN1A [69]. Decrease in miR-17-92 expression appears to be partly responsible for antiproliferative effect of butyrate, which is confirmed by the introduction of miR-17-92 cluster mimics. Use of miR-17-92 mimics reverses growth effects of butyrate and decreases PTEN, BCL2L11 and CDKN1A, which indicates antiproliferative effect of butyrate is mediated by changes in miRNA activity, with downregulation of the miR-17-92 cluster as a possible mechanism.

Butyrate is a strong inhibitor of VSMC proliferation, a critical factor in the development of atherosclerosis. Since the cellular effects that are stimulated by butyrate are also regulated by miRNAs and expression of miRNAs is regulated by epigenetic mechanisms including DNA methylation and histone modification [14], miRNA expression profiles of butyrate treated rat VSMC is determined using qRT-PCR platform based miRNA microarrays. Butyrate treatment altered the expression of 60 miRNAs significantly. Among these, members of the miR-17-92 cluster are some of the miRNAs that are downregulated in VSMC by butyrate. The miR-17-92 cluster is a polycistronic miRNA gene, which is referred as oncomir-1 in humans because of their oncogenic properties and overexpression in different cancers [70]. The cluster encodes six mature miRNAs: miR-17, -18a, -19a, -20a, 19b-1 and -92a-1 that are grouped within 800 base-pair region of human chromosome 13. Target genes for some of these miRNAs have been identified, which include cell cycle inhibitor CDKN1A (p21Cip1) and apoptotic PTEN and BCL2L11. Transcription of miR-17-92 cluster is activated by c-myc [71]. Earlier studies have shown butyrate causes downregulation of c-myc [72] and upregulation of CDKN1A in proliferation arrested VSMC [12, 19, 48]. It is possible by downregulating c-myc expression via epigenetic mechanisms, butyrate inhibits expression of members of miR-17-92 cluster with a corresponding increase in miR-17-92 target genes such as CDKN1A. Overall, studies in VSMC emphasize role of miRNAs in antiproliferative and chemoprotective effects of butyrate.

CONCLUSION

This chapter has provided synopsis of epigenetic mechanisms of butyrate through which butyrate regulates its many facets of cellular effects. Even though it is long known that butyrate alters gene expression via histone acetylation, even before the identification of enzymes that participate in histone acetylation status, HATs/HDACs, its role in DNA methylation and miRNA expression, is emerging quite recently. Besides histone acetylation, DNA methylation state at promoter regions appears to be modified by butyrate through the inhibition of expression of DNMT. To make this complicated, butyrate can also alter miRNA expression by changing its promoter methylation and histone acetylation state. These recent information suggest that all three epigenetic mechanism cross-talk to each other in the regulation of gene expression, which is essential for perfect cellular effects. Because these are emerging areas of research, several details of the mechanisms are still vague and not clear. The challenge is to assimilate how all three epigenetic mechanisms collaborate with each other in the mediation of beneficial effects of butyrate to improve health and prevent chronic diseases in a more natural way.

REFERENCES

[1] Gibson GR, Rastall RA, Roberfroid MB, *Prebiotics. Colonic Microbiota, Nutrition and Health.* Gibson GR, Roberfroid MB, editors. Dordrecht, The Netherlands Kluwer Academic Publishers; 1999.

[2] Ranganna K, Yatsu FM, Hayes BE. Butyrate, a small pleiotropic molecule with multiple cellular and molecular actions: Its role as an anti-atherogenic agent. *Recent Res Dev Mol Cell Biochem*. 2005; 2: 123–151.

[3] Ranganna K, Yatsu FM, Mathew OP. Insights into the pathogenesis and intervention of atherosclerosis. *Vasc Dise Prev*. 2006; 3: 375-390.

[4] Berni Canani R, Di Costanzo M, Leone L. The epigenetic effects of butyrate: potential therapeutic implications for clinical practice. *Clin Epigenetics.* 2012; 4(1):4.

[5] Mehnert JM, Kelly WK. Histone deacetylase inhibitors: biology and mechanism of action. *Cancer J.* 2007; 13(1):23-29.

[6] Davie JR. Inhibition of histone deacetylase activity by butyrate. *J Nutr.* 2003; 133(7 Suppl):2485S-2493S.

[7] Anderson JW. Whole grains protect against atherosclerotic cardiovascular disease. *Proc Nutr Soc.* 2003; 62(1):135-42.

[8] Hu FB. Plant-based foods and prevention of cardiovascular disease: an overview. *Am J Clin Nutr.* 2003; 78(3 Suppl):544S-551S.

[9] Kim YI. AGA technical review: impact of dietary fiber on colon cancer occurrence. *Gastroenterology.* 2000; 118(6):1235-1257.

[10] Esteller M. Epigenetics in cancer. *N Engl J Med.* 2008; 358(11):1148-1159.

[11] Kouzarides T. Chromatin modifications and their function. *Cell.* 2007; 128(4):693-705.

[12] Ranganna K, Yatsu FM, Mathew OP. Emerging epigenetic therapy for vascular proliferative diseases. In Atherogenesis, SampathParthasarathy (Ed.), 2011, ISBN: 978-953-307-992-9, InTech, Available from: *http://www.intechopen.com/articles/show/title/emerging-epigenetic-therapy-for-vascular-proliferative-diseases.*

[13] Mattick JS, Amaral PP, Dinger ME, Mercer TR, Mehler MF. RNA regulation of epigenetic processes. *Bioessays.* 2009; 31(1):51-59.

[14] Ranganna K, Mathew OP, Milton SG, Hayes BE. MicroRNAome of vascular smooth muscle cells: Potential for microRNA-based vascular therapies, current trends in atherogenesis, Prof. Rita Rezzani (Ed.), 2013, ISBN: 978-953-51-1011-8, InTech, DOI: 10.5772/54636. Available from: *http://www.intechopen.com/books/current-trends-in-atherogenesis/micrornaome-of-vascular-smooth-muscle-cells-potential-for-microrna-based-vascular-therapies.*

[15] Furrow RE, Christiansen FB, Feldman MW. Environment-sensitive epigenetics and the heritability of complex diseases. *Genetics.* 2011; 189(4):1377-1387.

[16] McKay JA, Mathers JC. Diet induced epigenetic changes and their implications for health. *Acta Physiol (Oxf).* 2011; 202(2):103-118.

[17] Feinberg AP. Epigenetics at the epicenter of modern medicine. *JAMA.* 2008; 299(11):1345-1350.

[18] Bergmann A, Lane ME. HIDden targets of microRNAs for growth control. *Trends Biochem Sci.* 2003; 28(9):461-463.

[19] Mathew OP, Ranganna K, Yatsu FM. Butyrate, an HDAC inhibitor, stimulates interplay between different posttranslational modifications of histone H3 and differently alters G1-specific cell cycle proteins in vascular smooth muscle cells. *Biomed Pharmacother.* 2010; 64(10):733-740.

[20] Robertson KD. DNA methylation and human disease. *Nat Rev Genet.* 2005; 6(8):597-610.

[21] Simmons, D. Epigenetic influence and disease. *Nature Education* 2008; 1(1): 6.

[22] Theresa Phillips. The role of methylation in gene expression*: Nature Education* 2008; 1(1): 116.

[23] Szyf M. Epigenetics, DNA methylation, and chromatin modifying drugs. *Annu Rev Pharmacol Toxicol.* 2009; 49:243-263.

[24] Wajed SA, Laird PW, DeMeester TR. DNA methylation: an alternative pathway to cancer. *Ann Surg.* 2001; 234(1):10-20.

[25] Esteller M. Epigenetic lesions causing genetic lesions in human cancer: promoter hypermethylation of DNA repair genes. *Eur J Cancer.* 2000; 36(18):2294-2300.

[26] Fang M, Chen D, Yang CS. Dietary polyphenols may affect DNA methylation. *J Nutr.* 2007; 137(1 Suppl):223S-228S.

[27] Li G, Ji Y, Liu C, Li J, Zhou Y. Reduced levels of p15INK4b, p16INK4a, p21cip1 and p27kip1 in pancreatic carcinoma. *Mol Med Rep.* 2012; 5(4):1106-1110.

[28] de Haan JB, Gevers W, Parker MI. Effects of sodium butyrate on the synthesis and methylation of DNA in normal cells and their transformed counterparts. *Cancer Res.* 1986; 46(2):713-716.

[29] Cosgrove DE, Cox GS. Effects of sodium butyrate and 5-azacytidine on DNA methylation in human tumor cell lines: variable response to drug treatment and withdrawal. *Biochim Biophys Acta.* 1990; 1087(1):80-86.

[30] Saunthararajah Y, DeSimone J. Clinical studies with fetal hemoglobin-enhancing agents in sickle cell disease. *Semin Hematol.* 2004; 41(4 Suppl 6):11-16.

[31] Fathallah H, Weinberg RS, Galperin Y, Sutton M, Atweh GF. Role of epigenetic modifications in normal globin gene regulation and butyrate-mediated induction of fetal hemoglobin. *Blood.* 2007; 110(9):3391-3397.

[32] Xiong Y, Dowdy SC, Podratz KC, Jin F, Attewell JR, Eberhardt NL, et al. Histone deacetylase inhibitors decrease DNA methyltransferase-3B messenger RNA stability and down-regulate de novo DNA methyltransferase activity in human endometrial cells. *Cancer Res.* 2005; 65(7):2684-2689.

[33] van der Ploeg LH, Flavell RA. DNA methylation in the human gamma delta beta-globin locus in erythroid and nonerythroid tissues. *Cell.* 1980; 19(4):947-958.

[34] Atweh GF, Sutton M, Nassif I, Boosalis V, Dover GJ, Wallenstein S, et al. Sustained induction of fetal hemoglobin by pulse butyrate therapy in sickle cell disease. *Blood.* 1999; 93(6):1790-1797.

[35] Spurling CC, Suhl JA, Boucher N, Nelson CE, Rosenberg DW, Giardina C. The short chain fatty acid butyrate induces promoter demethylation and reactivation of RARbeta2 in colon cancer cells. *Nutr Cancer.* 2008; 60(5):692-702.

[36] Fialova B, Smesny Trtkova K, Paskova L, Langova K, Kolar Z. Effect of histone deacetylase and DNA methyltransferase inhibitors on the expression of the androgen receptor gene in androgen-independent prostate cancer cell lines. *Oncol Rep.* 2013; 29(5):2039-2045.

[37] Taverna SD, Li H, Ruthenburg AJ, Allis CD, Patel DJ. How chromatin-binding modules interpret histone modifications: lessons from professional pocket pickers. *Nat Struct Mol Biol.* 2007; 14(11):1025-1040.

[38] Milton SG, Mathew OP, Yatsu FM, Ranganna K. Differential cellular and molecular effects of butyrate and trichostatin a on vascular smooth muscle cells. *Pharmaceuticals* (Basel). 2012; 5(9):925-943.

[39] Strahl BD, Allis CD The language of covalent histone modifications. *Nature.* 2000; 403(6765):41-45.

[40] Walker GE, Wilson EM, Powell D, Oh Y. Butyrate, a histone deacetylase inhibitor, activates the human IGF binding protein-3 promoter in breast cancer cells: molecular mechanism involves an Sp1/Sp3 multiprotein complex. *Endocrinology.* 2001; 142(9):3817-3827.

[41] Yang J, Kawai Y, Hanson RW, Arinze IJ. Sodium butyrate induces transcription from the G alpha (i2) gene promoter through multiple Sp1 sites in the promoter and by

activating the MEK-ERK signal transduction pathway. *J Biol Chem.* 2001; 276(28):25742-25752.

[42] Siavoshian S, Segain JP, Kornprobst M, Bonnet C, Cherbut C, Galmiche JP, et al. Butyrate and trichostatin A effects on the proliferation/differentiation of human intestinal epithelial cells: induction of cyclin D3 and p21 expression. *Gut.* 2000; 46(4):507-514.

[43] Ma X, Ezzeldin HH, Diasio RB. Histone deacetylase inhibitors: current status and overview of recent clinical trials. *Drugs.* 2009; 69(14):1911-34.

[44] Rajendran P, Ho E, Williams DE, Dashwood RH. Dietary phytochemicals, HDAC inhibition, and DNA damage/repair defects in cancer cells. *Clin Epigenetics.* 2011; 3(1):4.

[45] Williams EA, Coxhead JM, Mathers JC. Anti-cancer effects of butyrate: use of micro-array technology to investigate mechanisms. *Proc Nutr Soc.* 2003; 62(1):107-115.

[46] Mariadason JM, Corner GA, Augenlicht LH. Genetic reprogramming in pathways of colonic cell maturation induced by short chain fatty acids: comparison with trichostatin A, sulindac, and curcumin and implications for chemoprevention of colon cancer. *Cancer Res.* 2000; 60(16):4561-4572.

[47] Wu S, Li RW, Li W, Li CJ. Transcriptome characterization by RNA-seq unravels the mechanisms of butyrate-induced epigenomic regulation in bovine cells. *PLoS One.* 2012; 7(5):e36940.

[48] Ranganna K, Yousefipour Z, Yatsu FM, Milton SG, Hayes BE. Gene expression profile of butyrate-inhibited vascular smooth muscle cell proliferation. *Mol Cell Biochem.* 2003; 254 (1-2):21-36.

[49] Ito T. Role of histone modification in chromatin dynamics. *J Biochem.* 2007; 141(5):609-614.

[50] McManus KJ, Hendzel MJ. The relationship between histone H3 phosphorylation and acetylation throughout the mammalian cell cycle. *Biochem Cell Biol.* 2006; 84(4):640-657.

[51] Edmondson DG, Davie JK, Zhou J, Mirnikjoo B, Tatchell K, Dent SY. Site-specific loss of acetylation upon phosphorylation of histone H3. *J Biol Chem.* 2002; 277(33):29496-29502.

[52] Eberlin A, Grauffel C, Oulad-Abdelghani M, Robert F, Torres-Padilla ME, Lambrot R, et al. Histone H3 tails containing dimethylated lysine and adjacent phosphorylated serine modifications adopt a specific conformation during mitosis and meiosis. *Mol Cell Biol.* 2008; 28(5):1739-1754.

[53] Ducasse M, Brown MA. Epigenetic aberrations and cancer. *Mol Cancer* 2006; 5: 60.

[54] Fischle W, Wang Y, Allis CD. Histone and chromatin cross-talk. *Curr Opin Cell Biol.* 2003; 15(2):172-183.

[55] Garcia BA, Hake SB, Diaz RL, Kauer M, Morris SA, Recht J, et al. Organismal differences in post-translational modifications in histones H3 and H4. *J Biol Chem.* 2007; 282(10):7641-7655.

[56] Mali P, Chou BK, Yen J, Ye Z, Zou J, Dowey S, et al. Butyrate greatly enhances derivation of human induced pluripotent stem cells by promoting epigenetic remodeling and the expression of pluripotency-associated genes. *Stem Cells.* 2010; 28(4):713-720.

[57] Kuroiwa-Trzmielina J, de Conti A, Scolastici C, Pereira D, Horst MA, Purgatto E, et al. Chemoprevention of rat hepatocarcinogenesis with histone deacetylase inhibitors: efficacy of tributyrin, a butyric acid prodrug. *Int J Cancer.* 2009; 124(11):2520-2527.

[58] Esteller M. Non-coding RNAs in human disease. *Nat Rev Genet.* 2011; 12(12):861-874.

[59] Alexander RP, Fang G, Rozowsky J, Snyder M, Gerstein MB. Annotating non-coding regions of the genome. *Nat Rev Genet.* 2010; 11(8):559-571.

[60] Derrien T, Guigó R, Johnson R. The Long Non-Coding RNAs: A New Player in the "Dark Matter". *Front Genet.* 2012; 2:107.

[61] Ambros V. The functions of animal microRNAs. *Nature.* 2004; 431(7006):350-355.

[62] Hwang HW, Mendell JT. MicroRNAs in cell proliferation, cell death, and tumorigenesis. *Br J Cancer.* 2006; 94(6):776-80.

[63] Jovanovic M, Hengartner MO. miRNAs and apoptosis: RNAs to die for. *Oncogene.* 2006; 25(46):6176-87.

[64] Qi J, Yu JY, Shcherbata HR, Mathieu J, Wang AJ, Seal S, et al. microRNAs regulate human embryonic stem cell division. *Cell Cycle.* 2009; 8(22):3729-3741.

[65] Scott GK, Mattie MD, Berger CE, Benz SC, Benz CC. Rapid alteration of microRNA levels by histone deacetylase inhibition. *Cancer Res.* 2006; 66(3):1277-1281.

[66] Bandres E, Agirre X, Bitarte N, Ramirez N, Zarate R, Roman-Gomez J, et al. Epigenetic regulation of microRNA expression in colorectal cancer. *Int J Cancer.* 2009; 125(11):2737-2743.

[67] Li C-J, Li RW, Elsasser TH. MicroRNA (miRNA) expression is regulated by butyrate-induced epigenetic modulation of gene expression in bovine cells. *Genetic and Epigenetics* 2010; 3:23-32.

[68] Hu S, Dong TS, Dalal SR, Wu F, Bissonnette M, Kwon JH, et al. The microbe-derived short chain fatty acid butyrate targets miRNA-dependent p21 gene expression in human colon cancer. *PLoS One.* 2011; 6(1):e16221.

[69] Humphreys KJ, Cobiac L, Le Leu RK, Van der Hoek MB, Michael MZ. Histone deacetylase inhibition in colorectal cancer cells reveals competing roles for members of the oncogenic miR-17-92 cluster. *Mol Carcinog.* 2013; 52(6):459-474.

[70] He L, Thomson JM, Hemann MT, Hernando-Monge E, Mu D, Goodson S, et al. A microRNA polycistron as a potential human oncogene. *Nature.* 2005; 435(7043):828-833.

[71] Mendell JT miRiad roles for the miR-17-92 cluster in development and disease. *Cell.* 2008; 133(2):217-222.

[72] Ranganna K, Joshi T, Yatsu FM. Sodium butyrate inhibits platelet-derived growth factor-induced proliferation of vascular smooth muscle cells. *Arterioscler Thromb Vasc Biol.* 1995; 15(12):2273-2283.

In: Butyrate: Food Sources, Functions and Health Benefits
Editor: Cong-Jun Li
ISBN: 978-1-63117-657-9
© 2014 Nova Science Publishers, Inc.

Chapter 14

Butyrate: A Dietary Inhibitor of Histone Deacetylases and an Epigenetic Regulator

Cong-Jun Li*[*,1], *Robert W. Li, Ransom L. Baldwin and Theodore H. Elsasser

Bovine Functional Genomics Laboratory, Agricultural Research Service, US Department of Agriculture, Beltsville Agricultural Research Center, Maryland, US

Abstract

The short-chain fatty acids (SCFAs, acetate, propionate and butyrate), also known as volatile fatty acids (VFA), are produced in the gastrointestinal tract by microbial fermentation. Consumption of dietary fibers has been shown to have positive metabolic health effects, such as increasing satiety, and lowering blood glucose and cholesterol levels. At the cellular level, butyrate induces cell cycle arrest and apoptosis. These effects are associated with SCFAs, particularly butyrate.

The mechanisms of action of butyrate are different and many of these involve an epigenomic regulation of gene expression through the inhibition of histone deacetylases (HDACs). Epigenomics is the study of both heritable and non-heritable changes in the regulation of gene activity and expression that occur without change in the DNA sequence. This dynamic and rapidly developing discipline is making its impact across biomedical science.

Inhibition of HDACs results in hyperacetylation of histones, thereby modifying the chromatin and chromosomal (epigenomic) landscape. Chromatin modification has clearly emerged as a very important mechanism in regulating the transcriptional status of the genome. Butyrate-induced biological effects provide an example of epigenomic regulation and provide a basis for understanding the full range of the biological roles and molecular mechanisms that butyrate may play in cell growth, proliferation, and energy metabolism. This chapter is concentrated on recent research advances regarding the

[*] Corresponding author: congjun.li@ars.usda.gov, Tel: (301) 504-7216.

[1] Disclaimer: Mention of a product, reagent or source does not constitute an endorsement by the USDA to the exclusion of other products or services that perform a comparable function. The US Department of Agriculture is an equal opportunity provider and employer.

epigenetic effects of butyrate in essential biological activities. Discoveries from our own research endeavors in related areas are also reviewed.

INTRODUCTION

The short-chain fatty acids (SCFAs, acetate, propionate and butyrate), also known as volatile fatty acids (VFA) are produced in the gastrointestinal tract by microbial fermentation of carbohydrates, mostly dietary fibers, and endogenous substrates, such as mucus. The major source of butyrate is the fermentation of dietary fibers. In addition to milk as the major source of butyrate from food, butyrate can also be found in butter and cheese [1, 2].

It is now well established that microbial fermentation in the gastrointestinal tract contributes to the energy balance of all mammalian species [3, 4]. This can be of great advantage to animals and humans, since no digestive enzymes exist for breaking down cellulose or other complex carbohydrates. The large number of bacterial species, the complex nature of their interactions, and the end products of their fermentation processes are all likely to have significance in human and animal health.

SCFAs are produced in the largest amounts in herbivorous animal species, and especially in the fore stomach of ruminants. The principal SCFAs in either the rumen or large intestine are acetate, propionate and butyrate, and they are produced in ratios ranging from approximately 75:15:10 to 40:40:20. Absorption of SCFAs at their site of production is rapid, and large quantities are metabolized by the ruminal or large intestinal epithelium before reaching the portal blood.

Most of the butyrate is converted to ketone bodies or CO2 by the epithelial cells, and the liver removes nearly all of the remainder. Propionate is similarly removed by the liver, but it is largely converted to glucose. Although species differences exist—principally peripheral tissues, especially fat and muscle—use acetate. Considerable energy is obtained from SCFAs in herbivorous species, and far more research has been conducted on ruminants than on other species. Significant amount of SCFAs, however, are now known to be produced in omnivorous species, such as pigs and humans. Current estimates show that SCFAs contribute approximately 70 percent to the caloric requirements of ruminants, such as sheep and cattle, approximately 10 percent for humans, and approximately 20–30 percent for several other omnivorous or herbivorous animals [4].

In addition to the energy or nutritional contributions of SCFAs to the body, they may indirectly influence cholesterol synthesis and even help regulate insulin or glucagon secretion. SCFA production and absorption have very significant effects on epithelial cell growth, blood flow, and the normal secretory and absorptive functions of the large intestine, cecum, and rumen. The absorption of SCFAs and sodium, for example, seems to be interdependent, and the release of bicarbonate usually occurs during SCFA absorption.

SCFAs are also produced in the lower digestive tract of humans and all other animal species. Intestinal fermentation resembles that which occurs in the rumen with respect to the metabolic pathways involved in anaerobic degradation of organic matter, and in the concentrations of SCFA end products [5]. The amount, type and balance of the main dietary macronutrients (carbohydrates, proteins and fats) greatly affect the large intestinal microbiota. The human colon contains a dense population of bacterial cells that outnumber host cells tenfold.

Bacteroidetes, Firmicutes and Actinobacteria are the three major phyla that inhabit the human large intestine, and these bacteria possess a fascinating array of enzymes that can degrade complex dietary substrates. Certain colonic bacteria are able to metabolize a remarkable variety of substrates, whilst other species carry out more specialized activities, including primary degradation of plant cell walls. Microbial metabolism of dietary carbohydrates results mainly in the formation of short-chain fatty acids and gases. The major bacterial fermentation end products are acetate, propionate and butyrate [6]. The amount of fiber in the diet affects the amount of SCFAs produced, and thus the contribution of SCFAs to the energy needs of the body could become considerably greater as dietary fiber increases.

Pigs and some species of monkeys most closely resemble humans, and current research should be directed toward examining the fermentation processes and SCFA metabolism in those species. The production of these SCFAs tends to lower colonic pH. These weak acids influence the microbial composition and directly affect host health, with butyrate being the preferred energy source for colonocytes. Certain bacterial species in the colon survive by cross-feeding, using either the breakdown products of complex carbohydrate degradation or fermentation products, such as lactic acid for growth. Microbial protein metabolism results in additional fermentation products, some of which are potentially harmful to host health [6]. Diet is a major factor driving the composition and metabolism of the colonic microbiota. Thus, rumen bacteria are useful for understanding the dynamics and potential interactions of human intestinal bacteria.

It has been recognized for a long time that consumption of dietary fibers has many positive metabolic health effects, such as increasing satiety, and lowering blood glucose and cholesterol levels. These effects may be associated with short-chain fatty acids, particularly propionic and butyric acids, formed by the microbial degradation of dietary fibers in the colon, and by their capacity to reduce low-grade inflammation [7].

In the last decade, multiple beneficial effects of butyrate at the intestinal and extraintestinal levels have been demonstrated. The mechanisms of action of butyrate are different, and many of these involve an epigenetic regulation of gene expression through the inhibition of histone deacetylases. There is a growing interest in butyrate because its impact on epigenetic mechanisms could lead to more specific and efficacious therapeutic strategies for the prevention and treatment of different diseases, ranging from genetic/metabolic conditions to neurological degenerative disorders [8]. This chapter is concentrated on recent data regarding the epigenetic effects of butyrate in essential biological activities.

BUTYRATE AND CELL FUNCTION: CELL CYCLE, APOPTOSIS AND HISTONE DEACETYLASE INHIBITORY ACTIVITY

Butyrate Induces Cell Cycle Arrest

Beyond their nutritional impact, SCFAs (especially butyrate) modulate cell differentiation, proliferation, motility, and in particular, induce cell cycle arrest and apoptosis. However, a majority of previous studies focused on the therapeutic potential of butyrate for cancer, and thus, used cancer cell lines as research models [9].

The cell cycle regulatory effects of butyrate at the cellular and molecular levels in normal bovine cells have not been studied until recent years [10–12]. During the last two decades, we have come to realize that lipids function as both energy stores and signaling molecules. They play pivotal roles in regulating a wide variety of cellular processes. As a particular group of lipids, short-chain fatty acids have been studied intensively [3, 13]. It is now well established that microbial fermentation in the gastrointestinal tract contributes to the energy balance of all mammalian species [3, 4]. Short-chain fatty acids contribute up to 70 percent of the energy requirements of ruminants [4, 14, 15]. Among these short-chain fatty acids, butyrate is the major source of energy for colonocytes [16, 17].

While acetate and propionate hold prominent positions in providing energy to ruminant metabolism, butyrate, low in its relative concentrations, appears to be involved in metabolism beyond its role as a nutrient. Roles for butyrate have been established in cell differentiation, proliferation, motility, and, in particular, induction of cell cycle arrest and apoptosis [18–20].

Apoptosis is a genetically regulated cellular suicide mechanism that plays a crucial role in development and in the defense of the homeostasis of animals [21]. The mechanism(s) by which butyrate induces cellular differentiation and suppresses growth have been elucidated. Similarly, the mechanism through which butyrate and other short-chain fatty acids induce the cell cycle regulatory and apoptotic effects, and the mechanism by which the decision between cell death and survival is arbitrated, are gradually being understood.

Some definitive studies in cattle have addressed the capabilities for nutrients to modulate gene expression and proteomic outcomes as a means of arresting metabolic stress. The cell cycle regulatory and apoptotic effects of butyrate and other short-chain fatty acids at the cellular and molecular levels in normal bovine cells have been studied, and would serve as a principle launch point to validate the need for further study of these phenomena in cattle [10, 22].

Butyrate Blocks DNA Replication and Cell Cycle Checkpoints

When cells were treated with 2.5 to 10.0 millimolar (mM) butyrate for 24 hours, cell morphology became distorted. Cells with large vacuoles, and with ragged membranes, lacking distinct intracellular organelles, and having increased spaces between cells, were readily visible and recurrent. Flow cytometry analysis of the cell population profiles for DNA content and 5-Bromo-2´-Deoxyuridine (BrdU) labeling also confirmed that the cells were arrested at the growth 1(or gap 1) phase (G1) and G1/S (synthesis phase) boundaries The incorporation of the BrdU label suggested that DNA synthesis was blocked by butyrate treatment [22].

Epidemiological, animal and interventional studies suggest the protective effects of dietary fiber in chronic diseases such as bowel disorders and colorectal cancer, cancer of other tissues, cardiovascular disease, diabetes, obesity and hypertension are linked to the bioactivity of butyrate [23]. Butyrate elicits many cytoprotective, chemopreventive and chemotherapeutic activities, mainly through the arrest of cell proliferation, induction of apoptosis or stimulation of cell differentiation by selectively altering gene expression [9, 24–26, 27, 28–32].

The biological activity of butyrate-induced cell cycle arrest has been studied since the early 1970s [33, 34]. Recent advances in molecular biology indicate that this product of large bowel microbial fermentation of dietary fiber might evoke the above-mentioned effects by indirect action on genes. Butyrate was shown to inhibit histone deacetylase activity, allowing DNA binding of several transcription factors. Higher genomic activity leads to the higher expression of proapoptotic genes, higher levels of their protein products and elevated sensitivity to death ligand-induced apoptosis. Cancer cells might be arrested in the G1 phase of the cell cycle in a cyclin-dependent kinase inhibitor 1 (p21/WAF1)-dependent manner [24]. Butyrate also induces cell cycle arrest and apoptosis.

In a previous study [10], the potential biological roles of butyrate were investigated using the established Madin-Darby bovine kidney (MDBK) epithelial cell line. The study focused on determining whether normal bovine cells in a standard cell culture condition were sensitive to the growth inhibitory effects of butyrate. The data suggested that sodium butyrate could induce apoptosis and cell cycle arrest in MDBK cells. Up to 38 percent of cells became apoptotic after 24 hours of treatment with 10.0 mM of butyrate. Butyrate also blocked the surviving cells at two distinct stages of the G1/S boundaries and gap 2 (G2)/mitosis (M).

Ruminant species have evolved to metabolize the short-chain fatty acids, acetate, propionate and butyrate, to fulfill up to 70 percent of their nutrient energy requirements. The inherent VFA dependence of ruminant cells was exploited to add a level of increased sensitivity to the study of the role of butyrate gene-response elements in regulatory biochemical pathways. Global gene expression profiles of the bovine kidney epithelial cells regulated by sodium butyrate were investigated with high-density oligonucleotide microarrays. The detailed mechanisms by which butyrate induces cell growth arrest and apoptosis were analyzed using the Ingenuity Pathways Knowledge Base (IPKB). The functional category and pathway analyses of the microarray data revealed that four canonical pathways (Cell cycles: G2/M DNA damage checkpoint, and pyrimidine metabolism; G1/S checkpoint regulation and purine metabolism) were significantly perturbed.

The development of the next-generation sequencing (NGS) has provided novel tools for expression profiling and genome analysis [35–37]. As a vital step towards a comprehensive understanding of the molecular mechanism of butyrate-induced acetylation, as well as its biological effects, next-generation sequencing technology was used to profile the transcriptome in normal cells and butyrate treated cells. Four canonical pathways (Cell cycle G2/M DNA damage checkpoints, purine metabolism, pyrimidine metabolism, and G1/S checkpoint regulation) previously identified by the microarray experiment were also confirmed by the RNA-sequence analysis. The biologically relevant networks and pathways of these genes were also identified. IGF2, TGFB1, TP53, E2F4, and CDC2 were established as being centered in these genomic networks [38]. Those findings will be discussed later in this chapter.

Butyrate Induces Apoptosis

Apoptosis was an idea more than 50 years ago as an explanation for a little-recognized mechanism of controlled cell deletion, which appears to play a complementary but opposite role to mitosis in the regulation of animal cell populations [39, 40]. It is an active, inherently programmed phenomenon (therefore, it is also called programed cell death).

Butyrate-induced apoptosis was first reported during the early 1990s. Sodium butyrate induces apoptosis in human colonic tumor cell lines, and the cellular tumor antigen p53 (p53) tumor-suppressor gene is not required to mediate signals for the induction of apoptosis. This is the first implication for the possible role of dietary fiber in the prevention of large-bowel cancer [41]. Since then, butyrate as an HDAC inhibitor has being clinically evaluated as an anti-neoplastic therapeutic, primarily because of its ability to impose cell cycle arrest, differentiation, and/or apoptosis in many tumor cell types, and for its favorable safety profile in humans. Furthermore, HDAC inhibitors could be used in combination with certain established antitumor therapeutics, such as those that target transcription, to augment clinical efficacy, and/or reduce toxicity.

The molecular pathways of butyrate and related next-generation synthetic SCFAs in mediating these effects have not been fully elucidated, but HDAC inhibition is associated with the regulation of critical cell cycle regulators, such as cyclin D, p21/WAF1, and p27/KIP1. It is anticipated that a better understanding of this critical intersection between SCFAs, HDACs, and cell cycle control will lead to the design of novel treatment strategies for neoplasias [18].

The butyrate-induced apoptosis was mostly confirmed in the cancer cell lines. Few definitive studies, if any, have addressed the capabilities of short-chain fatty acids as signaling molecules to modulate cellular functions and apoptosis in normal cell lines. Therefore, an important question is whether normal cells in a standard cell culture condition are sensitive to the growth inhibitory effects of butyrate. Investigation of the cell cycle regulatory and apoptotic effects of butyrate in a bovine cell line confirmed that butyrate not only induced apoptosis but also induced cell cycle arrest at the G1/S boundary and G2/M in MDBK cells. The cell responses were concentration-dependent [10].

These results are also consistent with the growing body of evidence suggesting that disruption of the coordination between the regulation of DNA synthesis and cyclin-dependent kinase activity is an important feature of apoptosis. This disruption causes the unscheduled activation of cyclin-dependent kinases in cells with non-replicated or partially replicated chromosomes.

All three major components of short-chain fatty acids (acetate, propionate and butyrate) induce apoptosis and inhibit cell proliferation. However, butyrate was the most potent in the induction of apoptosis and the inhibition of cell proliferation [42, 43]. Rates of short-chain fatty acid production and absorption in ruminants are much higher than in other animals and humans, which has been calculated to be about 5.0-mol/kg dry matter intake [4]. The principal short-chain fatty acids in either the rumen or large intestine are acetate, propionate and butyrate. The concentrations of short-chain fatty acids in the rumen are highly variable, and the total amount present usually fluctuates between 60.0 to 150.0 mM. Butyrate concentrations in the digestive tracts and blood of sheep are established between 0.5 to 13.0 mM [4]. The results of terminal deoxynucleotidyl transferase dUTP nick end labeling (TUNEL) assay and the activation of caspase-3 upon butyrate treatment also strongly argue that cell death is due to apoptosis [10].

Gene-environment interactions are so numerous and biologically complicated that it can be challenging to understand their roles in cancer. However, dietary fiber and colorectal cancer prevention may represent a tractable model system. As the products of fiber fermentation by colonic bacteria, butyrate has differential effects depending on its concentration and the metabolic state of the cell. Low to moderate concentrations, which are present near the base of colonic crypts, are readily metabolized in the mitochondria to stimulate cell proliferation via energetics. Higher concentrations, which are present near the lumen, exceed the metabolic capacity of the colonocyte.

Unmetabolized butyrate enters the nucleus and functions as an HDAC inhibitor that epigenetically regulates gene expression to inhibit cell proliferation and induce apoptosis as the colonocytes exfoliate into the lumen. Butyrate may therefore play a role in normal homeostasis by promoting turnover of the colonic epithelium [6]. Because cancerous colonocytes undergo the Warburg effect [44], their preferred energy source is glucose instead of butyrate. Consequently, even moderate concentrations of butyrate accumulate in cancerous colonocytes and function as HDAC inhibitors to inhibit cell proliferation and induce apoptosis [6].

Butyrate, Histone Acetylation and Cellular Functions

While acetate and propionate hold prominent positions with respect to the provision of energy in ruminant metabolism, butyrate, low in concentration relative to other SCFAs, appears to be involved in metabolism in ways that differ from its role as a nutrient. It has also proven to be a strong regulator of genomic activities. SCFAs—especially butyrate—participate in metabolism both as nutrients and as inhibitors of histone deacetylases (HDACs). Butyrate treatment enhances histone acetylation by inhibiting HDACs activities.

After the discovery of histone acetylation in the 1960s [45, 46] it was suggested that this post-translational modification of histones could provide an enzymatic mechanism for modulating the interactions between histones and DNA in ways that affect the structure and function of chromatin, with acetylated histones losing much of their capacity for inhibiting RNA synthesis [47]. This provided the first evidence that histone deacetylation was associated with transcriptional repression.

Correlations between gene activation for RNA synthesis and increased acetylation of the histones were confirmed during the 70s [48]. The simple postulation of such activity of histone modification was that acetylation of the lysine residues in the basic amino-terminal regions of the histones neutralizes their positive charges and would be expected to weaken their interactions with the phosphate groups of the DNA strand enveloping the nucleosome core [2]. Now, after the discovery of histone acetylation and methylation over 50 years [47], modifications of histones are strongly implicated in virtually all-genomic processes.

During late 1960s and early 1970s, histone deacetylation, the reverse action of histone acetylation, and the enzyme responsible for histone deacetylation, histone deacetylase (HDAC) were discovered [49, 50]. Thereafter, butyrate became one of the chemical compounds discovered with inhibitory activity against histone deacetylation during the late 1970s [1, 2, 51]. Adding butyrate into cell culture led to accumulation of multiacetylation of histones H3 and H4. In Hela cells and in avian erythrocytes, the multiacetylated forms of histones H3 and H4 are preferentially released during limited deoxyribonuclease I (DNase I) digestions, confirming their association with transcriptionally active regions of the chromatin [2].

The major biochemical change that occurs in cells treated with butyrate and other HDAC inhibitors is the global hyperacetylation of histones [10, 52, 53]. Clear evidence is beginning to link modifications in chromatin structure to cell cycle progression, DNA replication, and overall chromosome stability [54]. However, the molecular basis of these effects is poorly defined. The modulation of genome expression as a consequence of chromatin structural changes is considered a major mechanism. Data from bovine in vitro experiments show that as the direct result of hyperacetylation of histones induced by butyrate treatment at physiologic concentrations, cultured bovine cells are arrested in the early G1 phase, and DNA synthesis is eliminated as assayed by BrdU incorporation and flow cytometric analyses [10]. At a relatively high concentration, butyrate also induces apoptosis in an established bovine MDBK cell line. In isolated ruminal epithelial cells, DNA replication is also inhibited by butyrate treatment [55]. Butyrate as a histone deacetylase inhibitor can also alter histone methylation [56], suggesting the interplay between histone acetylation and histone methylation.

SCFAs are nutrients especially critical to ruminants. They are formed during microbial fermentation of dietary fiber in the gastrointestinal tract, and are directly absorbed at the site of production [16]. Ruminant species have evolved to metabolize SCFAs to fulfill up to 70 percent of their nutrient energy requirements. Because ruminants are so dependent on low-molecular weight volatile fatty acids for metabolic needs [4], cells derived from ruminants are presumed to be equipped to respond to SCFAs with increased sensitivity compared to other species [4].

The rumen epithelium is responsible for several physiologically important functions, including absorption, transport, SCFA metabolism, and protection. Moreover, at weaning, the calf rumen must transition from a pre-ruminant state to a fully functional rumen. For normal development of the ruminal epithelium to progress, viable ruminal fermentation must be established, implicating a requirement for the presence of SCFAs in the ruminal lumen to promote normal papillary development [57].

The mechanisms responsible for rumen development have not been completely characterized. Little is known about the genomic/epigenomic mechanisms contributing to these physiologic changes. The profound changes in gene expression in bovine cells induced by butyrate elucidate the pleiotropic effects of histone acetylation [11]. Epigenomics is an emerging area of scientific investigation, and it is still in its infancy with respect to livestock species. The most important next steps to understand the functional roles of histone modification in gene expression and rumen development are to comprehensively, quantitatively, and cost-effectively analyze histone-DNA interactions in the bovine genome that are responsive to SCFA modulation in order to reveal the "epigenetic code" as a unique set of genomic observations. To open up the epigenetic code will be the most important step to understand the gene regulation mechanism induced by butyrate.

The Epigenetic Regulatory Network of Histone Modifications

The Rapidly Emerging Field of Epigenomics

Epigenomics is the study of both heritable and non-heritable changes in the regulation of gene activity and expression that occur without an alteration in the DNA sequence. Epigenomics is an emerging area of scientific investigation that is confirming the complexity of the mechanisms used to determine the "how," "when," and "where" of gene expression in order to ensure the normal development, health and homeostasis of humans and animals.

During the last couple of decades, many publications have reported the use of HDAC inhibitors to study histone acetylation and gene regulation. An important question to be addressed by the study of histone modification is how modifications affect not only chromatin dynamics but also various cellular processes (e.g., DNA replication, RNA transcription) along the DNA-template. These processes can be influenced by a number of post-translational modifications of histones, including acetylation, methylation, phosphorylation and ubiquitination. These modifications may not act alone, but in concert and in a context-dependent manner to facilitate or repress chromatin-mediated processes [58].

Histone Modifications and Transcription Regulation

Genomic DNA is the ultimate template of animal heredity. However, despite the fact that genome projects have delivered high-quality genome sequence assemblies for humans and several species of animals, many challenges nevertheless remain in understanding the regulation and transduction of genetic information. Transcriptional regulation is a complex process. It involves not only the recruitment of polymerases and transcription factors to active promoters, but also changes to chromatin. One of the mechanisms that controls the state of chromatin structure is the modification of histones [59, 60].

The dynamic variability of nucleosomal architecture is primarily achieved via condensation or relaxation of the nucleosome. Epigenetic modification, such as DNA methylation and histone tail modifications (acetylation, methylation and phosphorylation) play major roles in the dynamic variability of nucleosomal architecture [61]. Chromatin is subject to a diverse array of post-translational modifications that largely impose various chemical groups on histone amino termini, regulating access to the underlying DNA. Distinct histone amino-terminal modification can generate synergistic or antagonistic interaction affinities for chromatin-associated proteins, which in turn dictate dynamic transitions between transcriptionally active or transcriptionally silent chromatin states [61].

The nuclear enzymes that modify the state of acetylation of lysines in the amino terminal tail of histones are known as HDACs, which lead to histone deacetylation and histone acetyltransferases (HATs), which cause histone hyperacetylation. Acetylation and deacetylation of lysine residues in the N termini of histones play fundamental roles in diverse chromatin-based processes. Acetylation may result in structural transitions, as well as specific signaling within discrete chromatin domains. Such roles have been established through genetic and biochemical analyses of individual sites of acetylation, as well as the discovery of HAT and HDAC as co-regulators in transcription, DNA replication, and DNA repair.

The sites of acetylation include at least four highly conserved lysines in histone H4 (K5, K8, K12 and K16), five in histone H3 (K9, K14, K18, K23 and K27), as well as less conserved sites in histone H2A and H2B [59]. Those modifications have been clearly linked to gene activation and active transcription in mammalian cells. Different sites of histone acetylation may target different aspects of gene expression [62–64]. The profound changes in gene expression also elucidate the pleiotropic effects of histone acetylation induced by butyrate in bovine cells.

At physiologic concentrations, butyrate regulates the expression of individual genes by inhibition of histone deacetylation and attendant chromatin remodeling [65, 9, 66]. Utilizing global gene expression profiling, recent studies indicate that butyrate induces significant changes in the expression of genes associated with the regulatory pathways critical to cell growth, immune response, and signal transduction [11]. A majority of these genes are repressed by butyrate and are associated with cell cycle control.

The generation of induced pluripotent stem cells (iPSCs) by somatic cell reprogramming involves global epigenetic remodeling [67]. It was found that butyrate can also greatly enhance derivation of human-induced pluripotent stem cells by promoting epigenetic remodeling and the expression of pluripotency-associated genes. More evidence indicates that chromatin-modifying enzymes such as histone acetylases and deacetylases function as modulators of reprogramming. Those specific chromatin-modifying enzymes function as either barriers to or facilitators of reprogramming. Those studies demonstrated that butyrate induced modification of chromatin can be exploited to more efficiently generate iPSCs with fewer exogenous transcription factors [67].

Transcirptome Profiling Reveals the Mechanisms of Butyrate-Induced Epigenomic Regulation

The completed profiling of global gene expression used a high-density oligonucleotide microarray [11, 38]. The study identified 450 genes in bovine kidney epithelial cells that were significantly regulated by sodium butyrate at a very stringent false discovery rate (FDR) of zero percent. The functional category and pathway analyses of the microarray data revealed that four canonical pathways (cell cycles: G2/M DNA damage checkpoint, pyrimidine metabolism, G1/S checkpoint regulation, and purine metabolism) were significantly perturbed. The biologically relevant networks and pathways of these genes were also identified, including genes such as IGF2, TGFB1, TP53, E2F4 and CDC2, which were established as central to these networks.

However, because they are restricted to probes designed to target the genes in a given species' genome, hybridization-based microarray technologies offer a limited ability to fully catalogue and quantify the diverse RNA molecules that are expressed from genomes over a wide range of levels [68], and they often fail to capture the full catalogue of transcripts and their variations.

The development of the next-generation sequencing (NGS) has provided novel tools for expression profiling and genome analysis [36, 37, 68]. As a vital step towards a comprehensive understanding of the molecular mechanism of butyrate-induced acetylation, as well as its biological effects, the next-generation sequencing technology was utilized in order to provide a more complete characterization of the RNA transcripts of MDBK cells. This study has generated comprehensive information on an experimental system that can be used in many functional genomics studies of bovine cells. The NGS results, with a comparative transcriptomic profiling approach, stretched far beyond the findings reported using microarray technologies [38, 69]. The phenomenal number of genes identified falls within a broad range of functional categories. The NGS profiling provided a very detailed molecular basis for the butyrate-induced biological effects [22].

Butyrate-Induced Gene Regulation Targets Proteins Involved in DNA Replication and Cell Cycle Regulation

The stable propagation of genetic information requires that the entire genome of an organism be faithfully replicated only once in each cell cycle [70]. In eukaryotes, this replication is initiated at hundreds to thousands of replication origins distributed over the genome, each of which must be prohibited from re-initiating DNA replication within a single cell cycle.

Initiation of DNA replication is a two-step process: First, initiation proteins are assembled onto the replication origin in a stepwise fashion to develop a pre-replication complex. Second, the initiation complex is activated by protein kinases, resulting in the establishment of replication forks. This process is tightly regulated [70] to ensure that initiation at a given replication origin occurs only once per cell cycle. In eukaryotic cells, cell cycle checkpoint regulation assures the fidelity of cell division. The G1 (first gap phase)/S cell cycle checkpoint controls the passage of eukaryotic cells from the G1 into the S phase. Mitogen-dependent progression through the G1 of the cell-division cycle is accurately regulated to ensure that normal cell division is synchronous with cell growth and that the initiation of DNA synthesis (the S phase) is timed precisely to avoid inappropriate DNA amplification. The G1/S checkpoint control is vital for normal cell division and involves the key components that include cell cycle kinases, CDK4/6-cyclin D and CDK2-cyclin E, and the transcription complex composed of the retinoblastoma protein (Rb) and transcription factor E2F. The activation of E2F is necessary for the G1/S transition.

To ensure that the genome is replicated once, and only once, each time a cell divides, DNA replication initiation events are restricted in at least two ways: First, pre-RCs that are assembled during the M to G1 phase transition are inactivated during S phase; and second, new pre-RCs cannot be assembled until G1 phase. In addition to blocking pre-RC assembly and activation at multiple steps such as the Cdc6, Cdt1, Mcm(2–7), and Cdk2 functions, the premier step in determining both where and when DNA replication begins is the assembly of functional origin recognition complex (ORC) on chromatin sites, and this step appears to be regulated by inactivating ORC during the G1 to S phase transition [71, 72] and then preventing re-establishment of ORC activity until mitosis is completed and, in the metazoan, a nuclear membrane is reassembled [73, 74, 75].

Although these studies suggest that ORC activity in mammalian cells is regulated by cell-cycle-dependent changes in origin recognition complex subunit 1 (Orc1) function (ORC cycle), it has been suspected for a long time that histone acetylation may also affect the initiation of DNA replication [76, 77, 78]. However, at present neither the enzymes nor the steps involved are known [79].

Even though it is likely that other gene products targeted by butyrate treatment may play functional roles in the cell cycle arrest, epigenetic constraints imposed by chromatin structure, such as hyperacetylation induced by butyrate, may regulate aspects of DNA replication and origin selection by ORC proteins at the levels of RNA transcription and protein translation of ORC1 [80].

The first clear evidence that the activity of a six-subunit "origin recognition complex" (ORC) in mammalian cells is regulated by cell cycle-dependent changes in the affinity of the largest subunit 1 (Orc1) for chromatin has been reported [71, 81]. Evidence has since confirmed these findings and extended them to show that mammalian Orc1 is selectively ubiquitinated and phosphorylated during the S-to-M phase transition, while Orc subunits 2 to 5, which constitute a stable core complex, remain tightly bound to chromatin throughout cell division [82].

In addition, a second mechanism prevents the assembly of a functional ORC until the completion of mitosis: the selective association of Orc1 with Cdk1 (Cdc2)/cyclin A during the G2/M phase of cell division. This association accounted for the appearance in M-phase cells with hyperphosphorylated Orc1 that was subsequently dephosphorylated during the M-to-G1 transition [73]. The rebinding of Orc1 to chromatin follows the same time course as the degradation of cyclin B, suggesting that the exit from mitosis triggers Orc1 binding to chromatin. In fact, the inhibition of Cdk activity in metaphase cells resulted in the rapid binding of Orc1 to chromatin, and NGS profiling shows that all six subunits of ORC are down-regulated by butyrate-induced histone acetylation, adding yet another layer of regulation of ORC activities via the modified expression of those genes. In our previous microarray profiling [38], some of the components of this pathway were found to be perturbed by butyrate-induced gene regulation; however, Orc1 was the only one of the six ORC complex genes that was detected to be a down-regulated gene. In the present report, Orc1 is still the most significantly down-regulated gene, but the other ORC components (Orc2 to Orc6) are also identified as down regulated. This result certainly indicates the superb sensitivity of deep RNA sequencing [22].

Significant up-regulation of both BTG1 and BTG2 was also reported. The BTG family member-2 (BTG2) has antiproliferative activity, and the expression of BTG2 in cycling cells induces the accumulation of hypophosphorylated, growth-inhibitory forms of retinoblastoma protein (Rb) and leads to G1 arrest through the impairment of DNA synthesis. These up-regulated antiproliferation activities are strengthened by the extensive repression of cyclin-dependent kinase and cell cycle-related genes that are clearly associated with the cell growth arrest induced by butyrate [22].

Cyclin/CDK inhibitor p21/waf1 is required for butyrate-mediated growth inhibition of human cancer cells. Butyrate and other SCFAs induce growth arrest in colon cancer cells through a process requiring the induction of the G1 cell cycle inhibitor p21/waf1 [83]. The activity of a variety of protein cyclins and their associated cyclin-dependent kinase (CDK) is required for the cell cycle progresses in mammalian cells. Cyclin/cdk inhibitor proteins such as p21/waf1 inhibit these complexes. The balance between the activation and inhibition of cyclin-cdk activities determines the cell cycle progression. Butyrate also induces up-regulated expression of p21/waf1 in "normal" MDBK cells. In contrast, cyclins E and E2F were significantly down regulated by butyrate-induced histone acetylation [10, 80].

Since cancer cells are characterized by abnormalities in cell cycle regulation, the result that butyrate also induces up-regulated expression of cyclin-kinase inhibitor p21/waf[1] in MDBK cells indicate that p21/waf1 may have a very similar function in both cancer cells and normal cells. It also underlies the possibility that in addition to the beneficial effects of butyrate and other HDAC inhibitors, which induce growth arrest in colon cancer, it may also cause some side effects on normal cells [80]. All of these perturbations of gene expression in the G1/S cell cycle checkpoint pathways are consistent with the observed biological effects of butyrate, which induces cell cycle arrest at the G1/S boundary [84].

Functional Interplay between TP53 and HDACs

Among SCFAs, butyrate induces the highest histone acetylation. It was believed that butyrate inhibits class I and class IIa HDACs, but not class IIb (HDAC6 and HDAC10). However, more recent studies established more evidence that butyrate not only inhibits the HDACs activities, it also affects many other epigenetic-related enzymes by regulating the expression of the respective genes encoding HDACs attributable to the potential of butyrate to alter epigenetic landscapes.

In addition, cross talking between upstream and downstream regulators such as TP53 and HDACs set up another layer of regulation network. HDACs are active components of transcriptional regulation complexes. HDACs down-regulate the functions of p53, the TP53 gene product. It was suggested that interactions of p53 and HDACs likely result in p53 deacetylation, thereby reducing its transcriptional activity [85]. Inhibitors of HDAC can restore the p53 pathway [86]. Butyrate, an HDAC inhibitor, can activate the TP53 pathway. In return, activation of TP53 may directly or indirectly regulate the expression of HDACs [22].

RNA-sequencing data revealed that the expression of HDACs was modulated by butyrate. In particular, HDACs 7, 8, 9 and 10 were down regulated and HDACs 3, 5 and 11 were up regulated. The downstream analysis also indicates inhibition of the activities of HDACs 2, 4, 6 and 9. The mechanism and biological relevance of HDAC inhibitors in the regulation of expression of HDACs is not clear, but may possibly indicate the existence of an auto-regulatory feedback loop for the expression of several HDACs after their activities are inhibited. It will be of great interest to understand the connections between the inhibition of HDAC activities and the regulation of expression of these genes.

The dynamic Canonical Pathways are well characterized metabolic and cell signaling pathways. Canonical Pathways are distinct from networks. The p53 (TP53) tumor suppressor protein is a key transcriptional regulator that responds to a variety of cellular stresses such as DNA damage, UV irradiation, and hypoxia. P53 regulates key cellular processes such as DNA repair, cell-cycle progression, angiogenesis, and apoptosis. These p53-dependent pathways shut down damaged cells, either through apoptosis or cell-cycle arrest. Loss of p53 function is thought to be a contributing factor in the majority of cancer cases. Many butyrate-induced differentially expressed genes are involved in the TP53 signaling pathway. The RNA sequencing data strongly supports that TP53 signaling pathways are crucially involved in the cellular functions that were moderated by the butyrate treatment. These differentially expressed genes underlie the butyrate-induced modifications of the cellular functions, such as cell cycle arrest, cell survival and apoptosis, etc.

Butyrate-Induced Cascade of Histone Modifications

Butyrate, as a histone deacetylase inhibitor, can also decrease histone methylation [56], suggesting interplay between histone acetylation and histone methylation. An emerging possibility is that histone modifications can influence one another. In other words, there may be "cross-talk among histone modification" [58]. Consistently, KDM5B, a specific histone demethylase (H3-trimethyl-K4), was significantly up regulated by butyrate treatment.

However, JSRID2, which is directly related to histone methylation and responsible for maintaining the methylation level on histone H3 lysine 27 trimethylation (H3K27me3) [87, 88], was also significantly up regulated. JARID2 possesses an in vitro methyl-protective activity, stabilizing Polycom Repressive Complex 2 (PRC2)-catalyzed H3K27me3 by protecting it from the activity of H3K27 demathylases [89].

This data may indicate that different histone marks (modifications) are differentially regulated and that, in turn, differentially regulated histone marks regulate different biological functions [90].

On the other hand, a reversal of DNA methylation by butyrate has also recently been reported to occur by the regulation of DNA (cytosine-5) methyltransferase 1 (DNMT1) through ERK signaling [91]. We found that three DNA methyltransferases (DNMTs), including DNMT1, DNMT3A and DNMT3B, were significantly down-regulated by the butyrate treatment [22].

While DNMT1 functions in the establishment and regulation of tissue-specific patterns of methylated cytosine residues, DNMT3A and DNMT3B function in the *de novo* methylation of DNA [92–94]. These DNMTs are regulated by several mechanisms in terms of their expression and catalytic activity. However, for the first time, our data directly indicated that histone modification has a role in the regulation of the expression of DNMTs, thereby affecting the level of DNA methylation.

A recent study [95] revealed direct evidence that butyrate can mediate differential CpG island (CGI) methylation. Butyrate causes methylation of genes related to several functional categories in a time-dependent manner. The analysis of differentially methylated regions showed many genes to be affected 24 hours upon butyrate treatment. One overrepresented group of affected genes was related to the "intracellular signaling cascade." A closer view showed involvement of pathways such as the mitogen-activated protein kinase (MAPK), Ca^{2+} and the canonical Wnt/β-catenin signaling system. Butyrate-mediated effects on these signal transduction pathways have been reported before in human cell lines [96, 97] and, among others, may lead to the observed apoptotic events and the negative impact on cell cycle progression.

A butyrate-mediated regulation of apoptosis, gene expression, cell cycle, transport, growth and proliferation was shown on other cellular levels and in other cell types as well [22, 98]. Canonical Wnt/β-catenin signaling is the core component differentially methylated. Butyrate-mediated DNA methylation within the canonical Wnt/β-catenin pathway ranges from members of Wnt biogenesis and signal transduction in the cytoplasm to transcriptional regulation in the nucleus.

Generally, the influence of butyrate on Wnt signaling has been stated before on other cellular levels (e.g., by measuring Wnt activity or Wnt target gene expression upon butyrate treatment) [99, 100]. However, such a far-reaching influence of butyrate-mediated DNA methylation changes on the Wnt signal transduction system has not been shown before. Altogether, butyrate inhibits enzymes that alter nucleosome structure or position are at the very center of gene and genome regulation. Understanding how, and to what extent, these diverse activities collaborate and control each other to shape the genome for dynamic regulation is a major challenge.

A new study provides an important step in this direction by illustrating the cooperative nature of ATP-dependent chromatin-remodeling systems in mammalian cell chromatin [101]. Studies in yeast illustrate how various nucleosome-remodeling factors have overlapping and complementary functions to shape chromatin over and around genes (e.g., in regulating the progression of RNA polymerase II) [102, 103]. Recent studies have indicated that a cascade of histone modifications, which includes histone phosphorylation and deacetylation, is required to induce chromatin condensation in mitosis [104].

Butyrate-Induced Histone Acetylation Regulates miRNA Expression, and in Turn, miRNAs May Interfere with Butyrate-induced Modulation of Gene Expression and Cellular Function

MicroRNAs are a class of highly conserved, small non-coding RNAs (~22 nucleotides) that regulate gene expression post-transcriptionally [105]. MicroRNAs (miRNAs) bind to complementary sequences in the 3'-untranslated regions (3' UTRs) of target messenger RNA transcripts (mRNAs), usually resulting in gene silencing [106]. The miRNAs are encoded by specific genes in the genome, which are transcribed as primary transcripts called primary miRNAs. While Histone modification and miRNA are the two different epigenetic pathways for regulation of gene expression, in recent years, some evidence has suggested that these two pathways may cross talk and interfere with each other [107]. Butyrate-induced histone acetylation may regulate miRNA expression, and in turn, miRNAs may interfere with butyrate-induced modulation of gene expression and cellular functions.

MicroRNA was first discovered from *C. elegans* in 1991 and was demonstrated as a novel mechanism for gene regulation. Lin-4 is a heterochronic gene in *C. elegans* that is required for proper cell fate specification in larval development. Genetic evidence indicated that the lin-4 gene product negatively regulated the heterochronic lin-14 targeting the 3' UTR. [108]. During the first 10 years after microRNA discovery, only a handful of publications appeared each year on the subject. Little was known about the mechanism of how microRNAs function to lead to the translational repression of target mRNA. From 1991 to 1997, this novel mechanism was largely ignored and assumed to be a worm-specific anomaly. However, let-7 was cloned from *C. elegans* [109, 110] and was also found to be conserved in Drosophila and in humans [109]. Since then, the level of microRNA research has increased to become a microRNA revolution.

MicroRNAs are regulated by a variety of stimuli such as gene amplification, gene deletion, cellular stress, and inflammation, as well as by epigenetic mechanisms. The mechanism of microRNA silencing of mRNA is based on the interaction between microRNAs and mRNAs. These interactions include competition for the nuclear cap-binding protein complex, which is an RNA-binding protein complex that binds to the 5' cap inside the nucleus; deadenylation and mRNA degradation; mRNA sequestration; and ribosome drop-off. Many different microRNAs exist and each can target many mRNAs, which can be involved in various cellular processes such as cell division, cell death, DNA repair, differentiation, and epigenetic mechanisms. Therefore, the expression of miRNA can have a profound effect in regulating gene expression. Under certain cellular conditions, microRNA can also increase the translation of target genes. It was recently reported that butyrate alone could enhance the transcription factor-dependent up-regulation of the miR302/367 cluster. In turn, miR302/367 can greatly enhance the efficiency of induced pluripotent stem cell (iPSC) generation. Using a promoter reporter assay, it was confirmed that butyrate remarkably enhanced the transcriptional activity of the four transcription factors in the miR302/367 promoter. Notably, attenuation of miRNA302/367 using a miRZip impairs the ability of the butyrate in promoting reprogramming.

Collectively, these findings suggest that butyrate promotes reprogramming at least partly through the induction of the miR302/367 cluster expression [111]. A study performed in colon cancer cells also concluded that microbe-derived SCFAs regulate host gene expression involved in intestinal homeostasis as well as carcinogenesis through modulation of miRNAs [112].

SCFA induced transcriptional reprogramming is achieved through various and complex mechanisms not fully understood, including histone deacetylation, transcription factor or regulator (including HDAC1) deacetylation followed by chromatin remodeling, and have a positive or negative outcome regarding transcription initiation. While only a low percentage of protein-coding genes are affected by the action of HDAC inhibitors, it was found that about 40 percent of noncoding microRNAs are up regulated or down regulated. Moreover, a whole new world of long noncoding RNAs is emerging, revealing a new class of potential targets for HDAC inhibition. HDAC inhibitors might also regulate transcription elongation and have been shown to impinge on alternative splicing [113, 114].

In bovine cells, MicroRNA microarray profiling of miRNAs and statistical tests, as well as clustering analysis, show that butyrate induces profound changes in miRNA expression. The 35 transcripts were significantly ($p < 0.05$) differentially expressed. Among these, expression of 11 transcripts was very significant ($p < 0.01$) [53]. These observations reflect cross-talk between miRNA and histone acetylation. Deep RNA-sequence also reveals a significant amount of information regarding non-coding RNA (ncRNA) [22]. There are 24 ncRNAs that are differentially expressed due to the butyrate treatment. Those ncRNAs belong to different types of ncRNAs, including snoRNA (small nucleolar RNA), snRNA (splicesomal RNA), and some miscRNAs. Particularly, the expression of 10 snoRNAs (five down-regulated and five up-regulated) was found to be disrupted by the butyrate treatment. The snoRNAs are intermediate-sized ncRNAs (60-300 bp). They are components of small nucleolar ribonucleoproteins (snoRNPs), which are complexes that are responsible for the modification and processing of ribosomal RNA [115]. More importantly, a large proportion of snoRNAs have been found to be further processed into smaller molecules, such as microRNAs (miRNAs) [116].

A recent and very interesting report also identified the important growth regulatory role for colonic epithelial miRNAs in mediating the effects of the microbe-derived short-chain fatty acid butyrate on host gene expression [112]. In that report, it was found that in HCT-116 cells, butyrate suppressed many of the same miRNAs increased in human colon cancers. One of these miRNAs, miR-106b, was found to target p21. Butyrate and miR-106b treatment of a p21 three prime undertranslated region (3' UTR) luciferase reporter construct in HCT116 cells indicates that butyrate-stimulated p21 expression is inhibited in translation in part by miR-106b. This partial inhibition by miR-106b confirms previous reports that butyrate also regulates p21 expression via a miRNA independent mechanism, through its inhibition of HDAC.

Understanding the regulatory mechanisms controlling miRNA expression is crucial because miRNA can have extensive effects through regulation of a variety of genes that are essential for cell functions and that are involved in the most crucial cellular processes. MicroRNA and epigenetic regulation present a very complicated interplay because miRNA can regulate the expression of components of the epigenetic machinery, by targeting molecules involved in methylation or acetylation of DNA and histones [117].

In bovine cells, butyrate-induced epigenetic modulation of gene expression resulted in profound changes in miRNA expression; in turn, miRNA modulate epigenetic regulation induced by butyrate by regulating expression of the genes targeted by differentially expressed miRNA. Functional network analysis indicated that differentially expressed miRNAs target some important gene networks. All of these findings indicate that a complicated interaction between the two different regulation machineries that use miRNA and histone acetylation results in a highly integrated regulation mechanism.

It is worth mentioning that histone deacetylase inhibitors (HDACi) are an emerging class of novel anti-cancer drugs that cause growth arrest, differentiation and apoptosis of tumor cells. The short-chain fatty acids like butyrate are among the first class of HDACi to be identified [118]. Since then, a great effort has been devoted to develop HDAC inhibitors as antineoplastic drugs, and some HDAC inhibitors are showing encouraging efficacy in cancer patients [119, 120]. There are also many other beneficial effects of HDACi, such as their therapeutic implications in the innate immune system [121]; in the generation of the anti-tumor immune response [122]; modulation of antigen-presenting cells by HDAC inhibitors [123]; as well as their anti-parasite activities [124], which have been studied intensively [125].

Butyrate Induces the Distinctive Epigenomic Landscape Modification

Chromatin modification has clearly emerged as a very important mechanism in regulating the transcriptional status of the genome [126]. Butyrate-induced biological effects in bovine cells provide an example of epigenetic regulation and provide a basis for understanding the full range of the biological roles and molecular mechanisms that butyrate may play in animal cell growth, proliferation, and energy metabolism.

Experimental approaches to understanding the biology of histone acetylation have generally been oversimplified as a result of focusing on one or two lysines, or by the examination of only a few genomic loci at a time. A comprehensive and high-resolution co-localization analysis of all histone acetylation for the entire bovine genome is required in order to understand the functional correlation of various histone lysine acetylations in processes such as transcription and DNA replication [127].

Utilizing next-generation sequencing technology, combined with ChIP (Chromatin Immunoprecipitation) technology, histone modification (acetylation) induced by butyrate was analyzed. A high-resolution whole-genome map of the epigenomic landscape revealed distinctive changes induced by butyrate. The enriched binding regions in the proximal promoter (within 5 kb upstream or at the 5'-untranslated region (UTR) from the transcriptional start site (TSS)), and the exon, intron, and intergenic regions (defined by regions 25 kb upstream and 10 Kb downstream from the TSS) were analyzed. A *de novo* search for the binding motif of the ChIP-sequence datasets discovered numerous motifs from each of the data sets. These consensus sequences indicated that histone modification at different locations changes the histone H3 and H4 binding preferences. Nevertheless, a high degree of conservation in histone binding was also presented in these motifs [127].

This first extensive epigenomic landscape mapping in bovine cells offers a new framework and a great resource for testing the role of epigenomes in cell function and transcriptomic regulation. For example, we investigated how butyrate regulated the expression of IGFs, IGF receptors and IGFBP. And specifically, we assessed the major histone modification status associated with the expression of IGF2/H19 genes using RNA-sequence and ChIP-sequence technologies [128]. Insulin-like growth factor 2 (IGF2) is an imprinted gene with the parental allele expressed and the maternal allele silenced. IGF2 activity is further controlled through differential expression of receptors and IGF-binding proteins (IGFBPs) that determine protein availability [12].

To illustrate the fundamental association of the chromatin modification landscape that may play a role in the activation of the IGF2 gene, a high-resolution map of the major chromatin modification at the IGF2/H19 locus was constructed by mining our RNA-sequence and ChIP-sequence data. ChIP-sequence data reveals that IGF2 may be regulated by dispersed epigenomic domains, which show a strong correlation between the structure of the IGF2 gene and the clustered imprinting gene H19 [128].

CONCLUSION

Histone modification has emerged as a very important mechanism regulating the transcriptional status of the genome. Butyrate, as a natural microbial fermentation product in the gastrointestinal tract, is an important nutrient in ruminants. In humans, the colonic microbiota converts dietary fiber to produce prodigious amounts of butyrate that benefits the host through metabolic, nutritional and chemopreventative effects. Additionally, butyrate functions as an inhibitor of histone deacetylases (HDACs), which are critical epigenetic regulators [10, 11, 126]. Therefore, butyrate can regulate gene expression epigenetically by increasing global histone acetylation.

The relationship between genetics and epigenetics offers wide-open insights into transcription regulation. In the near future, with the rapid development of biotechnologies, epigenomic approaches will help us to characterize genome-wide epigenetic landscapes that are targets for dietary regulation elements such as butyrate. The discovery and characterization of these novel epigenetic landscape and epigenetic mechanisms will help us to understand how butyrate modulate these epigenetic regulatory mechanisms. This is a great research opportunity and exploring this area will provide a better perception of the role of butyrate in changing epigenetic patterns. It certainly will have important impacts on functional genomic research in animals and humans. In the meantime, we have to become conscious that epigenetics and epigenomics are much more complicated and more vibrant than previously thought. Standardized platforms, procedures, and even reagents are increasingly required for epigenomics research and for the development of maps of the epigenomic landscapes. Substantial international collaboration is essential to accomplish this goal.

REFERENCES

[1] Boffa, L.C., et al., Suppression of histone deacetylation in vivo and in vitro by sodium butyrate. *J Biol Chem,* 1978. 253(10): p. 3364-6.

[2] Vidali, G., et al., Butyrate suppression of histone deacetylation leads to accumulation of multiacetylated forms of histones H3 and H4 and increased DNase I sensitivity of the associated DNA sequences. *Proc Natl Acad Sci U S A,* 1978. 75(5): p. 2239-43.

[3] Andoh, A., T. Tsujikawa, and Y. Fujiyama, Role of dietary fiber and short-chain fatty acids in the colon. *Curr Pharm Des,* 2003. 9(4): p. 347-58.

[4] Bergman, E.N., Energy contributions of volatile fatty acids from the gastrointestinal tract in various species. *Physiol Rev,* 1990. 70(2): p. 567-90.

[5] Fleming, S.E. and D.S. Arce, Volatile fatty acids: their production, absorption, utilization, and roles in human health. *Clin Gastroenterol*, 1986. 15(4): p. 787-814.

[6] Bultman, S.J., Molecular Pathways: Gene-environment interactions regulating dietary fiber induction of proliferation and apoptosis via butyrate for cancer prevention. *Clin Cancer Res*, 2013.

[7] Jakobsdottir, G., M. Nyman, and F. Fak, Designing future prebiotic fiber to target the metabolic syndrome. *Nutrition,* 2013.

[8] Berni Canani, R., M. Di Costanzo, and L. Leone, The epigenetic effects of butyrate: potential therapeutic implications for clinical practice. *Clin Epigenetics,* 2012. 4(1): p. 4.

[9] Myzak, M.C. and R.H. Dashwood, Histone deacetylases as targets for dietary cancer preventive agents: lessons learned with butyrate, diallyl disulfide, and sulforaphane. *Curr Drug Targets,* 2006. 7(4): p. 443-52.

[10] Li, C.J. and T.H. Elsasser, Butyrate-induced apoptosis and cell cycle arrest in bovine kidney epithelial cells: involvement of caspase and proteasome pathways. *J Anim Sci,* 2005. 83(1): p. 89-97.

[11] Li, R.W. and C. Li, Butyrate induces profound changes in gene expression related to multiple signal pathways in bovine kidney epithelial cells. *BMC Genomics,* 2006. 7: p. 234.

[12] Li, R.W. and C.J. Li, Effects of butyrate on the expression of insulin-like growth factor binding proteins in bovine kindery epithelial cells. *The Open Veternary Science Journal,* 2007. 2007(1): p. 14-19.

[13] Hague, A., A.J. Butt, and C. Paraskeva, The role of butyrate in human colonic epithelial cells: an energy source or inducer of differentiation and apoptosis? *Proc Nutr Soc,* 1996. 55(3): p. 937-43.

[14] Siciliano-Jones, J. and M.R. Murphy, Production of volatile fatty acids in the rumen and cecum-colon of steers as affected by forage:concentrate and forage physical form. *J Dairy Sci*, 1989. 72(2): p. 485-92.

[15] Sharp, W.M., R.R. Johnson, and F.N. Owens, Ruminal VFA production with steers fed whole or ground corn grain. *J Anim Sci,* 1982. 55(6): p. 1505-14.

[16] Bugaut, M., Occurrence, absorption and metabolism of short chain fatty acids in the digestive tract of mammals. *Comp Biochem Physiol B,* 1987. 86(3): p. 439-72.

[17] Roediger, W.E., Role of anaerobic bacteria in the metabolic welfare of the colonic mucosa in man. *Gut,* 1980. 21(9): p. 793-8.

[18] Chen, J.S., D.V. Faller, and R.A. Spanjaard, Short-chain fatty acid inhibitors of histone deacetylases: promising anticancer therapeutics? *Curr Cancer Drug Targets,* 2003. 3(3): p. 219-36.

[19] Gassull, M.A. and E. Cabre, Nutrition in inflammatory bowel disease. *Curr Opin Clin Nutr Metab Care,* 2001. 4(6): p. 561-9.

[20] Scheppach, W., H.P. Bartram, and F. Richter, Role of short-chain fatty acids in the prevention of colorectal cancer. *Eur J Cancer,* 1995. 31A(7-8): p. 1077-80.

[21] Johnson, I.T., Anticarcinogenic effects of diet-related apoptosis in the colorectal mucosa. *Food Chem Toxicol,* 2002. 40(8): p. 1171-8.

[22] Wu, S., et al., Transcriptome characterization by RNA-seq unravels the mechanisms of butyrate-induced epigenomic regulation in bovine cells. *PLoS One,* 2012. 2012.

[23] Kim, N.S. and G.M. Lee, Overexpression of bcl-2 inhibits sodium butyrate-induced apoptosis in Chinese hamster ovary cells resulting in enhanced humanized antibody production. *Biotechnol Bioeng,* 2000. 71(3): p. 184-93.

[24] Mehnert, J.M. and W.K. Kelly, Histone deacetylase inhibitors: biology and mechanism of action. *Cancer J,* 2007. 13(1): p. 23-9.

[25] Davie, J.R., Inhibition of histone deacetylase activity by butyrate. *J Nutr,* 2003. 133(7 Suppl): p. 2485s-2493s.

[26] Dashwood, R.H., M.C. Myzak, and E. Ho, Dietary HDAC inhibitors: time to rethink weak ligands in cancer chemoprevention? *Carcinogenesis,* 2006. 27(2): p. 344-9.

[27] Myzak, M.C., E. Ho, and R.H. Dashwood, Dietary agents as histone deacetylase inhibitors. *Mol Carcinog,* 2006. 45(6): p. 443-6.

[28] Russo, G.L., et al., Protective effects of butyric acid in colon cancer. *Adv Exp Med Biol,* 1999. 472: p. 131-47.

[29] Hamer, H.M., et al., Review article: the role of butyrate on colonic function. *Aliment Pharmacol Ther,* 2008. 27(2): p. 104-19.

[30] Hamer, H.M., et al., Butyrate modulates oxidative stress in the colonic mucosa of healthy humans. *Clin Nutr,* 2009. 28(1): p. 88-93.

[31] Zeitlin, P.L., Future pharmacological treatment of cystic fibrosis. *Respiration,* 2000. 67(4): p. 351-7.

[32] Ferrante, R.J., et al., Histone deacetylase inhibition by sodium butyrate chemotherapy ameliorates the neurodegenerative phenotype in Huntington's disease mice. *J Neurosci,* 2003. 23(28): p. 9418-27.

[33] Wright, J.A., Morphology and growth rate changes in Chinese hamster cells cultured in presence of sodium butyrate. *Exp Cell Res,* 1973. 78(2): p. 456-60.

[34] Ginsburg, E., et al., Growth inhibition and morphological changes caused by lipophilic acids in mammalian cells. *Proc Natl Acad Sci U S A,* 1973. 70(8): p. 2457-61.

[35] Ozsolak, F. and P.M. Milos, Single-molecule direct RNA sequencing without cDNA synthesis. Wiley interdisciplinary reviews. *RNA,* 2011. 2(4): p. 565-70.

[36] Kahvejian, A., J. Quackenbush, and J.F. Thompson, What would you do if you could sequence everything? *Nature biotechnology,* 2008. 26(10): p. 1125-33.

[37] Shendure, J. and H. Ji, Next-generation DNA sequencing. *Nature biotechnology,* 2008. 26(10): p. 1135-45.

[38] Li, C.J., et al., Pathway analysis identifies perturbation of genetic networks induced by butyrate in a bovine kidney epithelial cell line. *Funct Integr Genomics,* 2007. 7(3): p. 193-205.

[39] Kerr, J.F., History of the events leading to the formulation of the apoptosis concept. *Toxicology,* 2002. 181-182: p. 471-4.
[40] Kerr, J.F., A.H. Wyllie, and A.R. Currie, Apoptosis: a basic biological phenomenon with wide-ranging implications in tissue kinetics. *Br J Cancer,* 1972. 26(4): p. 239-57.
[41] Hague, A., et al., Sodium butyrate induces apoptosis in human colonic tumour cell lines in a p53-independent pathway: implications for the possible role of dietary fibre in the prevention of large-bowel cancer. *Int J Cancer,* 1993. 55(3): p. 498-505.
[42] Hague, A. and C. Paraskeva, The short-chain fatty acid butyrate induces apoptosis in colorectal tumour cell lines. *Eur J Cancer Prev,* 1995. 4(5): p. 359-64.
[43] Emenaker, N.J., et al., Short-chain fatty acids inhibit invasive human colon cancer by modulating uPA, TIMP-1, TIMP-2, mutant p53, Bcl-2, Bax, p21 and PCNA protein expression in an in vitro cell culture model. *J Nutr,* 2001. 131(11 Suppl): p. 3041S-6S.
[44] Warburg, O., On the origin of cancer cells. *Science,* 1956. 123(3191): p. 309-14.
[45] Phillips, D.M., The presence of acetyl groups of histones. *Biochem J,* 1963. 87: p. 258-63.
[46] Allfrey, V.G., R. Faulkner, and A.E. Mirsky, Acetylation and Methylation of Histones and Their Possible Role in the Regulation of Rna Synthesis. *Proc Natl Acad Sci U S A,* 1964. 51: p. 786-94.
[47] Allfrey, V.G. and A.E. Mirsky, Structural Modifications of Histones and their Possible Role in the Regulation of RNA Synthesis. *Science*, 1964. 144(3618): p. 559.
[48] Ruiz-Carrillo, A., L.J. Wangh, and V.G. Allfrey, Processing of newly synthesized histone molecules. *Science,* 1975. 190(4210): p. 117-28.
[49] Inoue, A. and D. Fujimoto, Enzymatic deacetylation of histone. *Biochem Biophys Res Commun,* 1969. 36(1): p. 146-50.
[50] Inoue, A. and D. Fujimoto, Histone deacetylase from calf thymus. *Biochim Biophys Acta,* 1970. 220(2): p. 307-16.
[51] Candido, E.P., R. Reeves, and J.R. Davie, Sodium butyrate inhibits histone deacetylation in cultured cells. *Cell,* 1978. 14(1): p. 105-13.
[52] Riggs, M.G., et al., n-Butyrate causes histone modification in HeLa and Friend erythroleukaemia cells. *Nature,* 1977. 268(5619): p. 462-4.
[53] LI, C.J., W.R. Li, and T.H. Elsasser, MicroRNA (miRNA) expression in regulated by butyrate-induced epigenetic modulation of gene expression in bovine cells. *Genetics & Epigentics,* 2010. 2010(3): p. 23-32.
[54] Wolffe, A.P. and D. Guschin, Review: chromatin structural features and targets that regulate transcription. *J Struct Biol,* 2000. 129(2-3): p. 102-22.
[55] Baldwin, R.L., The proliferative actions of insulin, insulin-like growth factor-I, epidermal growth factor, butyrate and propionate on ruminal epithelial cells in vitro. *Smal Ruminant Research,* 1999. 32: p. 261-268.
[56] Marinova, Z., et al., Histone deacetylase inhibition alters histone methylation associated with heat shock protein 70 promoter modifications in astrocytes and neurons. *Neuropharmacology,* 2011. 60(7-8): p. 1109-15.
[57] Lane, M.A. and B.W. Jesse, Effect of volatile fatty acid infusion on development of the rumen epithelium in neonatal sheep. *J Dairy Sci,* 1997. 80(4): p. 740-6.
[58] Berger, S.L., The complex language of chromatin regulation during transcription. *Nature,* 2007. 447(7143): p. 407-12.

[59] Kurdistani, S.K. and M. Grunstein, Histone acetylation and deacetylation in yeast. *Nat Rev Mol Cell Biol,* 2003. 4(4): p. 276-84.
[60] Ito, T., Role of histone modification in chromatin dynamics. *J Biochem,* 2007. 141(5): p. 609-14.
[61] Jenuwein, T. and C.D. Allis, Translating the histone code. *Science,* 2001. 293(5532): p. 1074-80.
[62] Kurdistani, S.K., S. Tavazoie, and M. Grunstein, Mapping global histone acetylation patterns to gene expression. *Cell,* 2004. 117(6): p. 721-33.
[63] Shahbazian, M.D. and M. Grunstein, Functions of site-specific histone acetylation and deacetylation. *Annu Rev Biochem,* 2007. 76: p. 75-100.
[64] Bhaumik, S.R., E. Smith, and A. Shilatifard, Covalent modifications of histones during development and disease pathogenesis. *Nat Struct Mol Biol,* 2007. 14(11): p. 1008-16.
[65] Parab, S., B.B. Nankova, and E.F. La Gamma, Differential regulation of the tyrosine hydroxylase and enkephalin neuropeptide transmitter genes in rat PC12 cells by short chain fatty acids: concentration-dependent effects on transcription and RNA stability. *Brain Res,* 2007. 1132(1): p. 42-50.
[66] Della Ragione, F., et al., Genes modulated by histone acetylation as new effectors of butyrate activity. *FEBS Lett,* 2001. 499(3): p. 199-204.
[67] Onder, T.T., et al., Chromatin-modifying enzymes as modulators of reprogramming. *Nature,* 2012. 483(7391): p. 598-602.
[68] Ozsolak, F. and P.M. Milos, RNA sequencing: advances, challenges and opportunities. *Nature reviews. Genetics,* 2011. 12(2): p. 87-98.
[69] Tabuchi, Y., et al., Genetic networks responsive to sodium butyrate in colonic epithelial cells. *FEBS Lett,* 2006. 580(13): p. 3035-41.
[70] Bell, S.P. and A. Dutta, DNA replication in eukaryotic cells. *Annu Rev Biochem,* 2002. 71: p. 333-74.
[71] Li, C.J. and M.L. DePamphilis, Mammalian Orc1 protein is selectively released from chromatin and ubiquitinated during the S-to-M transition in the cell division cycle. *Mol Cell Biol,* 2002. 22(1): p. 105-16.
[72] Tatsumi, Y., et al., The ORC1 cycle in human cells: I. cell cycle-regulated oscillation of human ORC1. *J Biol Chem,* 2003. 278(42): p. 41528-34.
[73] Li, C.J., A. Vassilev, and M.L. DePamphilis, Role for Cdk1 (Cdc2)/cyclin A in preventing the mammalian origin recognition complex's largest subunit (Orc1) from binding to chromatin during mitosis. *Mol Cell Biol,* 2004. 24(13): p. 5875-86.
[74] Tatsumi, Y., et al., Association of human origin recognition complex 1 with chromatin DNA and nuclease-resistant nuclear structures. *J Biol Chem,* 2000. 275(8): p. 5904-10.
[75] Thome, K.C., et al., Subsets of human origin recognition complex (ORC) subunits are expressed in non-proliferating cells and associate with non-ORC proteins. *J Biol Chem,* 2000. 275(45): p. 35233-41.
[76] Brown, J.A., S.G. Holmes, and M.M. Smith, The chromatin structure of Saccharomyces cerevisiae autonomously replicating sequences changes during the cell division cycle. *Mol Cell Biol,* 1991. 11(10): p. 5301-11.
[77] Lipford, J.R. and S.P. Bell, Nucleosomes positioned by ORC facilitate the initiation of DNA replication. *Mol Cell,* 2001. 7(1): p. 21-30.
[78] Simpson, R.T., Nucleosome positioning can affect the function of a cis-acting DNA element in vivo. *Nature,* 1990. 343(6256): p. 387-9.

[79] Iizuka, M., et al., Regulation of replication licensing by acetyltransferase Hbo1. *Mol Cell Biol,* 2006. 26(3): p. 1098-108.

[80] Li, C.J. and R.W. Li, Butyrate induced cell cycle arrest in bovine cells through targeting gene expression relevant to DNA replication apparatus. *Gene Regul Syst Bio,* 2008. 2: p. 113-23.

[81] Li, C.J., et al., Selective activation of pre-replication complexes in vitro at specific sites in mammalian nuclei. *J Cell Sci,* 2000. 113 (Pt 5): p. 887-98.

[82] DePamphilis, M.L., The 'ORC cycle': a novel pathway for regulating eukaryotic DNA replication. *Gene,* 2003. 310: p. 1-15.

[83] Archer, S., et al., Butyrate inhibits colon carcinoma cell growth through two distinct pathways. *Surgery,* 1998. 124(2): p. 248-53.

[84] Vermeulen, K., D.R. Van Bockstaele, and Z.N. Berneman, The cell cycle: a review of regulation, deregulation and therapeutic targets in cancer. *Cell Prolif,* 2003. 36(3): p. 131-49.

[85] Dimova, D.K. and N.J. Dyson, The E2F transcriptional network: old acquaintances with new faces. *Oncogene,* 2005. 24(17): p. 2810-26.

[86] Condorelli, F., et al., Inhibitors of histone deacetylase (HDAC) restore the p53 pathway in neuroblastoma cells. *Br J Pharmacol,* 2008. 153(4): p. 657-68.

[87] Pasini, D., et al., Characterization of an antagonistic switch between histone H3 lysine 27 methylation and acetylation in the transcriptional regulation of Polycomb group target genes. *Nucleic Acids Res,* 2010. 38(15): p. 4958-69.

[88] Pasini, D., et al., JARID2 regulates binding of the Polycomb repressive complex 2 to target genes in ES cells. *Nature,* 2010. 464(7286): p. 306-10.

[89] Jones, M.A., et al., Jumonji domain protein JMJD5 functions in both the plant and human circadian systems. *Proc Natl Acad Sci U S A,* 2010. 107(50): p. 21623-8.

[90] Xu, C., et al., Binding of different histone marks differentially regulates the activity and specificity of polycomb repressive complex 2 (PRC2). *Proc Natl Acad Sci U S A,* 2010. 107(45): p. 19266-71.

[91] Sarkar, S., et al., Histone deacetylase inhibitors reverse CpG methylation by regulating DNMT1 through ERK signaling. *Anticancer research,* 2011. 31(9): p. 2723-32.

[92] Kinney, S.M., et al., Tissue-specific distribution and dynamic changes of 5-hydroxymethylcytosine in mammalian genomes. *J Biol Chem,* 2011. 286(28): p. 24685-93.

[93] Kinney, S.R. and S. Pradhan, Regulation of expression and activity of DNA (cytosine-5) methyltransferases in mammalian cells. *Prog Mol Biol Transl Sci,* 2011. 101: p. 311-33.

[94] Jurkowska, R.Z., T.P. Jurkowski, and A. Jeltsch, Structure and function of mammalian DNA methyltransferases. *Chembiochem,* 2011. 12(2): p. 206-22.

[95] Wippermann, A., et al., Establishment of a CpG island microarray for analyses of genome-wide DNA methylation in Chinese hamster ovary cells. *Appl Microbiol Biotechnol,* 2013.

[96] Bertos, N.R., A.H. Wang, and X.J. Yang, Class II histone deacetylases: structure, function, and regulation. *Biochem Cell Biol,* 2001. 79(3): p. 243-52.

[97] Zhang, Y., et al., Butyrate induces cell apoptosis through activation of JNK MAP kinase pathway in human colon cancer RKO cells. *Chem Biol Interact,* 2010. 185(3): p. 174-81.

[98] Chang, M.C., et al., Butyrate induces reactive oxygen species production and affects cell cycle progression in human gingival fibroblasts. *J Periodontal Res,* 2013. 48(1): p. 66-73.

[99] Bordonaro, M., D.L. Lazarova, and A.C. Sartorelli, Butyrate and Wnt signaling: a possible solution to the puzzle of dietary fiber and colon cancer risk? *Cell Cycle,* 2008. 7(9): p. 1178-83.

[100] Shin, H., et al., Change in gene expression profiles of secreted frizzled-related proteins (SFRPs) by sodium butyrate in gastric cancers: induction of promoter demethylation and histone modification causing inhibition of Wnt signaling. *Int J Oncol,* 2012. 40(5): p. 1533-42.

[101] Morris, S.A., et al., Overlapping chromatin-remodeling systems collaborate genome wide at dynamic chromatin transitions. *Nat Struct Mol Biol,* 2014. 21(1): p. 73-81.

[102] Petty, E. and L. Pillus, Balancing chromatin remodeling and histone modifications in transcription. *Trends Genet,* 2013. 29(11): p. 621-9.

[103] Varga-Weisz, P.D., Chromatin remodeling: a collaborative effort. *Nat Struct Mol Biol,* 2014. 21(1): p. 14-6.

[104] Wilkins, B.J., et al., A cascade of histone modifications induces chromatin condensation in mitosis. *Science,* 2014. 343(6166): p. 77-80.

[105] Bartel, D.P., MicroRNAs: target recognition and regulatory functions. *Cell,* 2009. 136(2): p. 215-33.

[106] Bartel, D.P., MicroRNAs: genomics, biogenesis, mechanism, and function. *Cell,* 2004. 116(2): p. 281-97.

[107] Kim, J. and D.P. Bartel, Allelic imbalance sequencing reveals that single-nucleotide polymorphisms frequently alter microRNA-directed repression. *Nat Biotechnol,* 2009. 27(5): p. 472-7.

[108] Arasu, P., B. Wightman, and G. Ruvkun, Temporal regulation of lin-14 by the antagonistic action of two other heterochronic genes, lin-4 and lin-28. *Genes Dev,* 1991. 5(10): p. 1825-33.

[109] Pasquinelli, A.E., et al., Conservation of the sequence and temporal expression of let-7 heterochronic regulatory RNA. *Nature,* 2000. 408(6808): p. 86-9.

[110] Reinhart, B.J., et al., The 21-nucleotide let-7 RNA regulates developmental timing in Caenorhabditis elegans. *Nature,* 2000. 403(6772): p. 901-6.

[111] Zhang, Z. and W.S. Wu, Sodium butyrate promotes generation of human induced pluripotent stem cells through induction of the miR302/367 cluster. *Stem Cells Dev,* 2013. 22(16): p. 2268-77.

[112] Hu, S., et al., The microbe-derived short chain fatty acid butyrate targets miRNA-dependent p21 gene expression in human colon cancer. *PloS one,* 2011. 6(1): p. e16221.

[113] Delcuve, G.P., D.H. Khan, and J.R. Davie, Roles of histone deacetylases in epigenetic regulation: emerging paradigms from studies with inhibitors. *Clin Epigenetics,* 2012. 4(1): p. 5.

[114] Delcuve, G.P., D.H. Khan, and J.R. Davie, Targeting class I histone deacetylases in cancer therapy. *Expert Opin Ther Targets,* 2013. 17(1): p. 29-41.

[115] Esteller, M., Non-coding RNAs in human disease. *Nat Rev Genet,* 2011. 12(12): p. 861-74.

[116] Scott, M.S. and M. Ono, From snoRNA to miRNA: Dual function regulatory non-coding RNAs. *Biochimie,* 2011. 93(11): p. 1987-92.

[117] Iorio, M.V., C. Piovan, and C.M. Croce, Interplay between microRNAs and the epigenetic machinery: An intricate network. *Biochim Biophys Acta,* 2010.

[118] Leder, A. and P. Leder, Butyric acid, a potent inducer of erythroid differentiation in cultured erythroleukemic cells. *Cell,* 1975. 5(3): p. 319-22.

[119] Gallinari, P., et al., HDACs, histone deacetylation and gene transcription: from molecular biology to cancer therapeutics. *Cell research,* 2007. 17(3): p. 195-211.

[120] Khan, O. and N.B. La Thangue, HDAC inhibitors in cancer biology: emerging mechanisms and clinical applications. *Immunology and cell biology,* 2012. 90(1): p. 85-94.

[121] Suliman, B.A., D. Xu, and B.R. Williams, HDACi: molecular mechanisms and therapeutic implications in the innate immune system. *Immunology and cell biology,* 2012. 90(1): p. 23-32.

[122] Leggatt, G.R. and B. Gabrielli, Histone deacetylase inhibitors in the generation of the anti-tumour immune response. *Immunology and cell biology,* 2012. 90(1): p. 33-8.

[123] Woan, K.V., et al., Modulation of antigen-presenting cells by HDAC inhibitors: implications in autoimmunity and cancer. *Immunology and cell biology,* 2012. 90(1): p. 55-65.

[124] Andrews, K.T., A. Haque, and M.K. Jones, HDAC inhibitors in parasitic diseases. *Immunology and cell biology,* 2012. 90(1): p. 66-77.

[125] Fairlie, D.P. and M.J. Sweet, HDACs and their inhibitors in immunology: teaching anticancer drugs new tricks. *Immunology and cell biology,* 2012. 90(1): p. 3-5.

[126] Goldberg, A.D., C.D. Allis, and E. Bernstein, Epigenetics: a landscape takes shape. *Cell,* 2007. 128(4): p. 635-8.

[127] Shin, J.H., et al., Genome-wide ChIP-seq mapping and analysis reveal butyrate-induced acetylation of H3K9 and H3K27 correlated with transcription activity in bovine cells. *Functional & integrative genomics,* 2012.

[128] Shin, J.H., et al., Butyrate Induced IGF2 Activation Correlated with Distinct Chromatin Signatures Due to Histone Modification. *Gene Regul Syst Bio,* 2013. 7: p. 57-70.

[129] Goncalves, P. and F. Martel, Butyrate and colorectal cancer: the role of butyrate transport. *Curr Drug Metab,* 2013. 14(9): p. 994-1008.

INDEX

#

3-hydroxy-3- methylglutaryl CoA synthase 2, 34
4-phenylbutyrate (4-PB), 113
5-hyrdoxymethylcytosine (5-hmC), 181

A

acarbose, 18
access, 28
accounting, 5
acetate, 2, 7, 15, 26, 29, 52, 55, 56, 57, 58, 59, 60, 65, 81, 85, 92, 93, 100, 105, 134, 148, 159, 162, 168, 177, 178, 179, 180, 181, 186, 201, 204, 205, 212, 213, 220, 233, 234, 235, 236, 237, 238, 239
acetoacetate, 34, 202
acetoacetyl CoA thiolase, 34
acetylation, 3, 36, 187
acetylcholine, 36
acetyl-CoA, 3, 32, 210
acid, 2, 7, 10, 12, 14, 17, 21, 22, 23, 25, 28, 33, 52, 53, 54, 55, 56, 59, 62, 63, 64, 65, 66, 68, 185, 186, 187
Acidaminococcus sp, 6
acute lung injury, 32
adaptation, 13, 17, 37, 185
adenocarcinoma, 33, 54, 62, 65
adenomas, 19, 136, 139, 145, 152, 155
adenomatous polyposis coli (APC), 135, 149
adenylate cyclase/cAMP signaling pathway, 162
adhesion, 25, 29, 33
adiponectin, 60
adipose, 2, 13, 58, 59, 60, 61, 65, 67, 68
adipose tissue, 13, 58, 59, 60, 61, 65, 67, 68
adiposity, 58, 63, 187
adults, 185
adverse effects, 29
aerobic metabolism, 32
age, 10, 15, 186
Agricultural Research Service, viii, ix, x, xi
airway inflammation, 55
alcohol consumption, 33
allergy, 3, 14
alters, 1, 28, 68
amino, 26
amino acid(s), 26
anaerobe, 22
anaerobic bacteria, 7, 21
anaphylaxis, 82, 88
anexin A1 (AnxA), 31
angiogenesis, 72, 164, 219, 220, 224, 245
antiatherogenic, 111, 224
antibiotic, 10, 15, 22, 37
anticancer drug, 33
Anticarcinogenic, 21, 43, 78, 112, 252
antigen, 30
Anti-inflammatory, 3, 29, 103, 105, 187
anti-inflammatory cytokine, 28, 30, 52, 54, 64, 83, 98, 107, 183
antioxidant, 21, 28, 32, 64
antioxidant effect, 32
antitumor, 34
AP-1, 94, 95, 103
APC, 3
apoptotic pathways, 53
appetite, 52, 53, 58, 60, 62, 65, 66, 67, 187
apples, 19
Arabinoxylan (AX), 8
arabinoxylooligosaccharides (AXOS), 8
ARA-C, 33
arrest, 33
ARS, 1
arthritis, 28, 55
Asia, 47
asthma, 28
Astrocytoma, v, 109, 110, 114, 115, 116, 117, 118, 122, 124

ATP, 25, 26, 28, 32
atrophy, 37
Austria, ix, xi
autophagy, 3, 13, 28, 30, 53, 62, 110, 116, 117

B

Bacilli, 178
bacteria, 1, 2, 3, 5, 6, 7, 8, 9, 10, 11, 12, 13, 14, 15, 16, 17, 22, 30, 35, 56, 62, 64, 65, 186, 187
bacterial fermentation, 26, 63
bacterial infection, 56
bacterial strains, 1, 4, 12
bacterium, 15, 16, 21, 22, 23, 64
Bacteroides, 6, 54, 84
Bacteroidetes, 178, 235
Bacteroidetes vulgatus, 178
basement membrane, 33
bcd (butyryl-CoA dehydrogenase), 3
BCL2L11, 227, 228
beneficial effect, vii, 13, 32, 33, 36, 38
benefits, 3, 7, 8, 12, 17, 52, 56, 57
Bifidobacteria, 10, 57, 65, 83
Bifidobacterium spp, 178
bioavailability, 1, 11
biodiversity, 35
bioinformatics, vii
biological roles, vii
biological sciences, 16
biosynthesis, 1, 2, 6, 7, 10, 11, 12, 57, 66
biotechnology, 15, 20, 23
Blautia, 85, 86
blood, 8, 9, 38, 53, 62, 65
body composition, 185
body fat, 58, 65, 66, 67
body weight, 58
bone, 9, 28
bone marrow, 28
bowel, 8, 10, 13, 16, 17, 18, 20, 25, 34, 37, 51, 52, 54, 55, 56, 57, 58, 60, 61, 62, 63, 64
brain, 66, 186
Brazil, ix, 25
burn, 32
butyrate kinase, 4, 14, 159, 170, 179, 186
butyrate oxidation, 34
butyryl triglyceride (tributyrin), 11
butyryl-CoA, 3, 15, 158, 159, 177, 178, 179, 180, 181, 186, 202
  acetate CoA transferase, 159
butyrylphosphate, 159

C

C. rodentium, 95, 96, 98
cabbage, 16
CACO, 57
caecum, 15
calcium, 36
calorie, 7, 17
cAMP, 37, 168
cancer, vii, 9, 12, 13, 14, 19, 26, 28, 29, 30, 31, 32, 33, 34, 53, 61, 63, 65, 68
cancer cells, 28, 29, 31, 32, 33, 65
capsule, 16
carbohydrate(s), 1, 3, 7, 9, 12, 13, 25, 51, 52, 57, 64
carbohydrate metabolism, 7
carbon, 25
carboxylic acid(s), 63, 186
carcinogen, 8, 18
carcinogenesis, 19, 64
carcinoma, 13, 63
cardiovascular disease, 52
caspases, 30, 31, 123
Cathelicidin, 111
cattle, 5, 23
CD103, 83, 88
CD4+, 83, 84, 88
CDKN1A, 227, 228
cecum, 2, 4, 5, 6, 7, 8
celecoxib, 33
cell biology, 16
cell cycle, 33, 53
cell death, 28, 30, 33, 62, 63
cell differentiation, 25
cell division, 64
cell fate, 186
cell line(s), 21, 30, 31, 33, 54, 57, 65, 66
cell metabolism, 28
cell surface, 53
cellular reprogramming, 189, 191, 193, 197
cellulose, 9
central nervous system, 58
Central nervous system tumors, 110
challenges, 55
chemokine(s), 25, 29, 32, 55, 60, 105
chemotactic proteins, 29
chemotaxis, 13, 29, 54
chemotherapy, 33, 34, 38
chicken, 5, 6, 15, 16, 22
children, 10, 20, 22
chloroform, 56
cholera, 37
cholesterol, 57, 66
choline, 36

chromatography, 67
cigarette smoke, 3
circulation, 3, 53, 55, 60
cisplatin, 33, 73, 76, 154
Citrobacter rodentium, 55, 166
clinical application, 21
clinical trials, 9, 10, 19
clostridial genera, 86
Clostridium cluster IV, 177, 181
Clostridium cluster XIVa, 16, 177, 178, 180, 181
Clostridium leptum cluster, 178
Clostridium perfringens/butyricum, 84
clusters, 5, 35
coenzyme, 185
colectomy, 6
colitis, 3, 8, 10, 14, 18, 20, 21, 25, 26, 28, 30, 31, 32, 34, 35, 36, 37, 54, 55, 64, 85, 89, 98, 99, 104, 107, 108, 166, 167, 179, 187
colonic epithelium, 26, 28, 134, 181, 239
colorectal adenocarcinoma, 54
colorectal cancer(s) (CRCs), v, 25, 26, 31, 33, 39, 45, 51, 52, 64, 68, 133, 134, 147, 155
commercial, 12
community(s), 6, 15, 16
composition, 5, 7, 9, 15, 21, 26, 52, 62, 64
compounds, 1, 7, 9, 12
consensus, 35
conservation, 14
consumption, vii, 8, 10, 16, 19, 21, 52, 54, 57, 61, 62
contradiction, 60
control group, 8, 58
controversies, 37
corticosteroids, 34
counterbalance, 16
CREB-binding protein (CBP), 134, 140
crotonoyl-CoA, 159
crt (crotonase), 3
CT, 18
culture, 6, 7, 9, 10, 17, 22, 59
customers, 187
CVD, 57, 59
cyclooxygenase, 32
cysteine, 31
cystic fibrosis, 35
cytochrome, 30, 33
cytochrome c, 30, 33, 148
cytokine(s), 25, 28, 29, 30, 31, 34, 35, 52, 54, 55, 58, 60, 68, 83, 84, 96, 99, 105, 167, 175, 183
cytoplasm, 30

D

deacetylation, 32
death receptors, 30
deficiency, 52
deficit, 6
degenerate, 185
degradation, vii, 7, 14, 30, 62
dendritic cell, 56, 187
Department of Agriculture, viii, ix, x, xi, 12
deposition, 57, 65
derivatives, 9
detoxification, 34
developing countries, 2
diabetes, 10, 62, 66, 185
diarrhea, 3, 10, 14, 22, 34, 35, 37
diet, 2, 8, 9, 10, 14, 15, 18, 33, 36, 52, 56, 57, 58, 59, 61, 62, 63, 64, 66, 67, 68, 185, 186
diet composition, 67
dietary fiber(s), vii, 7, 13, 17, 25, 26, 62, 86, 92, 93, 184, 233, 235
dietary intake, 13, 60
dietary supplementation, 53, 58
diffusion, 2, 26, 27, 36
digestibility, 17
digestion, 7, 8, 16, 25, 37, 52, 56, 57, 61
discomfort, 36
disease rate, 52
diseases, vii, 2, 8, 13, 26, 28, 31, 37, 38, 51, 53, 185
disorder, 34
distribution, 3, 5, 14, 186
diversification, 186
diversity, 5, 10, 22, 185
DNA, 8, 16, 18, 32, 33, 44, 64, 68, 186, 187
DNA damage, 8, 18, 32, 33, 64, 68
DNA methylation, 33, 69, 70, 71, 75, 94, 113, 122, 159, 164, 177, 179, 181, 183, 186, 187, 219, 220, 221, 222, 223, 226, 227, 228, 229, 230, 241, 246, 255
DNA methyltransferase (DNMT), 221
DNA-binding proteins (MBDs), 222
DNA-methyltransferases (Dnmts), 181
dogs, 5
dominance, 6
donors, 5
down-regulation, 34
drinking water, 53, 55, 56, 57, 60, 61
drug targets, 21
drugs, 17, 35
D-tagatose, 7, 17
duodenum, 11
dysbiosis, 14, 16, 35, 81, 83, 84, 176

E

ecology, 15, 17, 20, 21, 186

ecosystem, 5, 6, 20
ectoderm, 190
effluent, 16
electron, 3, 22
embryonic stem cells, 191
emulsions, 11
endoderm, 190
endothelial cells, 29, 30
endothelial dysfunction, 29
endothelium, 29
endotoxemia, 185
enemas, 11, 20, 21, 32, 35, 36, 37, 54, 64
energy, vii, 1, 2, 7, 13, 17, 26, 28, 31, 52, 53, 54, 58, 59, 62, 66, 67, 185, 187
energy expenditure, 58, 59, 66, 67
energy supply, 54
enteric nervous system (ENS), 36
enterocytes, 33, 34, 92, 110, 208, 210
enteroendocrine, 53, 58, 63, 101, 158, 162, 163, 164, 166, 174, 175
environment, 13, 19, 64, 185
environmental influences, 34
enzymatic activity, 34
enzyme(s), 7, 25, 28, 32, 33, 34, 38, 56
epidemiology, vii
epigenetic modification, 187
epithelia, 2, 13
epithelial cells, 1, 2, 13, 14, 35, 37, 53, 57, 64, 65
epithelium, 2, 26, 28, 32, 35, 57, 108, 135, 158, 195, 199, 200, 201, 202, 203, 204, 205, 206, 207, 208, 209, 210, 211, 212, 213, 214, 216, 234, 240, 253
equal opportunity, 12
ERK (extracellular regulated kinase), 184
etfA (ETF-α), 3
ethanol, 55
etiology, 34
etoposide, 33
Eubacterium, 4, 5, 22, 23, 35, 85, 177, 180
Eubacterium rectale/Roseburia spp, 177
Eubacterium rectale-Roseburia, 5
eubiosis, 84
evidence, 1, 19, 22, 38, 52, 53, 57, 61, 187
excretion, 1, 2, 8, 19, 37
experimental condition, 29, 59
exposure, 3, 60
extravasation, 29

F

F. prausnitzii, 5, 6, 180
Faecalibacterium, 4, 5, 15, 22, 35, 45, 86, 110, 176, 177, 178, 180, 181
Faecalibacterium prausnitzii, 4, 5, 15, 22, 35, 110, 176, 177, 178, 181
fat, 10, 11, 28, 57, 58, 65, 66, 67, 185
fatty acids, vii, 1, 2, 7, 12, 13, 17, 18, 19, 20, 26, 36, 37, 51, 52, 62, 63, 64, 65, 66, 67, 185, 186, 187
FDA, x, 7
feces, 2, 4, 6, 7, 10, 14, 15, 16, 21, 23
fermentable carbohydrates, 62
fermentation, 1, 2, 3, 5, 10, 16, 17, 18, 19, 20, 22, 25, 26, 51, 52, 54, 55, 56, 57, 60, 63, 65, 81, 92, 100, 109, 110, 126, 133, 134, 152, 155, 157, 158, 163, 167, 168, 169, 171, 172, 178, 204, 207, 219, 220, 233, 234, 235, 236, 237, 238, 240, 250
fiber(s), vii, 2, 5, 16, 26, 33, 61, 66
fibroblasts, 30
fibrosarcoma, 31
filters, 35
Firmicutes, 5, 11, 15, 177, 178, 235
flora, 15, 17
fluid, 37
fluorescence, 22
food, vii, 7, 10, 18, 19, 20, 26, 57, 58, 59, 66
food additive, 7
Food allergy, 82, 87, 88
Food and Drug Administration, x
food intake, 58, 59, 66
formation, 3, 14, 15, 26, 28, 29
Foxp3, 64, 81, 82, 84, 85, 86, 88
fructooligosaccharides, 7, 105
fructo-oligosaccharides (FOS), 7, 95
fructose, 7, 9
functional food, 37
fungi, 187
fusion, 2

G

gastrointestinal tract, 1, 13, 17, 18, 34, 37, 38, 56, 60, 61, 64
gel, 35
gene promoter, 28
gene regulation, 26
gene transfer, 14
genes, 1, 2, 3, 5, 6, 13, 14, 15, 25, 26, 28, 30, 54, 57, 60, 64, 68, 185, 186, 187
genome, vii, 3
genomics, vii
genus, 5, 6, 16, 23
Georgia, x, xi, xii
gingival, 4, 23
glial fibrillary acidic protein (GFAP), 116
Glioblastoma, 43
glucagon, 53, 66

glucose, 22, 26, 28, 35, 37, 53, 60, 65, 66, 67, 185
glucose tolerance, 65
glucuronic acids, 7
GLUT4, 60
glutamate, 34
glutamine, 26, 28, 34
glutathione, 32, 33
glutathione/glutathione S-transferase (GST), 32
glutathione-S-transferase (GST), 32
glutathione-sulfhydryl-transferase (GST), 112
glycerol, 22, 38
glycogen synthase kinase-3 beta (GSK-3beta), 135
glycolysis, 26, 28, 31
glycoproteins, 35
goblet cells, 35
GPR109A, 53, 63, 94, 101, 102, 158, 162, 167, 169, 171, 172
GPR41, 2, 27, 28, 52, 53, 55, 56, 57, 58, 59, 60, 63, 65, 66, 67, 91, 92, 93, 94, 96, 99, 100, 101, 111, 158, 162, 166, 171, 172, 174, 175, 181, 186, 187
GPR43, 2, 12, 13, 27, 28, 52, 53, 55, 56, 57, 58, 59, 60, 63, 65, 67, 91, 92, 93, 94, 96, 98, 99, 100, 101, 102, 158, 162, 166, 167, 169, 171, 172, 174, 175, 181, 186
G-protein coupled receptors (GPR), 53
graduate students, viii
grain cereals, 109
granules, 30
Great Britain, 21
growth, vii, 23, 25, 30, 33, 53, 187
growth factor, 25, 30

H

habitat(s), 1, 4, 5, 12
half-life, 37, 55
hbd (β-hydroxybutyryl-CoA dehydrogenase), 3
HDAC, 2, 3, 28, 31, 33, 53, 54, 55, 56
HDAC, histone deacetylase, 160
headache, 37
health, vii, 3, 7, 8, 9, 12, 16, 17, 26, 28, 52, 56, 57, 61, 62, 185, 186, 187
health effects, vii, 9, 53
heat shock protein, 25, 30
Helicobacter pylori, 113
hemicellulose, 9
hemoglobinopathies, 2
hepatic portal system, 8
heterogeneity, 5
high fat, 58
high-mobility group box 1 protein (HMGB1), 32
high-risk populations, 8
histone(s), vii, 1, 2, 3, 25, 28, 30, 31, 32, 34, 36, 37, 53, 62, 187
histone acetylases, 110, 112, 119, 121, 122, 124, 242
histone acetyltransferases, 28, 31, 224, 241
HM, 13, 17, 21
homeostasis, vii, 25, 26, 52, 54, 64, 65, 67, 83, 84, 89, 92, 107, 110, 137, 168, 169, 175, 184, 187, 216, 236, 239, 241, 248
hormone(s), 14, 20, 34, 52, 58, 59, 63, 64, 66, 186, 187
horses, 2, 5
host, 1, 2, 4, 5, 9, 12, 30, 52, 53, 62, 63, 64, 187
HSP25, 94
HSP70, 94
human, 4, 5, 6, 7, 8, 9, 10, 12, 13, 14, 15, 16, 17, 18, 19, 20, 21, 22, 23, 26, 31, 32, 52, 53, 54, 57, 60, 61, 62, 63, 64, 65, 66, 67, 68, 185, 186, 187, 188
human health, 52, 54
human milk, 20
human subjects, 60, 62
Hydrogen peroxide, 111
hydrolysis, 18
hygiene, 185
hyperacetylation, 28, 32, 73, 74, 94, 102, 126, 196, 233, 239, 241, 243
hypercholesterolemia, 2
hypersensitivity, 37, 64
hypocaloric diet, 178
hypothalamus, 66
hypothesis, 52, 53, 57, 59, 185

I

IBD, 3, 9, 10, 34, 35, 53, 54, 64
ICAM, 29
ideal, 9
identification, 6, 12, 17
IFN, 31, 34, 187
IgE, 83, 87, 88, 89
IL-10, 30, 81, 83, 97, 98, 99, 167, 178, 183
IL-1β, 30, 97, 98
immune cells, 28, 31, 53, 54, 60, 68, 83, 91, 96, 99, 157, 158, 160, 161, 163, 166, 167, 168
immune defense, 37
immune function, 2
immune response, 34, 53, 54, 55, 56
immune suppressive, 81
immune system, 52, 55
immunity, 2, 18
immunomodulator, 25
immunoregulatory, 90
in vitro, 1, 3, 6, 7, 10, 16, 19, 25, 29, 32, 33, 52, 53, 54, 55, 56, 57, 60, 61, 67, 187

in vivo, 18, 29, 52, 53, 55, 56, 57, 67
incidence, 33
India, 14
individuals, 2, 3, 5, 6, 7, 8, 15, 18, 34, 35, 52, 58, 60, 186
indoleamine 2,3-dioxygenase, 164, 168
Induced Pluripotent Stem Cell (iPSC), 189
induction, 13, 29, 31, 32, 33, 35, 36, 55, 56, 57, 63, 64, 187
industrialization, 33
infants, 3, 14
infection, 2, 3, 14, 30, 55, 57, 65
infectious agents, 29
inflammation, 2, 11, 21, 26, 28, 29, 30, 31, 32, 34, 35, 37, 52, 53, 54, 55, 57, 60, 64, 65, 67, 68, 185, 187
Inflammatory bowel disease (IBD), 3, 14, 16, 19, 21, 34, 35, 51, 53
inflammatory cell migration, 29
inflammatory cells, 31
inflammatory disease, 36, 52, 61, 187
inflammatory mediators, 28
inflammatory responses, 12, 25, 32, 65, 68
inflammatory stimulus, 31
ingestion, 8
ingredients, vii
inhibition, 25, 28, 31, 32, 33, 37, 53, 54, 55, 56, 58, 59, 63, 66
inhibitor, 1, 2, 3, 28, 31, 33, 34, 56
inhibitor of histone deacetylases, 2, 134, 159, 250
initiation, 68
innate immunity, 30
iNOS (Nitric oxide synthases), 184
insulin, 2, 53, 57, 58, 61, 66, 67, 187
insulin resistance, 2, 57, 67, 187
insulin sensitivity, 57, 58, 61, 66
integrin(s), 30, 33
integrity, 14, 18, 26, 34, 37
intercellular adhesion molecule (ICAM), 29
internalization, 2, 13
intervention, 62
intestinal barrier, 2, 25, 32, 35, 36, 104, 210
Intestinal epithelial cells, 91
intestinal immunity, 82, 91
intestinal obstruction, 34
intestinal tract, 16
intestine, 4, 5, 7, 9, 15, 17, 19, 21, 23, 26, 34, 35, 37, 38, 52, 56, 62, 63, 64, 66, 81, 82, 85, 91, 92, 93, 94, 95, 97, 98, 99, 100, 101, 110, 111, 148, 155, 161, 168, 169, 170, 174, 185, 186, 201, 203, 206, 207, 208, 210, 216, 234, 235, 238
intravenously, 37, 57, 58
inulin, 7, 8, 9, 11, 17, 19, 109, 110, 180
ions, 35
Iran, 47
Ireland, 21
iron, 19
irrigation, 21, 35
irritable bowel syndrome, 11, 21
Italy, ix, x, xii, xiii

J

JAK/STAT, 184
Japan, xi, xii, 51

K

keratinization, 203, 205
ketogenesis, 34, 200, 202, 203, 210, 212, 213
ketone, 26, 171, 202, 212, 234
kinetics, 68
Klebsiella, 84
Krebs cycle, 32

L

lactate, 10, 19, 21, 22, 26, 93, 101, 162, 165, 170, 171, 173, 174, 202, 203, 206
lactic acid, 7, 17, 26
Lactobacillus, 10, 19, 20
Lactobacillus gasseri, 179
landscape, vii
large intestine, 7, 15, 17, 19, 34, 62, 186
lead, vii, 30, 37
Leahy, 22
leptin, 59, 60, 67, 101, 166, 172, 177, 181, 182
lesions, 8, 11, 34
leukemia, 21
leukocyte(s), 29, 30, 55, 63, 96, 97, 105
leukocyte migration, 97
LFA, 30
liberation, 3
life changes, 10
ligand, 32
lipases, 11
lipid metabolism, 60
lipids, 11, 59, 60
lipolysis, 52, 53, 59, 63
lipopolysaccharide (LPS), 54
liquid phase, 15
liver, 9, 12, 34, 55, 57, 58, 66
liver disease, 9
low risk, 8
low-grade inflammation, 185

LPS, 29, 31, 36, 55, 96, 97, 98, 183
lumen, 3, 26
lung cancer, 38
Luo, 63
lymph, 28, 55
lymph node, 28, 55
lymphocytes, 31, 53, 64, 185

M

macrophages, 30, 31, 60
majority, 3, 5, 6, 9, 33
malignant cells, 25, 26, 31, 32, 34
management, 9
manufacturing, 11
MAPK, 16, 28, 57, 154, 246
marrow, 28
Maryland, 1
mass, 17, 37, 66, 67
mass spectrometry, 67
mast cells, 63
MB, 19
MBD2, 189, 195, 198
measurement, 58
median, 38
medical, 10, 21
medication, 17
medicine, 19
Megasphaera elsdenii, 4, 7, 19, 23
melanoma, 74, 78, 79, 117, 118, 128
mellitus, 66
mesoderm, 190
mesothelioma, 13
Metabolic, 39, 46, 48, 50, 62
metabolic disorder(s), 185
metabolic pathways, 54
metabolic syndrome, 53, 59, 60
metabolites, 53, 57, 62, 65
metabolized, 3, 32, 34, 38
methuosis, 117, 128
methyl group, 186
methylation, 33, 186, 187
methyl-malonyl-CoA, 202
Mexico, xi
mice, 6, 8, 10, 15, 23, 26, 28, 31, 32, 33, 34, 35, 55, 56, 57, 58, 59, 65, 66, 67, 185
microbe-associated molecular patterns (MAMPs), 96
microbial community, 16
microbial dysbiosis, 177
microbiome, 5, 12, 13, 52, 62, 64, 84, 87, 88, 108, 152, 185
microbiota, 1, 2, 3, 9, 10, 12, 14, 15, 17, 18, 19, 20, 21, 22, 26, 34, 35, 51, 52, 54, 55, 56, 62, 63, 64, 65, 66, 68, 81, 83, 84, 85, 86, 89, 102, 109, 110, 138, 149, 151, 152, 175, 176, 177, 178, 179, 180, 181, 184, 185, 186, 187, 234, 235, 250
microflora, 17, 20, 82, 83, 84, 89, 135, 220
microorganisms, 9
microRNA (miRNA), 220
migration, 28, 33, 60, 65
mitochondria, 2, 30, 32, 111, 117, 120, 200, 203, 238
mitogen, 28, 29
modelling, 21
models, 3, 8, 10, 16, 25, 30, 31, 32, 35, 36, 54, 55, 57, 66
modifications, 187
molar ratios, 2, 52
molecular biology, vii
molecules, 25, 26, 27, 29, 32, 35, 36
monocarboxylate co-transporter-2 (MCT2), 36
monolayer, 36
Moon, 22
morphogenesis, 30
motif, 32
motor neurons, 36
mRNA, 60, 186
MUC2, 35, 95, 104
mucin, 6, 16, 35
mucosa, 8, 11, 13, 18, 21, 25, 31, 32, 33, 34, 35, 37, 54, 56, 60, 64
mucositis, 25, 26, 33
mucus, 35
muscle relaxation, 36
mutations, 33
myosin, 35

N

NAD/NADH, 202
nanoparticles, 11, 38
n-butanoic acid, 158
necrosis, 34
nervous system, 36
neuroimaging, 187
neuroinflammation, 112
neurological disease, 186
neuronal proliferation, 112
neurons, 36, 67
neutrophils, 2, 28, 30, 31, 44, 46, 53, 55, 60, 65, 187
next generation, 61
NFκB, 94, 97
nitric oxide(NO), 28, 29, 36
nitric oxide synthase, 29
non-cancerous cells, 12
non-digestible oligosaccharides, 7
NRP, 33

nuclear factor kappa beta (NFkB), 54
nucleic acid, 5
nucleus, 3, 25, 28, 31
null, 31
NuRD, 170, 189, 193, 195
nutrient(s), vii, 18, 26, 34, 37, 52, 62, 187
nutrition, vii, 10, 12, 13, 14, 16, 17, 18, 19, 20, 21, 37, 54, 61, 186, 187

O

obesity, 3, 7, 10, 14, 33, 52, 53, 57, 58, 60, 61, 63, 65, 66, 67, 68, 111, 145, 155, 185, 186, 187
oligofructoses (OF), 7
oncogenesis, 62
operon, 3
oral cavity, 4, 23
organelles, 30
organ(s), 2, 34, 55, 57, 61
overweight, 58, 60, 68, 185
oxidation, 2, 18, 26, 28, 32, 34, 41, 54, 212, 216
oxidative stress, 2, 11, 25, 29, 32, 33, 35, 64, 111, 123, 137, 252
oxygen, 26

P

p15INK4b, 222, 225, 230
p16INK4a, 222, 230
p21cip, 73
p21Waf1/Cip1, 94
pain, 11, 21, 34, 36
papillary growth, 204
parakeratosis, 204
participants, 61
pathogenesis, 13, 34
pathogens, 30
pathology, 3
pathways, 3, 6, 30, 53, 54, 64, 73, 75, 81, 85, 94, 103, 106, 130, 137, 143, 144, 145, 146, 154, 158, 159, 160, 162, 165, 174, 179, 187, 196, 203, 209, 220, 231, 234, 237, 238, 242, 244, 245, 246, 247, 251, 255
PBMC, 53
PCR, 6, 15
peptide(s), 13, 36, 53, 58, 66
perforation, 34
perfusion, 36, 58
peripheral blood, 53, 54, 65, 188
peripheral blood mononuclear cell(s) (PMBC), 53, 54, 65, 188
peristalsis, 36
permeability, 29, 32, 34
peroxidation, 29
peroxisome proliferator-activated receptor α (PPAR-α), 30
peroxynitrite, 29
pertussis, 56, 60
pH, 12, 17, 18, 19
pharmacokinetics, 12, 67
pharmacology, 13, 21
phenotype, 36
phenylacetate (NaPA), 184
phenylbutyrate (NaPB), 184
phosphorylation, 28, 29, 187
phosphotransbutyrylase, 4, 159, 179
phylum, 5, 11
physical activity, 61
Physiological, 13, 18, 26, 32, 48
physiology, vii, 12, 19, 187
pigs, 2, 7, 17, 54, 56, 64
pilot study, 19, 20
PKC, 94, 103
placebo, 9, 10, 11, 21, 32, 36, 64
plasma levels, 58
plasma membrane, 26, 27
platelet aggregation, 29
platelet endothelial cell adhesion molecule-1 (PECAM-1), 30
playing, 53
plexus, 36
pluripotent, 190, 191, 195, 196, 197, 198, 226, 231, 242, 247, 256
PM, 13, 18
polymer(s), 1, 7, 9
polymer chain, 1, 7, 9
polymerization, 8, 9
polypeptide, 63
polysaccharides (NSP), 5, 9, 18, 49, 52, 62
population, 5, 10, 19, 52
portal vein, 55, 56, 58
potato, 8
preparation, 20
preterm infants, 36
prevention, vii, 13, 25, 33, 38, 53, 60, 61, 62
proapoptotic protein, 94
probiotic(s), 2, 3, 6, 9, 10, 12, 16, 18, 19, 20, 21, 38, 86, 87
pro-biotics, 1
producers, 1, 5, 6, 7, 18, 35
pro-inflammatory, 25, 28, 29, 30, 31, 54, 60
promoter, 13
propagation, 68
propionate, 2, 14, 26, 29, 30, 52, 55, 56, 57, 58, 59, 60, 63, 66, 67, 81, 85, 92, 93, 100, 101, 105, 111,

127, 134, 148, 159, 162, 164, 168, 171, 179, 181, 182, 186, 201, 202, 204, 205, 212, 213, 214, 220, 233, 234, 235, 236, 237, 238, 239, 253
propionyl-CoA, 202
protection, 26, 35
protein kinase C, 94, 96, 150
protein kinases, 28
proteins, 5, 28, 29, 30, 34, 35, 36, 67
Proteobacteria, 178
proteomics, 61
psychiatric disorders, 186
Psyllum, 109
PTEN, 227, 228
pyrosequencing, 6, 84, 89
pyruvate, 26, 93, 113, 128, 170, 202

Q

quality of life, 10, 20

R

Rac1/2 GTPases, 94
Radiation, 40
RANTES, 32
reactive oxygen, 30, 32, 54
reactive oxygen species (ROS), 32, 54, 98
reality, 11
receptors, 1, 2, 25, 27, 28, 30, 33, 37, 52, 53, 55, 56, 58, 60, 62, 63, 67, 91, 94, 96, 99, 101, 102, 111, 115, 135, 158, 162, 163, 166, 168, 169, 171, 172, 173, 174, 177, 181, 182, 186, 187, 215, 250
recovery, 16, 25, 35
rectum, 2, 15, 34
recurrence, 5
redox, 202
regeneration, 34
Regulatory T cells (Tregs), 81
relevance, 13, 55, 186
remission, 10, 11, 20, 21, 32, 34, 35, 64
repair, 33, 64
repressor, 13
requirements, 22
researchers, vii
resection, 37
resistance, 67
resolution, 31, 55
respiration, 3
response, 2, 15, 30, 34, 54, 55, 56, 59, 62, 64, 65, 66
retinoblastoma (RB), 222
risk, 5, 14, 19, 33, 51, 52, 59, 61, 64, 68
RNA(s), 1, 13, 186
rodents, 61
Roseburia, 4, 5, 6, 16, 23, 45, 86, 176, 178, 180
routes, 36, 37, 38, 57
rumen, 5, 10, 15, 23, 199, 200, 201, 202, 203, 204, 205, 206, 207, 208, 209, 210, 211, 212, 213, 214, 216, 234, 235, 238, 240, 251, 253
ruminal development, 200, 201, 204, 217

S

S-adenosylhomocystein (AdoHcy), 181
S-adenosylmethionine (SAM), 181
saliva, 23
Salmonella, 36, 40
salts, 58, 59
science, 19
secrete, 58
secretion, 20, 25, 29, 30, 31, 34, 37, 52, 55, 59, 65, 66, 188
segregation, 57
selectivity, 36
sensing, 62, 187
sensitivity, 36, 58, 64
sensors, 187
sequencing, 61, 186
serotonin, 37
serum, 9, 10, 19, 58, 65
services, iv
sheep, 5
short bowel syndrome, 10, 20, 25, 37
Short chain fatty acids, 12, 26, 62, 81, 92, 100, 104, 148, 155, 186, 199
showing, 52, 54, 56
signaling pathway, 36, 187
signalling, 55, 57, 60
simulation, 20
skeletal muscle, 65
small intestine, 4, 7, 9, 23, 26, 34, 37, 38, 52
smooth muscle, 29, 32, 36
smooth muscle cells, 29, 32, 94, 224
sodium, 2, 8, 11, 18, 20, 21, 26, 32, 35, 37, 58, 59, 61, 65, 67, 187
sodium butyrate (NaB), 184
solid tumors, 38
solution, 32
somatic cells, 189, 190, 197, 198, 226
sorbitol, 7
species, 2, 4, 5, 6, 10, 13, 15, 21, 22, 30, 32, 52, 54, 62, 63
spleen, 28, 55
Spring, 65, 185
stabilization, 29, 38

starch, 7, 8, 9, 16, 18, 19, 26, 36, 52, 56, 57, 62, 64, 65, 66, 68
starch polysaccharides, 9, 19, 52
state, 60
stimulation, 29, 59
stimulus, 31
stomach, 7, 11, 34
stress, 2, 11, 25, 29, 32, 33, 35, 64
stress response, 64
stroke, 2
structure, 7, 28, 64
substitutes, 17
substitution, 8
substrate(s), 1, 2, 5, 7, 26, 28, 32
sucrose, 7
sulfate, 8, 18, 20, 26
Sun, 13, 41, 45, 68
supplementation, 26, 33, 37, 58, 61
suppression, 53, 54, 63
susceptibility, 34, 66
symbiosis, 184, 200
symptoms, 6, 10, 21, 34, 35, 54, 55, 59
synbiotics, 1, 2, 9, 10, 12, 19, 20, 88
syndrome, 10, 20, 25, 37, 67, 68
synergistic effect, 10, 12
synthesis, 14, 28, 29, 35, 58, 66

T

T cell, 31, 52, 54, 60, 63, 65
T regulatory cells, 54
target, 2, 6, 28, 33
TGF-β, 83, 85
therapeutics, 13, 16, 21
therapy, 10, 20, 21, 33, 35, 64, 187
thl (thiolase), 3
thymus, 55, 56
tissue, 26, 31, 58, 59, 60, 67
TNF, 30, 31, 34, 54, 60, 62
TNF-alpha, 60, 62
TNF-α, 30
total energy, 2
toxic effect, 38
toxicity, 11
toxin, 37, 56, 60
trade, 12
transcription, 14, 28, 54
transcription factor(s), 28, 54, 72, 81, 85, 111, 120, 121, 149, 153, 192, 210, 243, 248
transcriptome, 1, 2, 159, 164, 209, 216, 224, 237
translocation, 2, 13, 34, 36
transmission, 36
transport, 2, 12, 36, 37
Transporters, vi, 62, 92, 157, 159, 163, 172
treatment, vii, 15, 20, 21, 25, 26, 30, 31, 32, 34, 35, 37, 55, 58
trial, 9, 10, 11, 20, 21, 64, 68
tricarboxylic acid, 54
tricarboxylic acid cycle, 54
trichostatin A, 34, 56, 65, 188
trinitrobenzene sulfonic acid, 55, 166
tumor, 3, 9, 12, 14, 33, 63, 65, 67, 188
tumor necrosis factor, 65, 67, 188
tumorigenesis, 2, 30, 70, 72, 76, 135, 138, 139, 140, 148, 232
type 2 diabetes, 13, 60, 185, 187
type II diabetes, 185

U

UDP-glucuronosyl transferases, 33
ulcerative colitis, 3, 14, 20, 21, 25, 26, 30, 31, 32, 34, 35, 54, 64, 98, 107, 108, 110, 148, 184, 187
underlying mechanisms, 53, 56, 60
United States, viii, ix, x, xi, xii, xiii, 62
uric acid, 32
USDA, 1, 12

V

vaccine, 15
Valproic acid (VPA), 112
variations, 3
vascular cell adhesion molecule (VCAM), 29
vascular inflammation, 29
vasculature, 26
vasodilator, 29
vein, 56
vessels, 29
VLA, 30
Volunteers, 50

W

Warburg effect, 26, 31, 32, 137, 151, 197, 239
Washington, 61
water, 35, 37, 55
water absorption, 37
weight gain, 58, 66
weight loss, 34, 58, 67, 185
WHO, 185
Wnt signaling, 33, 149, 150, 151, 153, 154, 246, 256
WNT/catenin, 134, 135, 136, 137, 138, 139, 140, 141, 142, 143, 144, 145, 146

X

xylooligosaccharides (XOS), 7

Y

yeast, 10, 47
yield, 8, 9

β

β-lactoglobulin, 87
β-oxidation, 2, 32, 193